Seminars in
INFECTIOUS DISEASE

Seminars in
INFECTIOUS DISEASE

Volume I

Edited by

LOUIS WEINSTEIN, M.D., Ph.D.

Visiting Professor of Medicine, Harvard Medical School;
Physician, Peter Bent Brigham Hospital, Boston, Mass.

BERNARD N. FIELDS, M.D.

Professor of Microbiology and Molecular Genetics,
Harvard Medical School; Chief, Infectious Diseases Division,
Peter Bent Brigham Hospital, Boston, Mass.

Stratton Intercontinental Medical Book Corporation

ISBN 0-913258-54-7
Printed in U.S.A.

CONTENTS

FOREWORD

This volume is the first of a series entitled "Seminars in Infectious Disease" that will be published annually. The Editors have long recognized the need for yearly review of old and recently acquired knowledge in the area of infectious disease. Perhaps no other field of medicine has witnessed such dramatic changes as has this area. With the introduction of antibiotics and development of methods for the prevention of disease produced by several agents that have, on occasion, been involved in major epidemics, many foresaw the end of concern with infectious agents. However, this view has been repeatedly proved wrong by the rapid appearance and recognition of such problems as bacterial resistance to antibiotics, limitations of the vaccines that have been used in the approach to the control of many of the most common and important viral infections, and recognition of altered presentations of viral disease, for example, slow virus infection.

The papers in this first volume of "Seminars in Infectious Disease" illustrate several examples of old problems brought into fresh focus and newly emerging ones that have been defined only recently. Fever of obscure origin (Weinstein and Fields), one of the classical problems in infectious disease, has undergone a major change in approach since the introduction of newer noninvasive technics that allow recognition of occult infection and malignancy. The gonococcus has emerged as an epidemic agent of enormous frequency and increasing resistance to penicillin (Sparling and Lee). The rapid advances and understanding of the role of cyclic AMP has provided important new insights into bacterial disease of the intestine (Hornick). The multiplicity of new antibiotics and antifungal agents points to the continuing need for translating changes in the modification of old agents to clinical situations (Neu, A. J. Weinstein). As progress in the treatment of cancer and other chronic diseases has improved, the impact of damaging normal host defenses has created new types of serious infections that are difficult to diagnose and to treat (Pennington). A newly recognized disease in the human, babesiosis, is beginning to be studied and understood (Dammin). The report of the successful treatment of systemic herpes virus infection with Ara-A has prompted a serious review of the current status of antiviral agents (Richman and Oxman). Newer technology has provided important clues to the etiology of previously defined syndromes of viral gastroenteritis (Blacklow, Schreiber, Trier). Finally, important changes in the way we think about viral infections have influenced and often delayed our ultimate understanding of the mechanisms and control of these processes (Horstmann). The choice of these topical reviews has been strongly influenced by our view of the significance of each topic to their individual areas as well as to the entire field.

It is obviously impossible for most physicians, whether their efforts are directed primarily to clinical problems or their main interest is in the basic processes involved in the phenomena of infection, to keep abreast of all such important new developments. Thus, the goal of "Seminars in Infectious Disease" is to fill this need by presenting a series of papers in each volume that will bring up-to-date new information related to purely clinical problems, as well as focus on significant recent developments in the basic sciences related to the mechanisms involved in the infectious process. In addition, the current status of the prevention and treatment of infection will continue to be stressed. The primary thrust of many of the papers will be to narrow the gap between advances in our understanding of the mechanisms involved in the pathogenesis of infection, and the direct impact of new data on approaches to clinical problems. We hope to provide a forum useful to all physicians interested in the "art and science" of infectious disease.

Louis Weinstein, M.D., Ph.D.
Bernard N. Fields, M.D.

CHAPTER 1

FEVER OF OBSCURE ORIGIN

Louis Weinstein, M.D. and
Bernard N. Fields, M.D.

One of the most difficult and frustrating problems in clinical medicine is prolonged fever, the cause of which defies identification. A number of reports of this syndrome have been essentially etiologic catalogues. It is difficult to compare many of the recorded experiences because of variation in the panorama of diseases in different areas of the world and in different hospital settings, as well as the varying criteria used to select the cases. In two large series, rigid criteria have been employed to define fever of unknown origin (FUO) in order to eliminate readily diagnosable causes and short-lived causes of fever. Petersdorf and Beeson [47] selected cases on the basis of elevation of temperature to greater than 101°F on several occasions, lasting for 3 weeks or longer and remaining undefined after one week of investigation in the hospital. A temperature higher than 100.5°F present for at least 3 weeks was the criterion suggested by Sheon and Van Ommen [55]. Fever of unknown origin has been defined, for the purpose of this discussion, as an elevation of rectal temperature to at least 100°F for 3 weeks or longer, the cause of which has defied elucidation even after a searching history has been taken, a minutely detailed physical examination carried out and laboratory studies of blood, urine and radiograph of the chest have been performed.

Although not usually included in the syndrome of FUO, many persons seek medical help for low-grade fever (99.6 to 100, orally) that has persisted for months and, in some instances, for years. These individuals are usually otherwise healthy, but complain frequently of headache and generalized malaise when they know that their temperature is elevated. Often they wander from one physician to another for long periods, seeking solution of their problem, and, unfortunately, are often subjected to a host of frequently unnecessary, intensive, expensive and potentially dangerous investigations. Because this is a common syndrome, it has been included in this discussion, albeit it does not meet the classic criteria for the diagnosis of FUO.

From the Division of Infectious Diseases, Department of Medicine, Peter Bent Brigham Hospital, and the Department of Medicine, Harvard Medical School, Boston, Mass.

Thus, although the more stringent criteria adopted by Petersdorf and Beeson [47] and others have been useful in eliminating certain diseases from consideration, we feel it is both timely and worthwhile to expand these to include and to focus on the larger number of patients that often comes to the attention of physicians. In addition, where pertinent, the personal experiences of the authors will be used to provide illustrative cases, or alternatively, to present material not adequately documented in the literature. Thus, the references cited in the bibliography are not intended to be comprehensive, but rather to call attention to some diseases not recently described in this setting, as well as to review some of the newer diagnostic radiologic procedures that have improved the clinical evaluation of the problem.

The characteristics of the "fever curve" are, for the most part, of little or no help in identifying the cause of a prolonged fever. It may be persistently low grade (100–100.4), at high levels without much variation through the day, intermittent, remittent or episodic, with alternating periods of elevated and normal temperature for days or weeks. Although rigors may be present, they are not always an integral part of the syndrome, and are often associated with the use of antipyretics. It must be emphasized that, in general, the characteristics of an elevated temperature curve provide no clue to its etiology.

Because the differential diagnosis of fever of unknown origin usually involves consideration of a large number and variety of etiologic factors, there is a great tendency for physicians to approach the problem from all aspects at the same time. This is often nonproductive and, at times, risky. There are more than 100 causes of FUO; it is clear that all cannot be studied simultaneously, or even over an extended period. A systematic approach to the problem is required. This should include not only a highly detailed history and physical examination, but also a search for answers to five inquiries that we feel should be made at the very beginning of the study of a case of prolonged etiologically undefined fever before embarking on a more detailed and expensive evaluation. These are: (a) What is the patient's normal temperature? This applies primarily to cases in which the "fever" does not exceed 100 orally; (b) Is there a physiologic or functional cause for the elevated temperature? (c) Is the fever factitious?; (d) Are hypersensitivity or idiosyncratic reactions to therapeutic agents or other chemicals involved?; (e) Is there a relation between the occupation of the individual and the etiology of the fever?

"Normal" Temperature

It is frequently difficult or impossible to obtain information concerning the "normal" temperature of most patients who seek medical attention because of prolonged "low-grade" fever. Most individuals do not measure their temperature until they feel ill. Many do not have a thermometer, and make a determination of the presence or absence of fever on the basis of subjective sensation of "feverishness," or by feeling the forehead or the back of the neck. Many physicians and other persons are under the impression that "normal" daily, maximal oral and rectal temperatures are 98.6°F and 99.6°F, respectively [51]. It is surprising that these single numbers are accepted as "normal" when it is well known that quantitation of other bodily functions of man and animals yields a variable range of values. This is also true for temperature.

In a large number of school children, only 29.5% had oral temperatures of 98.6° or below [70]. However, in a group of 108 boarding school girls aged 12 to 17, the normal temperature was closer to 97.4° than to 98.4° [45]. Oral temperatures of medical students recorded between 8 and 9 A.M. have been noted to range between 96.5° and 99.3°, with a mean of 98.1°; 68 per cent had temperatures between 97.3 and 98.5° [25]. Study of patients visiting physicians' offices has indicated that 17 per cent had a maximal oral temperature of 98.6; in 42 per cent, it was higher than this, reaching 100°F in some instances [51]. Maximal daily temperature tends to be lower in elderly persons than in younger adults; it may be as low as 96.6° in the morning and not exceed 97.6° late in the day. Unless these variations are appreciated, physicians may misinterpret 99.6° as fever in a young adult and fail to recognize the possibility of disease in an older individual with a maximal temperature of 98.6–99°F.

Physiologic Causes for "Low-Grade Fever"

It is important to consider the possibility of functional causes in patients who seek attention because of "fever" up to 100°F. The time of determining temperature is important in determining its clinical importance; it may be elevated as much as one degree F, if taken shortly after a substantial meal. A recording of 100°F early in the morning is more suggestive of organic disease.

Ovulation: Many patients with low-grade FUO are women who note elevation of temperature to 100–100.2°F for 2 weeks every month. Inquiry usually reveals that the "fever" is present only during the 2 weeks prior to the onset of menstruation. It is clear that this is related to ovulation, and requires no investigation save for recording the temperature daily over 2 to 3 successive months to establish its relation to the menstrual cycle [62].

Smoking: Heavy smokers of cigarettes, cigars and pipes may have oral temperatures above "normal," particularly towards the end of the day.

This is also true for persons who chew large wads of gum over prolonged periods.

Exercise: An important physiologic cause of fever that may be repeated day after day and reach a level as high as 101° is strenuous exercise [5]. This has been well demonstrated in young men engaged in collegiate rowing, in those who run long distances and in football players. A counterpart of this syndrome is elevation of temperature to 103°F or higher in patients with tetanus, a disorder in which fever is usually either minimal or absent. However, in those with frequent episodes of severe generalized tonic seizures, temperature may rise to 104 or higher. This is probably associated with the sustained, intense muscular exercise induced by the spasms.

Essential Oral Hyperthermia: A relatively common cause of low-grade fever of unknown origin, especially in young girls and women, is essential oral hyperthermia. This syndrome is characterized by a lack of difference between the oral and rectal temperatures. The oral temperature has been observed to be as much as 0.5 degree F higher than the rectal one, in some cases. This phenomenon usually disappears over a variable period of time and, although of interest, is of no clinical consequence [41].

Psychogenic "Fever"

Maximal daily temperatures of up to or a little over 100°F may be psychogenic in origin and persist for months to years [16]. This phenomenon is common, and occurs most often in young women whose chief complaints are daily "fever" (rarely higher than 100°F), generalized malaise, aching muscles and joints and chronic fatigue. Patients with this syndrome are frequently hospitalized, at times for prolonged periods, and subjected to intense investigation [18,49,50]. Detailed inquiry into the possibility of provoking psychogenic factors may fail to disclose any pertinent information in many cases. However, in some, an anxiety-producing cause can be identified. This often proves to be unhappiness or stress in a job or at home. In some instances, the psychogenic basis for the "fever" is suggested by the appearance of the patient and her behavior as she is questioned about symptoms. Such patients are frequently overweight, despite attempts at "dieting." They often appear restless, and clench their hands while the history is being elicited. Most suggestive of psychogenic fever is the diary of daily temperatures (4 or more recordings a day), covering weeks to months, brought by many such patients on their first visit to a consultant. If the pulse has been determined at the same time, a dissociation between the height of the "fever" and the cardiac rate is practically always apparent. If the patient has been extensively studied previously, the main focus of the consultation should be directed to the possibility of a psychogenic cause. Such persons rarely need referral for psychiatric help. Two simple approaches to the diagnosis and solution of the problem are very often effective. The first involves removing patients, for at least a week, if possible, from the environment at home or place of employment that may be the provocative element, and to have them record temperature and pulse 4 times a day. If "fever" is absent during this period, the patient is asked to return to her usual pursuits and again keep a record of her temperature. The absence of fever during the first and third weeks, and its recurrence during the second one is highly suggestive of a psychogenic basis for the elevated temperature. This course suggests the need for removing the patient from the situation responsible, if this can be accomplished. However, this is not possible in many instances. In this case, the administration of a mild sedative is often helpful. Treatment with 5 mg of diezapam (Valium) every 12 hours, or 15 mg of phenobarbital in the morning, afternoon and before sleep, usually leads to disappearance of the "fever" within 3 to 4 days. Patients should be instructed to omit the drugs after 1 to 2 weeks, monitor the temperature, and resume treatment if low-grade "fever" recurs. The disappearance of the elevated temperature during periods of sedation and its return to normal when this is omitted is not only helpful to the physician diagnostically, but is reassuring to patients, many of whom have been living for weeks or months with the fear of unrecognized, potentially fatal disease.

A prime example of the role of emotional factors in the pathogenesis of low-grade elevation of temperature is *"admission fever."* Careful scrutiny of the charts of patients admitted to hospitals for study of nonfebrile disorders often shows the initial recording to be above 98.6 orally; the slope of the line connecting the first three recorded points is frequently down. This is a reflection of the anxiety and fear associated with hospitalization. The phenomenon can be produced in persons in a normal environment by the administration of a small dose of epinephrine.

Factitious Fever

All physicians who deal with the problem of prolonged etiologically-undefined fever are faced occasionally by a person who, for no discoverable reason, is elevating the temperature factitiously [46]. Levels are usually higher than those present when physiologic or psychogenic factors are involved; they may reach 104 to 105°F, or higher, and are seldom below 101 to 102°F. These individuals have usually been thoroughly studied on a number of occasions. They have often been hospitalized repeatedly and have undergone numerous extensive, expensive and occasionally potentially dangerous diagnostic maneuvers, without elucidation of the cause of the elevated temperature. In many instances, no illness has preceded the onset of the "fever"; in others, it has followed and increased in degree after a mild and self-limited infection of the upper respiratory tract. Many people with factitious fever, although healthy, complain of headache, generalized aching of muscles and great fatigue that they associate with the presence of the elevated temperature. However, a few may appear chronically ill, have lost weight and are anemic because of inadequate diets; others are overweight. The presence of emotional disturbance is, most often, not apparent.

The ruses employed to establish and maintain the fiction of a factitious fever are often very clever, and may escape detection by even the most highly experienced physicians for months to years. There are a few, however, that are employed most often. One presently popular approach is for patients to bring their own thermometers to the hospital. They manipulate the bulbs of these until they raise the level of mercury to the temperature they have selected. They then remove the thermometer inserted by the nurse, and replace it with the one that they have manipulated. Another commonly used method is to remove the thermometer placed by hospital personnel, heat the bulb over the lamp of the bedside light, immerse it in hot water or rub it vigorously with the fingers to produce a rise in the column of mercury, and then replace it in either the mouth or rectum.

There are several approaches to the detection of factitious fever. Probably the most effective is careful monitoring of the patient while the temperature is being taken. This must be done with the individual uncovered when a rectal thermometer is used, because some persons, when covered, still manage to manipulate the instrument while under observation. Another approach is redetermination of the temperature within a few minutes after fever has been recorded; this leaves no time for manipulation of the thermometer, because the procedure is carried out when it is not expected. In instances in which there is suspicion that thermometers are being "swapped," it is important to check the brand name of the intrument. Those used in hospitals usually carry a different trade mark than those available in drug or other stores. Palpation of the skin is often helpful; it may be cool when the "temperature" is 103–104°F. The first suspicion of factitious fever is often aroused by detection of dissociation between the pulse rate and temperature. Normally, an increase in temperature of one degree F is accompanied by an increase in the pulse rate of 20 per minute. In those with factitious fever, the pulse rate is often increasing while the temperature is falling, or vice versa. This must not be confused with the true bradycardia that may be present in typhoid fever and some viral infections. In these disorders, the pulse rate may remain stable or rise to a lesser degree than in normal individuals.

Organic Causes of Fever of Unknown Origin

Two lines of inquiry must be pursued before studies other than the history, physical examination and "routine" laboratory investigations are carried out in patients in whom an organic cause of FUO is suspected. These involve elucidation of information related to exposure to drugs and to the occupation of patients.

"Drug Fever"

Fever due to sensitization or to idiosyncratic reactions to drugs is common. It must be emphasized that the height and other features of the temperature curve are of no value in directing attention to the involvement of these agents as etiologic factors. The temperature may be low- or high-grade, sustained or intermittent. The presence of chills prior to elevation of the temperature does not rule out the possibility of "drug fever." Cessation of exposure to the responsible agent is not always followed by rapid defervescence. The rate at which the temperature returns to normal is related to the time required for a drug to be completely excreted or metabolized; this may require 3 to 4 weeks, in some instances. It must be emphasized that rash is frequently absent, and peripheral eosinophilia is uncommon in the fever induced by drugs and other chemical agents.

Almost all therapeutic agents may produce fever [1]. Among those often involved are the antibiotics, sulfonamides, nitrofurantoin, the tuberculostatic compounds (isoniazid, ethambutol, para-aminosalyalic acid), pronestyl, barbiturates, quinidine, propylthiuracil, Aldomet and atropine. The fever induced by iodine may persist for 3–4 weeks after its ingestion has been discontinued, because of the very slow rate at which it is excreted [6]. Even salicylates may be responsible for an increase in temperature that may reach hyperpyretic levels (105°F). This is usually related to overdosage of the drug; in some cases, manifestations consistent with diffuse encephalitis are simultaneously present. It is striking that digitalis is the only commonly used agent that has not been associated with fever. The best way to rule out a drug or chemical as the cause of an etiologically undefined fever is to stop its administration. If, by the end of a week, an elevated temperature is still present, there is little likelihood that, with the exception of iodine, it is drug-related.

Occupation

Careful inquiry into the occupation of patients may disclose the cause for episodic or continued fever of unknown origin. Two recent reports have described "polymer fume fever" in persons who worked in factories in which plastics were manufactured [34]. One of us has studied a case that exemplified this syndrome. The patient was a 35 year old man who had had fever (101–101.5°F) for 5 days a week for about a year, but was afebrile every weekend during this period. He was employed as an executive in a company that manufactured plastic products. Although he rarely entered the area of the factory where the materials used to make the plastics were present, he had occasionally noted "fumes" and "fine dust" in his office. He was instructed to absent himself from work for one week, return for a week, again remain at home for another week, and to record his pulse and oral temperature 4 times a day. Review of these records disclosed an absence of fever while he was at home, and a daily temperature up to 101 for the 5 days during which he worked.

A similar phenomenon was observed many years ago in men who worked in brass foundries [48]. The features of this syndrome were low-grade fever, substernal pain, malaise, chills, nausea and vomiting; these often appeared shortly after these individuals came to work Monday but no other morning. The disorder was known under several names, including "zinc fume fever," "Monday night chill and fever" or "brass founder's ague." Metal fume fever has been the general term applied to this phenomenon. If the men were absent any day of the week and always when they had Sunday off (the work week was 6 days some years ago), the typical manifestations recurred when they returned to work. Investigation disclosed that the syndrome was caused by an idiosyncratic reaction to zinc, one of the metals that, together with copper, makes brass. A similar reaction is thought to be caused by iron, nickel or aluminum. All patients engaged in occupations in which they may be exposed to any type of chemicals, drugs or dust, especially when there is prolonged exposure in poorly ventilated areas, and who present with fever of unknown origin should be advised to absent themselves from work, and to record their temperature during this period as well as during the time spent at their occupation.

Certain occupations expose individuals to the risk of infections that, in the early stages, may be featured by fever and no other signs or symptoms. Among such persons are (a) microbiologists engaged in either diagnostic or research activity involving bacteria, fungi and viruses, (b) nurses who may come in contact with a variety of transmissible diseases, the primary and, sometimes, the only feature of which is fever, and (c) people who handle garbage and human wastes or work in occupations in which they come in contact with contaminated meat and meat products. Two infections that may often present as fever of unknown origin are primary or disseminated tuberculosis and brucellosis [58]. Both of these diseases are important considerations in the differential diagnosis of FUO in *veterinarians*, even in those whose only contact with brucella is with the attenuated vaccine strain. Dogs, cats, cows and horses, may transmit not only tubercle bacilli and brucella, but also *Leptospira* (dogs) and *Toxoplasma gondii* (cats).

INFECTIOUS DISEASES

Because the number of infections, both common and rare, in which cryptic fever may be the only manifestation is very large, it is obviously impossible to initiate a search for all of them simultaneously, or even over an extended period. The approach to diagnosis must, therefore, be systematic and focused first on those disorders that are most frequently characterized by FUO. Only when these have been excluded should possible involvement of the less common or rare causes be investigated. Among the infections most often associated with fever of unknown origin are tuberculosis, subacute infective endocarditis and infections of the liver.

Tuberculosis

Although not always the case, the first and only manifestation of tuberculosis, whether primary, secondary or disseminated, may be fever, occasionally of high degree [42]. No other clinical or laboratory evidence of the disease may be present. In the early phase of primary tuberculosis, the presence of elevated temperature is often associated with failure to demonstrate any pulmonary lesions by radiographic examination. This is so because the Ghon lesion is still too small to be detected, and sentinel hilar lymphadenopathy has not yet developed. The tuberculin reaction is negative if infection has been present for less than 4 to 6 weeks. FUO may occasionally be the only feature of secondary tuberculosis.

Two patients with cryptic elevations of temperature, study of whom disclosed no positive findings save for a positive tuberculin reaction, have recently been described [7]. Radiographic examination of the lungs revealed no lesions. However, culture of gastric aspirate yielded *M. tuberculosis* in both cases. Treatment with tuberculostatic agents produced prompt defervescence.

Miliary or disseminated tuberculosis often presents as fever of unknown origin [47,54,55]. Radiographic study of the lungs reveals no lesions in more than two-thirds of cases. However, this does not indicate a lack of involvement of the pulmonary tissues. Study at necropsy often discloses multiple small lesions, the miliary tubercles. Although not enlarged or tender, autopsy at times discloses a number of easily visible lesions in the liver and spleen. This form of infection may progress for a considerable period without development of evidence of involvement of any organ. The presence of miliary tubercles in the retina may be an important clue to the diagnosis of disseminated disease. A chronic form of miliary tuberculosis has been observed [24]. Death may occur in the rapidly progressive disease before any clinical or laboratory indication of infection appears.

Although less common, other forms of tuberculosis may be featured by FUO that may persist for weeks to months and reach levels as high as 103–104°F. Attention has recently been refocused on tuberculous infection of the kidney as a cause of fever of unknown origin [11, and unpublished data]. Cases in which hematuria, pyuria or proteinuria are present in urine that is sterile when cultured by conventional methods should suggest this possibility. In a number of instances, however, there are no urinary abnormalities, but culture of the urine grows *M. tuberculosis* or, very rarely, one of the atypical mycobacteria.

We have recently had experience with two cases of fever of unknown origin that proved, on abdominal exploration, to be due to tuberculosis of mesenteric nodes. These patients had no symptoms other than elevated temperature, and no evidence of disease in other organs or tissues.

The possibility of chronic tuberculous salpingitis or endometritis should be considered in women with fever of unknown origin [28]. Although disorders of menstruation, including metrorrhagia, menorrhagia and the recent appearance of dysmenorrhea, are often present, information concerning these may not be elicited because inquiry is not made. An important feature of this type of tuberculous infection is premenstrual fever that disappears shortly after onset of the period.

Although almost always accompanied by a visible effusion, tuberculous pericarditis may occasionally come to the attention of physicians as instances of fever of unknown origin. Substernal pain, a frequent symptom of viral infection of the pericardium, is uncommon. When discomfort is present, it is usually represented by a sensation of heaviness or dull aching over the lower end of the sternum, frequently relieved by pressure over this area. Radiographic examination of the chest almost always suggests the diagnosis; biopsy of the pericardium proves it. Tuberculous pericarditis is often not suspected in older patients because they present with a picture of progressive cardiac failure and prolonged fever. Tamponade as the cause of the "heart failure" may be overlooked because of the absence of pain in the chest, unless radiographic study is carried out.

Infective Endocarditis

Most cases of subacute infective endocarditis do not meet the criteria for fever of unknown origin, as defined in this discussion, because of the presence of a murmur, the diagnostic localizing sign of this disease. However, this clue is absent in a small number of patients [33,67,68,69]. The temperature is commonly not very high (100.2 to 102). Fever may be present for weeks or months before the diagnosis is established. The absence of a murmur does not necessarily indicate that the involved valve was normal prior to infection. In these cases, the primary injury to one of the leaflets may have been mild and produced a degree of valvular distortion, inadequate to lead to the development of a murmur, but enough to result in the formation of a sterile platelet-fibrin thrombus, the basic lesion of this disorder. Patients with subacute infective endocarditis without detectable murmur, when treated, may follow one of three courses. The murmur will develop in most during the first 2 to 3 weeks of antimicrobial therapy. In a small number a murmur appears only 1 to 3 months after treatment has been completed. Rarely, a murmur may never be detected, even after many years of observation. One-third of individuals with infections involving the right side of the heart may be free of murmur when first examined; one often appears during therapy. This may be the case when the tricuspid valve is involved. The possibility of endocarditis may be overlooked because of failure of the murmur to change its character in patients with a small intraventricular septal defect. Murmurs may be absent before or after infection has occurred in persons in whom the defect is large, and in those in whom the disease involves the right ventricular wall at the point of impact of the jet stream. Failure to suspect the possibility of subacute infective endocarditis has become an increasing problem as the frequency of this disease has increased in older people. Many of these individuals have had a loud basal systolic murmur for a long time as a result of tortuosity and widening of the aorta. When they are seen by a physician because of fever of unknown origin, the possibility of endocarditis of the aortic valve is paid little attention because the previously known murmur has not changed its character.

Infections of the Liver

Some infectious disorders involving the liver may be associated with prolonged fever of unknown origin. The characteristics of the temperature curve that develops in this kind of disease are not diagnostic.

Anicteric viral hepatitis may be featured only by fever, without hepatic enlargement or tenderness [31]. Although this is probably the commonest presentation of this infection in young children, it may also appear in this form in adults. Fever of varying degree that occasionally persists for weeks may be the only symptom of hepatic amebic or pyogenic abscesses [4]. This may also be the case when infection is present in the *subdiaphragmatic* and *subhepatic* areas [30]. An uncommonly recognized entity in which fever, often in the range of 102 to 104°F, without other symptoms or signs may be present for weeks to months is bacterial hepatitis (unpublished data). The liver may or may not be enlarged and/or tender in this disease. There is no evidence of disorders of the biliary and intestinal tracts in these cases. However, serum levels of alkaline phosphatase are usually elevated. The organisms recovered from the liver of patients with this syndrome have included *Propionobacterium acnes*, green pigment-producing streptococci and *Actinomyces israeli*.

Juandice may occasionally be absent in patients with acute suppurative cholangitis. The disease presents as fever of unknown origin, the temperature often reaching 103 to 104°F, in these cases. The bouts of fever are episodic, last for a week or less and reappear at an interval as short as 3 to 4 weeks or as long as 3 to 4 months. There often are no other symptoms or signs. The diagnosis is overlooked, particularly in individuals whose elevated temperature returns to normal after a few days without treatment. However, antimicrobial therapy is often given, despite failure to identify the cause of the fever. When an appropriate drug, one that inhibits the common enteric gram-negative bacteria, is administered, defervescence occurs in a few days. Since the period of therapy is usually short, fever often recurs after a variable period. Radiologic study practically always discloses chronic cholecystitis and cholelithiasis and, in some instances, dilatation of the intrahepatic biliary tree.

Determination of the level of serum alkaline phosphatase is frequently of great diagnostic help in the study of patients with persistent fever of unknown origin. In addition to the disorders discussed above, the combination of elevated temperature and increased level of the enzyme suggests the possibility of disseminated tuberculosis, lymphoma, Hodgkin's disease, primary and metastatic hepatic neoplasms, hypernephroma, infectious mononucleosis (cases in which lymphadenopathy and pharyngitis are absent—"typhoidal form") and cytomegalovirus infection. Alterations in serum transaminases are frequently minor or absent in most of these disorders.

Miscellaneous Infections

A number of infections other than those already discussed may be accompanied by fever persisting for 3 or more weeks, in the absence of any signs or symptoms suggesting their etiology. These are relatively uncommon and should be considered only after the infections most often responsible for FUO have been eliminated. Poststreptococcal fever in children is often a mystifying syndrome [66]. It occurs in a small number of youngsters as a complication of inadequately treated or mild untreated streptococcal pharyngitis. The features of this disorder include low grade fever (99.6–100.6°F), decrease in appetite, loss of weight, easy fatiguability and slowly progressive anemia. Sore throat is usually absent. Culture of the pharynx frequently grows *Str. pyogenes*. Appropriate antimicrobial therapy leads to rapid disappearance of all symptoms.

Fever persisting for several weeks may be the only manifestation of typhoid fever. In some instances, the elevation of temperature is relatively small. Symptoms may be so mild that patients are not forced to bed, but go about their normal activities, complaining only of fatigue and persistent low-grade fever; this is the syndrome of "walking typhoid fever." The pattern of presentation of this disease has changed since the introduction of chloramphenicol [21].

Salmonella bacteremia, a specific syndrome caused most frequently by *Salmonella typhimurium* and *Salmonella choleraesuis* [53], is characterized by high-grade fever (up to 104°F or higher), with or without rigors, that may persist for weeks to months. There are usually no other abnormalities. The organisms are, as a rule, not present in the intestinal tract, but are always recoverable from the blood. A prominent feature of this syndrome is its rapid response to appropriate antimicrobial therapy (often given before the diagnosis is established) and relapse, often within 2 to 3 days after treatment has been discontinued. This may occur even after multiple courses of treatment.

The *typhoidal form of infectious mononucleosis* almost always presents as fever of unknown origin [59]. The diagnosis is established by demonstration of abnormal lymphocytes in the peripheral blood, a positive heterophile agglutination reaction and antihemagglutinen.

The only manifestation of abscesses in various areas of the body may be FUO. Perinephric collections of pus are often associated with high temperature alone [61]. The urinary sediment is often completely normal. Several weeks may elapse before a characteristic bulge in the flank over the involved kidney appears and becomes sufficiently large to alert the patient or physician. The most common presentation of renal carbuncle is fever that may be present for weeks. Pain is frequently absent, and the urine usually contains no inflammatory cells until the lesion drains into the collection system; this may not occur for several weeks. The only manifestation of pelvic abscess, a complication of hysterectomy or caesarian section, may be prolonged fever that may not appear until a week after operation. Abdominal symptoms may be absent and pelvic examination fail to disclose a mass, early in the course of the disease.

Prostatic abscess is an occasional cause of FUO, and in some cases may involve an otherwise normal gland. In others, however, prostatic massage or chronic prostatitis are the provoking factors. The absence of any symptoms except fever and the surprising lack of detectable enlargement and tenderness of the prostate in many patients are usually responsible for failure to consider this disease as a cause of fever of unknown origin. Bacteremia is not always present. Unless detected and treated with antibiotics and surgical drainage, death may occur.

Abscess of the spleen occasionally develops in the course of endocarditis, typhoid fever and brucellosis. The presence of the lesion may not be associated with an increase in the size of the already enlarged organ.

Although prolonged fever associated with chronic bronchiectasis usually presents no diagnostic dilemma, because of the demonstration of a pulmonary lesion and a cough productive of varying quantities of sputum, no abnormalities other than persistent fever may be present in an occasional case; radiographic study of the lungs discloses no lesions in these patients.

NEOPLASTIC DISEASES

Various tumors, both malignant and benign, are a common cause of fever of unknown origin. This underscores the necessity of considering neoplastic disease at the same time as infectious disorders as the background for an etiologically undefined persistent elevation of temperature. Focusing on completely ruling out the possibility of an infection, an approach that often consumes many days or even weeks, may be of little benefit to patients with tumors.

Some types of neoplasms are more frequently associated with FUO than others [10]. However, it must be emphasized that, even in these, the temperature may not be elevated. Although uncommon and usually not considered a feature of tumors, the onset of the febrile reaction may be abrupt and preceded by rigors. The neoplastic lesions most frequently associated with fever of unknown origin are lymphomas, Hodgkins disease, acute and chronic myelogenous and acute lymphatic leukemia, primary or metastatic tumors of the liver, carcinoma of the lung, hypernephroma [65] and metastatic carcinoma of the thyroid. Pel-Ebstein fever, for many years considered the diagnostic hallmark of Hodgkin's disease, has become much less common over the last 10 to 15 years. It has been suggested that this type of febrile response is present most often in patients who have concomitant brucellosis, and that this, rather than the tumor, is responsible for the "characteristic" behavior of the temperature. Chronic lymphatic leukemia is usually an afebrile disorder unless complicated by infection, an acute hemolytic episode or a "blast crisis." Although carcinoma of the lung is usually not a febrile disease, significant elevation of temperature may be present, in the absence of atelectasis or pneumonia. Among malignant lesions uncommonly characterized by FUO are carcinoma of the colon (often complicated by ulceration and secondary bacterial infection), prostate, ovary, breast, rectum, pancreas (without metastasis) and brain. Cerebral tumors lying in close proximity to the hypothalamus may be accompanied by high temperature or hyperpyrexia (> 105°F). An interesting feature of hypernephroma, in the absence of metastasis, is elevation of serum alkaline phosphatase. A rare cause of fever of unknown origin is pheochromocytoma. Febrile episodes have been observed only in patients with episodic hypertension. Increase in temperature to 102 to 103°F may be detected when the blood pressure is high, and disappear with a return to normotension (unpublished data).

The occasional association of benign tumors with fever of unknown origin has not been sufficiently appreciated. Among such lesions are leiomyoma of the stomach, small intestine and uterus (without necrosis or hemorrhage in fibroid lesions).

The possibility of complicating cryptic bacterial, viral, mycotic or parasitic infections must receive serious consideration in patients with neoplastic disease, despite the fact that the tumor itself may be responsible for the febrile reaction. The immunosuppression produced by many types of malignant lesions, often exaggerated by chemotherapy, increases susceptibility to invasion by any kind of microorganism. The difficult problem in these cases is identification of the cause of the fever. In some instances, the neoplastic disease alone is responsible, in others it is solely the superimposed infectious process, while in still others it is both. Rapid definition of the cause of the increased temperature and the application of specific therapy, where possible, is critical in these patients.

CONNECTIVE TISSUE DISEASE

Fever associated with disorders of connective tissue usually poses little diagnostic difficulty because of the common presence of other symptoms and signs of these diseases, such as involvement of joints, muscles, tendons, skin, lungs, heart or kidneys. However, in some instances, the only early manifestation may be FUO [26,47]. This may be the case in allergic vasculitis, various forms of polyarteritis and systemic lupus erythematosus (normal levels of complement and negative ANA and L.E. preparations). An example of this category is a patient who had a temperature of 102 to 103°F for at least 3 months, progressive anemia and marked loss of weight. Because all investigations, including invasive and noninvasive procedures as well as immunologic tests, had failed to identify the cause of the fever, exploratory laparotomy was undertaken. Liver, lymph nodes and both kidneys were biopsied. Histologic examination disclosed no evidence of disease in any of the organs except the left kidney, in which the classic abnormalities of polyarteritis nodosa were present; the right kidney was completely normal. Renal function had been found to be normal on a number of occasions, prior to surgery. Therapy with prednisone produced rapid defervescence. Study over the following year disclosed gradual involvement of other organs (unpublished data).

We have studied 3 young women who were found to have an uncommon form of connective tissue disease in which the only manifestation was fever (unpublished data). This is "atypical" lupus erythematosus, in which L.E. preparations are negative, antinuclear antibodies not detectable and levels of complement normal, early in the disease. However, titers of antibody to DNA and RNA are usually elevated. None of the signs of classic lupus appeared after 3 or more years in 2 of the patients. However, in the third one, severe lupus with intense cerebral involvement developed after about 3 years, during which she was treated with 20 mg of prednisone per day, remained afebrile and had negative L.E. preparations, normal levels of complement and moderately elevated titers of antibodies to DNA and RNA. The L.E. test became strongly positive, and high titers of antinuclear antibody were demonstrated during the acute episode. These abnormalities disappeared 2 months after recovery. Levels of serum complement remained normal during both the active and quiescent stages of the disease.

Two forms of rheumatoid arthritis may present as fever of obscure origin. Patients with severe juvenile rheumatoid arthritis may exhibit striking elevations of temperature over prolonged periods, before arthritis develops. In some instances, involvement of joints may not appear during the first episode of the disease. The presence of a variety of skin eruptions, including petechiae or purpura, in some cases may lead to a mistaken diagnosis of infection. The only manifestation of "atypical" rheumatoid fever may be prolonged fever. Although arthritis is absent early in this syndrome, some patients may complain of stiffness of the proximal interphalangeal joints of the hands in the morning. The cause of the elevated temperature often becomes apparent when arthritis finally develops after several weeks or months.

DISEASES OF THE INTESTINAL TRACT

The presence of prolonged, etiologically undefined fever usually does not suggest the intestine as the site of disease because, in most instances, dysfunction of this organ is accompanied by diarrhea and/or abdominal pain. However, it is well known that, in rare instances, signs and symptoms suggesting a disorder of the intestinal tract may be absent in both idiopathic ulcerative colitis and regional enteritis involving the small or large bowel; the only manifestation in such cases is prolonged low- to high-grade fever [32]. Two patients whom we have studied emphasize this point. The first was a 16 year old girl who had had fever (102–104°F, daily) for 2 months; she developed anemia and lost considerable weight over this period. Neither abdominal pain nor diarrhea had been present. Because treatment with a variety of antibiotics had failed to produce defervescence, she came to our attention. Sigmoidoscopic examination now disclosed the classic findings of idiopathic ulcerative colitis. Treatment with corticosteroids led to rapid return of temperature to normal, regression of anemia and gain in weight. The development of abdominal pain, fever and increase in severity of the colonic lesions during the following years confirmed the diagnosis. The second patient was a 15 year old boy who had had daily fever to 102–103°F, but no other symptoms or signs, for about 3 months. He had been studied extensively by several physicians but the cause of the elevated temperature could not be identified. When seen by one of us, his temperature was 102.8°F, white blood count 22,000 with a shift to the left; the sedimentation rate was high and the spleen palpable. No abdominal tenderness was detected. Close questioning failed to elicit even a hint of abdominal pain, diarrhea or involvement of joints. Radiographic study of the upper and lower intestinal tract revealed no abnormalities save for a "string sign," about 20 cm in length, in the terminal ileum. Therapy with salicylazosulfapyridine (Azulfidine) produced gradual defervescence and return of the white blood cell count and erythrocyte sedimentation rate to normal. The patient has remained afebrile and free of abdominal pain and intestinal dysfunction for almost 2 years. The spleen has decreased in size so that it is presently barely palpable. Recent radiographic study of the ileum has indicated a definite increase in width of the lumen in the involved area. An occasional patient with Whipple's disease may have fever for weeks before the characteristic manifestations of the disease appear.

DISORDERS OF HEAT-REGULATING MECHANISMS

Processes that alter water balance or disturb the mechanisms that control body temperature may be responsible for the development of a significant degree of fever that may persist for months to years. Chronic congestive cardiac failure is an example of a disorder of water balance that may be associated with prolonged, moderate elevation of temperature [28]. Unless this possibility is appreciated, the presence of rales at the bases of the lungs, together with fever, may be interpreted as evidence of pulmonary infection, and lead to unnecessary exposure to antimicrobial agents. Unlike young children, adults do not develop fever on the basis of dehydration. An increase in temperature (> 100°F) that persists for 3 weeks or more in the chronically dehydrated elderly person is usually due to infection, tumor or other cause of FUO.

Disorders that interfere with any of the mechanisms responsible for loss of heat from the body, especially radiation from the skin and sweating, may be responsible for fever of unknown origin that may persist for long periods, and, in some instances, for life. Among such diseases are *diffuse icthyosis, widespread and severe eczema, scleroderma, and congenital ectodermal dysplasia of the anhidrotic type* [41,44,60]. The fever associated with these disorders tends to be highest during the warm seasons of the year. Patients are usually unable to compensate completely for the ineffectiveness of the major dermal mechanisms involved in loss of heat by increasing the losses normally produced by breathing, urination and defecation.

Congenital ectodermal dysplasia of the anhidrotic type is a rare and very perplexing cause of fever of unknown origin when it is seen prior to the development of the characteristic epithelial defects. One of us has studied twin 10 month old girls with this disorder who had had temperatures of 102 to 104 daily since birth. Examination disclosed them to be well nourished, active and developed, emotionally and physically, to levels consistent with their age. Suspicion of the possibility of congenital ectodermal dysplasia was aroused by the ethnic background (French) of the youngsters. The following study was carried out. One of the babies was covered by a blanket during the night; her temperature reached 104.6 by morning, while her sister, who had been left uncovered during the same period, was essentially afebrile when she awoke. The process was reversed the following night. The next morning, it was noted that the child who had been covered the previous evening, when left uncovered, had only low-grade fever. In contrast, the other one, after being covered, had developed a high temperature. The diagnosis was confirmed by biopsy of the skin; no sweat glands could be identified.

Two types of central or neurologic disorders that may be associated with persistance of significant levels of fever are hypothalamic dysfunction and dorsolumbar sympathectomy [17]. Any disease involving the hypothalamus may lead to increased temperature for long periods. As pointed out above, tumors of the brain lying in close proximity to or invading this organ may be accompanied by high fever that may, at times, reach hyperpyrectic levels (> 105°F). The development and persistence of high-grade fever is an uncommon complication of the viral encephalitides, that may appear in the acute, or during the convalescent, phase of the infection. Poikilothermia may develop in a rare case. When lying uncovered in a cool room, the temperature of these patients may be as low as 94°F; it may increase to 102 to 103°F when they are covered. The inability to control body temperature in these cases is, as a rule, transient; it persisted for 2 months in a young boy with post-measles encephalitis studied by one of us. The fact that persons who have undergone dorsolumbar sympathectomy may have fever during periods of hot weather is well known.

METABOLIC DISORDERS

Among the metabolic disorders that may present as fever of unknown origin are hyperthyroidism, hypersecretion of etiocholanalone and the production of an abnormal pyrogenic metabolite of progesterone. While "etiocholanalone fever" [9] was, for many years, considered an important cause of FUO, recent evidence has indicated that this entity is probably rare [17]. We have studied an 18 year old woman with a history of episodic elevation of temperature to 102–103, lasting for 2 to 3 days and recurring over 5 years. Circulating levels of etiocholanalone were found to be 100-fold higher when fever was present than when it was absent. Identification of the cause of elevated temperature in patients with obvious clinical manifestations of hyperthyroidism poses no problem. However, an occasional case of "masked" disease may come to the attention of a physician because of prolonged fever (100–101°F). The cause of a daily temperature of 102–103°F for 2 weeks every month for more than a year in a young woman was suspected when it was noted that her febrile episodes began at about the expected time of ovulation, and persisted until the onset of the menses. Studies indicated that the fever was induced by the presence of an abnormal pyrogenic metabolite of progesterone in the urine during about 2 weeks prior to menstruation.

MISCELLANEOUS CAUSES OF FUO

In addition to the disorders discussed above, there is a large number in which prolonged, etiologically-obscure fever of significant degree may be present for long periods. Limited space does not permit discussion of all of them; only a few that have come to our attention are presented.

Fever of unknown origin, particularly in women, should raise the possibility of multiple pulmonary emboli, usually arising from thrombosed pelvic veins [15], if all other studies fail to disclose the cause of the elevation of temperature. This diagnosis is often not suspected because (a) the patient has not been pregnant or undergone pelvic surgery recently, (b) gynecologic examination reveals no abnormalities, (c) abdominal pain is absent and (d) radiographic study of the lungs discloses no lesions. Increase in temperature to 101–102°F may be persistent, or episodic (3–7 days) interspersed with afebrile periods of 3 to 8 or more weeks. A recently studied patient was a 38 year old woman who had had repeated bouts of fever for about 18 months. She had not been pregnant, and had not experienced abdominal pain, surgical treatment, pelvic infection or abnormal menstruation in the preceding 5 years. Extensive investigation failed to disclose the etiology of the elevated temperature. Arterial PO_2 was normal. Phlebography of the veins of the legs revealed no thrombi. Attempts to demonstrate involvement of pelvic veins by this method were unsuccessful. Despite the fact that the lungs appeared normal by conventional X-ray examination, scanning was carried out. This revealed multiple abnormal areas; pulmonary arteriography disclosed a number of "cut-offs" in small vessels. Treatment with heparin produced prompt defervescence; later, coumadin was given prophylactically. Follow-up for the next 2 years revealed no recurrence of fever. Another example of persistent high temperature due to pulmonary infarcts was a 35 year old man who was admitted to a hospital with nonproductive cough, a temperature of 103–105°F and a diffuse alveolar and interstitial infiltrate of the lungs. The white blood count was elevated. Culture of blood was sterile; sputum could not be obtained. Because treatment with a number of antimicrobial agents over a period of 2 weeks was without effect on either the temperature or the lesions in the lung, he was transferred to another hospital, where pulmonary scan and arteriography demonstrated clear-cut occlusion of a number of vessels. Phlebography of the legs disclosed deep vein thrombosis on the right. The administration of heparin led to defervescence within 24 hours; an umbrella was then inserted into the vena cava.

Hematomas in most sites, unless infected, are usually not accompanied by elevation of temperature over 99.6–100°F. However, uninfected hemorrhages in the subarachnoid and retroperitoneal spaces may be responsible for fever as high as 103 to 104°F. Because involvement of the subarachnoid space leads to the rapid development of severe headache, coma and signs of menigeal irritation, the issue of fever of unknown origin is usually not raised. However, slow leakage of blood into the retroperitoneal space, a problem primarily in patients with bleeding disorders or in those receiving anticoagulants, is associated with early appearance of high-grade fever. Patients with this problem often present with FUO because there are no manifestations indicating the presence of blood in this area. Evacuation of the hemorrhage is followed by rapid defervescence.

Patients with diffuse sarcoidosis may, on rare occasions, present with fever of unknown origin when there is no evidence of arthritis, lesions of the skin, hilar and other lymphadenopathy or pulmonary infiltration [47]. In some cases, biopsy of the scalene fat pad, even when enlarged nodes are not palpable, may provide the diagnosis.

A commonly overlooked cause of fever of unknown origin is subacute thyroiditis [41]. Most patients with this disorder have an increase in temperature to 99.6 to 100.6 daily, generalized malaise, overwhelming fatigue and recurrent episodes of sore throat for weeks to months. There is usually no detectable enlargement of the gland. The hallmark of this disease is tenderness, practically always over the isthmus and less commonly over the lobes. Examination of the pharynx discloses no abnormalities. Pain in the ears is a common complaint; this often starts in the anterior neck and radiates to the ears. Examination reveals normal auditory canals and tympanic membranes. The classic laboratory findings— high level of protein-bound iodine, low radioiodine uptake and antibody to thyroglobulin—are frequently absent. Demonstration of elevated titers of antibody to thyroglobulin and thyroidal microsomes yields the diagnosis. An outstanding example of daily fever (101–103°F) continuing for more than a year was a 56 year old woman, the cause of whose elevated temperature had not been identified, despite extensive study. When examined by one of us, the only positive findings were fever, slight tenderness limited to the thyroidal isthmus and an elevated sedimentation rate. No abnormalities of thyroid function were detected. Administration of 30 mg of Armour's thyroid extract was followed by a decrease of temperature from 102.5 to 102°F. The dose was increased by 30 mg every

48 hours. The temperature fell by 0.5°F with each increment of the drug, and reached normal when 150 mg was given. Therapy was stopped after one week of freedom from fever. The temperature rose gradually over the following month and reached a height of 101.5 to 102°F each day. Reinstitution of treatment with 150 mg of thyroid extract led to defervescence after 2 days; this was maintained over the next 6 months, after which the patient failed to return for study. Another more dramatic instance of the association of high-grade fever with acute thyroiditis was a 28 year old woman who developed her problem during an episode of severe serum sickness induced by penicillin. All manifestations of the allergic reaction had disappeared after therapy with prednisone for 2 weeks. Within one week after the drug was stopped, temperature rose to 102–106°F, but no other manifestations of serum sickness reappeared. Because attempts to define the cause of the elevated temperature were unsuccessful after 2 weeks of investigation at one hospital, she was admitted to another institution, where the only significant findings were fever (106.5) and tenderness of the thyroidal isthmus. A single dose of 15 mg of Armour's thyroid extract produced complete defervescence in 24 hours. This was increased to 150 mg per day and continued for 2 weeks, during which the patient remained afebrile. She was then discharged to the care of her family physician and lost to follow-up.

Familial Mediterranean fever (FMF) is characterized by unperiodic episodes of moderate to high fever alone, or often in association with diffuse abdominal pain and/or arthritis. It involves ethnic groups whose origin is in countries bordering the shores of the Mediterranean Sea [22]. The possibility of this disease should be considered only in patients with the appropriate genetic background, in whom no other cause for elevation of temperature can be identified. A therapeutic test may be of diagnostic help, in some instances. Initiation of treatment with colchicine when fever is present, and continuation of the drug after defervescence has occurred, will, in most cases, prevent recurrences. Therapy often needs to be administered over an extended period because the interval between repeated febrile episodes may be long. A recent experience with a native-born Israeli, who because of repeated episodes of fever and pain in the abdomen while in his homeland, had been told that he had familial Mediterranean fever underscores the importance of careful and thorough search for other causes of this syndrome, despite the support of a predisposing ethnic background. When this man first came to our attention with fever, the diagnosis of FMF was not questioned. However, during three subsequent febrile episodes, it was noted that pain and tenderness were most marked in the right upper quadrant of the abdomen. For this reason, cholecystography was carried out, revealing stones. The gall bladder was removed. Following this, there were no attacks of fever or other symptoms over the following 3 years.

One of the most fascinating and still etiologically undefined causes of recurrent episodes of elevated temperature is periodic fever. This is one of a large number of syndromes described by Reimann [52], the primary characteristic of which is the exact predictability of the time of their appearance. They are thought to represent dysfunction of normal "clock mechanisms." Patients with periodic fever are able to predict exactly when their temperature will rise. The number of days between recurrent febrile episodes, when divided by 7, always yields an equal number. Thus, fever recurs every 7, 14, 21, etc., days, usually at about the same time of day. The interval may change, without reason, and shift from a period of 14 to 7, 21 or 28 or more days. The only symptom is an increase in temperature that may reach 102°F and persist for 2 to 3 days. Extensive studies of persons with this syndrome have failed to disclose any etiologic factor. Episodes of recurrent fever recur over many years. The following experience emphasizes the point that every person suspected of having periodic fever should be studied for other possibilities. The patient was a 22 year old man who had experienced fever that began at 7 p.m. on Friday, reached a height of about 102°F, disappeared after 48 hours, and recurred at the same time exactly 7 days later. All clinical and laboratory examinations, including radiographic study of the chest, failed to disclose any clues. A record of temperature determined 4 times a day over 3 weeks confirmed the periodicity of the fever. When reexamined at the end of this period, radiography raised a question of slight enlargement of the mediastinal shadow; it was definitely enlarged 4 weeks later. Mediastinoscopy, with biopsy of enlarged nodes, established the diagnosis of Hodgkin's disease.

A number of patients with various types of leukemia or lymphoma who have appeared to respond favorably to chemotherapy may develop prolonged high-grade fever, in the absence of detectable evidence of infection. The fact that the neoplastic disease appears, by all criteria, to have been brought under control by treatment does not rule out the possibility that it may be responsible for the elevated temperature as a result of invasion of some organ or tissue, the location of which is not immediately apparent.

Biopsy of the liver in patients with fever of unknown origin occasionally discloses "granulomatous hepatitis" [56]. The histologic picture usually does not permit definition of etiology. Among the diseases associated with this syndrome are histoplasmosis, chronic granulomatous disease of childhood, Hodgkin's disease, tuberculosis, brucellosis, Crohn's disease, parasitic infestations, fungal infection, berylliosis, reaction to drugs (sulfonamides and others), Q fever, vasculitis (syndromes of polyarteritis), primary biliary cirrhosis, syphilis, some types of hypoglobulinemia and postnecrotic hepati cirrhosis. About 50–65 per cent of cases appear to be due to tuberculosis or sarcoidosis; in 20 to 26 per cent, the etiology cannot be defined. Recovery is spontaneous in some cases. It has been suggested that, in all instances in which a specific cause cannot be identified, treatment for tuberculosis be initiated. If this fails to produce defervescence after 6 weeks, prednisone is substituted.

APPROACHES TO THE DIAGNOSIS OF FEVER OF UNKNOWN ORIGIN

As defined in this discussion, the term "fever of unknown origin" has been restricted to patients in whom the most minutely detailed history and physical examination, "routine" studies of blood and urine and radiography of the chest yield normal findings. The importance of these initial investigations cannot be overemphasized. Thorough inquiry into *genetic background, epidemiologic experiences, exposure to infectious agents, industrial chemicals, drugs and animals, pursuit of a symptom that patients may pass over lightly* (e.g. a soft or loose stool "once in a while"), *occupation and character of the fever curve* may, at times, yield the answer to what has been an insoluble problem. The physical examination must be so detailed that, were the patient found in a coma or dead, he or she could be identified by a stranger to whom the written description was available.

Serologic Studies. These have proved, for the most part, to be of little or no value. The commonly requested "febrile" agglutinins (*S. typhi*, the paratyphoid bacilli and *Proteus* OX19 and others) have rarely been helpful in the experience of the writers. A single elevated titer for any organism, unless quite high, is not diagnostic. Serial study of titers of antibodies frequently does not lead to a diagnosis in persons who have had prolonged FUO, because significant increases cannot be detected. However, a 4- or more fold increase or decrease (initially elevated titer) in the concentration of a specific antibody establishes a diagnosis in brucellosis, toxoplasmosis, the typhoidal form of infectious mononucleosis, a rare instance of persistent cytomegalovirus infection and other infections.

Isolation of Infectious Agents. Because, as defined in this discussion, there are no identifiable sites of infection in patients with fever of unknown origin, cultures of only a few areas have proved diagnostically helpful. It must be emphasized that microbiologic studies must always include methods appropriate for the recovery of microaerophilic and anaerobic bacteria, fungi and mycobacteria. Cultures should not be discarded for 3 to 4 weeks, if negative; 6 to 8 weeks of incubation are required for mycobacteria. It is important to be aware that normal urine may yield tubercle *M. tuberculosis* or one of the atypical mycobacteria. These organisms have also been recovered from gastric aspirates obtained from patients with FUO with normal radiographs of the lungs. Diseases produced by viruses are very uncommonly accompanied by fever that persists for longer than 3 weeks. In instances in which a viral infection remains active for longer than this period of time it is often impossible to recover the specific agent because of the presence of specific neutralizing antibody; this is not the case when hepatitis B or cytomegalovirus is present.

Blood Culture. Culture of the blood is one of the most important approaches to elucidation of the cause of fever of unknown origin. Negative cultures do not always rule out the presence of circulating organisms. This may be due to the use of inappropriate technics. Blood obtained at the height of fever may fail to grow organisms because the mechanisms involved in clearing the blood stream are probably most active at this time. Although it has been suggested that the optimal time for drawing blood is 2 hours before the temperature rises, because this is the period required for endotoxin to activate leukocyte endogenous pyrogen, this is not always practical. A useful alternative is to monitor the temperature every 30 minutes before it has been noted previously to increase; culturing is started when there has been an increase of about one degree. One sample is obtained every 10 minutes until 6 have been drawn. The minimal quantity of blood drawn should be 10 ml; this should be inoculated into at least 100 ml of an appropriate liquid medium. Cultures should be incubated both aerobically and anaerobically. Although most organisms attain visible growth in 48 to 72 hours, a few need a longer period of incubation; Brucella may occasionally require as long as 4 to 6 weeks. No "negative" culture should be discarded until it has been observed for at least 10 days.

Biopsy. Because there are no identifiable areas for biopsy in patients with FUO as defined here, the possibility of this diagnostic approach is usually not considered. However, it is clear that, in some cases, histologic study of certain tissues may yield the diagnosis. Biopsy of the liver proves most helpful when there is chemical evidence of hepatic dysfunction; in many instances, only the level of serum alkaline phosphatase is elevated. However, even in cases in which there is no evidence of hepatic disease, examination of tissue may indicate the etiology of the elevated temperature. The presence of noncaseating granulomas in which acid-fast organisms cannot be detected does not rule out the diagnosis of tuberculosis. Examination of bone marrow (biopsy, not aspirate) may also be helpful. In the absence of urinary abnormalities and evidence of renal dysfunction, biopsy of the kidney is rarely entertained. However, this has established a diagnosis in some of our patients in whom the cause of prolonged fever had not been identified after extensive investigation. Among the diseases that have been detected by this means have been tuberculous pyelonephritis (normal urine), interstitial nephritis, acute diffuse glomerulonephritis (multiple normal urines), systemic lupus erythematosus (fever and leukopenia but negative ANA and L.E. preparations, normal level of complement and no urinary abnormalities) and polyarteritis nodosa (normal urine and renal function). If, during the period of observation, patients with FUO develop enlargement of lymph nodes or lesions of the skin, these must be biopsied.

All biopsied tissues must be cultured for anaerobic and facultatively anaerobic bacteria, fungi and mycobacteria. Among the organisms recovered from the liver in patients with FUO, sterile blood, elevated levels of serum alkaline phosphatase (not always present) and normal biliary tracts have been *Propionobacterium acnes,* green-pigment-producing streptococci, *Actinomyces israeli, M. tuberculosis, Candia albicans* and a variety of gram-negative enteric bacilli (cases of chronic cholangitis) (unpublished data). Culture of tissue obtained by biopsy of lymph nodes has established the diagnosis of infection by *Propiono-bacterium acnes* in one case and tuberculosis in a number of others. The importance of appropriate culture of biopsies has been emphasized by recovery of *M. tuberculosis* from the nasal turbinates in two patients. In one, turbinitis was the only demonstrable lesion, while in the other it was one of a number of manifestations of generalized infection (unpublished data).

"Readmission" of the Patient. Failure to delineate the cause of fever of unknown origin is related, in some instances, to a lack of re-inquiry into the historical background and/or repetition of the physical examination. There is a tendency for physicians to become as discouraged as patients, particularly when the cause of the prolonged elevation of temperature has defied identification despite the most intensive and extensive study. An important and often very helpful approach in this situation is "readmission" of the patient. This involves approaching such cases as if they were being seen for the first time, and is based on the observation that many of these individuals have not had a physical examination or search into the history of their illness after the initial one. In an appreciable number of instances, findings not present at the time of

admission—for example, enlargement of lymph nodes, hepatomegaly and/or splenomegaly, increase in size of the mediastinum, a murmur or abnormalities of blood and urine—may not appear until weeks or, at times, months after fever first developed. This may also involve repetition of some of the more sophisticated studies, including scanning and arteriography, that have failed to yield diagnostic clues earlier in the course of the disease. "Readmission" has proved diagnostically successful in a number of cases in which the cause of the fever had been obscure for a long time. It emphasizes the well documented experience that, in some intances, a specific diagnosis can be reached only by following the course of disease over a long period, during which studies are repeated.

Exploratory Laparotomy. The value of exploratory laparotomy in the diagnosis of fever of obscure origin has been emphasized by Geraci et al. [20], who reported that this procedure established the cause in 60 per cent of 70 patients, and by Keller and Williams [29], who obtained "positive" results in 82 per cent of 46 cases. The diseases present most often in these individuals were retroperitoneal lymphoma, hypernephroma, metastatic neoplastic lesions of the liver, and tuberculous peritonitis. This approach was found to be less productive by Sheon and Van Omman [55], who were able to identify the etiology of FUO in only 26 per cent of 30 patients subjected to exploration of the abdomen. The present availability of sophisticated scanning and arteriographic technics, lymphangiography and increased use of biopsy has sharply decreased the need for exploratory laparotomy. This procedure is now very little used to define the cause of FUO. It should be restricted, with rare exception, to cases in which abdominal symptoms of unknown cause are present, or when modern invasive and non invasive technics have demonstrated abnormality of an abdominal organ or lymph node. Baker and his colleagues [3] have made the following important comments related to the indications for exploratory laparotomy in search for cause of FUO:

"Our experience supports the value of exploratory laparotomy in patients with obscure fever. The procedure may enable the clinician to make a diagnosis which makes specific therapy possible. Wise judgment, however, is needed to determine the appropriate time for operation. If the clinical evidence at hand, whether obtained from the history, physical examination or some laboratory or x-ray maneuver, definitely indicates some type of intra-abdominal disorder, the decision for laparotomy is a relatively easy one. We must urge a word of caution, however, in the interpretation of symptoms and signs which seem to point to intra-abdominal disease in patients with obscure fevers. Many disorders, although originating outside of the abdominal cavity, may be accompanied by disturbances of bowel function, nausea, abdominal distention or vague abdominal pain, as well as by mild enlargement of the liver and spleen.

"In the absence of firm clinical evidence pointing to intra-abdominal disease, exploratory laparotomy should not be performed until all pertinent diagnostic studies have been completed. The diagnostic approach must include not only various laboratory, x-ray and other special procedures but also and above all else, a searching clinical observation during which the patient is thoughtfully requestioned and re-examined. Fever alone is no cause for haste. Too often fever becomes an alarm which results in action which would never be undertaken on calm, second thought."

Nucleide Scanning, Arteriography and Ultrasonography. The availability, within the last few years, of a variety of scanning procedures has proved, in many instances, to be of great help in the identification of the cause of fever of unknown origin. These techniques include gallium-67 and technetium-99m scanning, simultaneous liver-lung scan, ultrasonography, lymphangiography, selective arteriography and whole-body computed tomography. These are of particular value in defining occult infections in four sites; (a) the *liver*, (b) *subphrenic space* and *abdominal cavity*, (c) *pelvis* and (d) *bone.*

(a) Liver: The development of arteriography and radioactive scanning (both anterior and lateral) of the liver has made it possible to recognize abscesses in early stages of development. Furthermore, exact localization of the lesions permits the surgeon to select the safest approach to management [40].

(b) Subphrenic and Intra-abdominal Areas: The development of fever following a disease or surgical procedure that may be complicated by entry of intestinal bacteria into the peritoneal cavity raises the question of subphrenic, subhepatic and intra-abdominal abscesses. However, there is often a considerable delay in their recognition [39], and identification of the cause of the febrile response may be difficult [2]. Because "routine" radiologic studies are usually not helpful in the absence of detectable distortion or displacement of adjacent structures or extraintestinal gas [38], scanning procedures play an increasingly important diagnostic role. Gallium scintography has been noted to be accurate in localizing deep abdominal as well as subphrenic abscesses, especially when used in conjunction with ^{99m}TC-sulfur colloid. This helps to reduce the background problem in this region created by localization of ^{67}Ga in liver and spleen; the ^{99}TC sulfur colloid defines the limits of these organs [23,35,36]. However ^{67}Ga scanning does not distinguish between drainable fluid and inflammatory tissue [8].

Ultrasonography is particularly helpful in distinguishing these entities; it identifies the presence of fluid more accurately [27]. This technic is occasionally of critical importance in guiding surgical drainage [57], and in determining if a mass is cystic, solid of mixed [19].

(c) Pelvis: The exact role of ultrasonography in the demonstration of pelvic infections has not yet been defined. It appears to be of some value as an adjunct to clinical evaluation, when it may help to (1) confirm or disprove the presence of a pelvic mass, (2) distinguish between a unilocular and multilocular abscess, (3) assess the response to antibiotics and (4) distinguish between tubo-ovarian and pelvic abscess and other pelvic inflammatory masses [12,63]. ^{67}Ga scans are of less importance in this anatomic area because the continued uptake of the nucleide by the bowel tends to obscure the pelvis [13].

(d) Bone: Technetium-99 phosphate scanning of bone is especially useful in the early diagnosis of osteomyelitis. Radiographic abnormality tends to develop late in this disease [64]. Scanning probably is positive in the early stage of infection because of the increase in blood flow in the involved bone [27].

Lymphangiography may be a helpful procedure in the diagnosis of those lymphomas in which biopsy and histologic verification are feasible; this is often the case when abdominal lymph nodes are involved [14]. It must be pointed out, however, that results may occasionally be falsely positive or negative.

Among other, approaches to elucidation of the etiology of fever of unknown origin is selective angiography. This may be useful in the detection of renal, pancreatic and cardiac lesions.

Gallium-67 may be employed as an early approach to elucidation of the cause of FUO. Although this nucleide was initially used in the detection of tumors, it has been found to be of some diagnostic value in the detection of a wide variety of metabolically and mitotically active non-neoplastic lesions, including inflammatory masses, because of its tendency to concentrate in them. The mechanism by which this agent localizes in abscesses is unknown. There is some evidence that it is sequestered in neutrophilic leukocytes [8]. Scans should be examined early (4 hours) as well as late (24 to 48 hours). Detection of a "hot spot" after 48 hours suggests a tumor. The use of ultrasound in conjunction with gallium scanning increases the possibility of localization of an infectious process.

Ultrasonography has occasionally been helpful in demonstrating vegetations on cardiac valves in patients with infective endocarditis [14,43]. However, this technic has not been of much help when the disease is subacute, because the lesions on the valve are too small; it may be more useful in fungal and acute bacterial infections where the vegetations are considerably larger.

CONCLUDING REMARKS

Fever of unknown origin, the cause of which is not established over a prolonged period, is a trying experience not only for patients but also for physicians engaged in attempts to unravel its etiology. Because the problem may remain unsolved for long periods, it tends to induce a progressive loss of interest and even unconscious medical neglect, because the patients are now "chronic cases" and because they may come to represent a varying degree of diagnostic defeat for the physician. Despite the fact that its solution is very often difficult, its causes multiple and complex and the level of frustration which it produces is high, fever of unknown origin is one of the most fascinating and challenging problems in medicine. This is underscored by experiences with persons who have had elevated temperatures for months or several years, and then defervesce spontaneously and remain afebrile for the rest of their lives, and by the rare individual who dies without a diagnosis and in whom the most detailed autopsy fails to reveal the cause of the elevated temperature.

REFERENCES

1. Alexander HL: *In:* Reactions with Drug Therapy. Philadelphia, Saunders, 1955, pp 49–65.
2. Altermeier WA, Culbertson WR, Fuller WD, Shook CD: Intra-abdominal abscesses. Am J Surg 125: 70–79, 1973.
3. Baker RR, Tumulty PA, Shelley WM: Topics in clinical medicine. The value of exploratory laparotomy in fever of undetermined etiology. Johns Hopkins Med J 125: 159–169, 1969.
4. Barbour G, Juniper K: A clinical comparison of amebic and pyogenic abscesses of the liver in 66 patients. Am J Med 53: 323–334, 1972.
5. Bardswell NE, Chapman JE: Some observations upon the deep temperature of the human body at rest and after exercise. Br Med J 1: 1106–1110, 1911.
6. Barker WH, Wood WB Jr: Severe febrile iodism during treatment of hyperthyroidism. JAMA 114: 1029–1038, 1940.
7. Barza M, Weinstein L: Uncommon presentations of pulmonary tuberculosis in adults. Postgrad Med 51: 143–148, 1972.
8. Blair DC, Carroll M, Carr EA, Fekety FR: ^{67}Ga-citrate for scanning experimental staphylococcal abscesses. J Nucl Med 14: 99–102, 1973.
9. Bondy PA, Cohn GL, Hermann W, Crispell KR: The possible relationship of etiocholanalone to periodic fever. Yale J Biol Med 30: 395–405, 1958.

10. Browder AA, Huff JW, Petersdorf RG: The significance of fever in neoplastic disease. Ann Intern Med 55: 932–942, 1961.
11. Christenson WI: Genito-urinary tuberculosis. Medicine 53: 377–390, 1974.
12. Cochrane WJ, Thomas MA: Ultrasound diagnosis of gynecologic pelvic masses. Radiology 110: 649–654, 1974.
13. Deysine M, Robinson R, Rafkin H et al: Clinical infections detected by ^{67}Ga scanning. Am J Surg 180: 897–901, 1974.
14. Dillon JC, Feiginbaum H, Konecke LL et al: Echocardiographic manifestations of valvular vegetations. Am Heart J 86: 698–704, 1973.
15. Dunn LJ, Van Voorhis LW: Enigmatic fever and pelvic thrombophlebitis. Responses to anticoagulants. N Engl J Med 276: 265–268, 1967.
16. Falcon-Lesses M, Proger SH: Psychogenic fever. N Engl J Med 203: 1034–1036, 1930.
17. Fog M: General acquired anhidrosis: Report of a case and investigation of the heat regulation and circulation. JAMA 107: 2040–2045, 1936.
18. Freidman M: Hyperthermia as one manifestation of neurocirculatory asthenia. War Med 6: 221–227, 1944.
19. Friday RO, Barriga P, Crummy AB: Detection and localization of intra-abdominal abscesses by diagnostic ultrasound. Arch Surg 110: 335–337, 1975.
20. Geraci JE, Weed LA, Nichols DR: Fever of obscure origin—the value of abdominal exploration in diagnosis: report of seventy cases. JAMA 169: 1306–1315, 1959.
21. Gulati P et al: Changing pattern of typhoid fever. Am J Med 45: 544–549, 1968.
22. Heller H, Sohar E, Sherf L: Familial Mediterranean fever. Arch Intern Med 102: 50–71, 1958.
23. Hopkins GB, Kan M, Mende CW: Gallium-67 scintography and intra-abdominal sepsis. West J Med 125: 425–430, 1976.
24. Hoyle JC, Vaizey JM: Chronic Miliary Tuberculosis. London, H. Milford, 1937.
25. Ivy AC: What is the normal body temperature? Gastroenterology 5:326–329, 1945.
26. Jacoby GA, Swartz MN: Fever of undetermined origin. N Engl J Med 289:1407–1410, 1973.
27. Jonsson K: The role of lymphography in the investigation of patients with fever of unknown origin. Acta Med Scand 198:135–136, 1935.
28. Keefer CS, Leard SE: Prolonged and Perplexing Fevers. Boston, Little, Brown, 1955, pp 1–248.
29. Keller JW, William RD: Laparotomy for unexplained fever. Arch Surg 90:494–498, 1965.
30. Konvalinka CW, Olearczyk A: Subphrenic abscess. Curr Prob Surg Jan 1–51, 1972.
31. Krugman S, Ward R, Glies JP et al: Infectious hepatitis: Detection of virus during the incubation period and in clinically unapparent infection. N Engl J Med 261:729–734, 1959.
32. Lee FI, Davids DM: Crohn's disease presenting as pyrexia of unknown origin. Lancet 1:1205–1206, 1961.
33. Lerner P, Weinstein L: Infective endocarditis in the antibiotic era. N Engl J Med 274:199–205, 323–330, 388–393, 1965.
34. Lewis C, Kerby G: An epidemic of polymer fever. JAMA 191:375–379, 1965.
35. Littenberg RL, Taketa RA, Alazraki NP et al: Gallium-67 for localization of septic lesions. Ann Intern Med 79:403–406, 1973.
36. Lomas F, Dibos PE, Wagner HR Jr: Increased specificity of liver scanning with the use of [67]gallium citrate. N Engl J Med 286:1323–1329, 1972.
37. Maklad NF, Doust BD, Baum JK: Ultrasonic diagnosis of postopertive intra-abdominal abscess. Radiology 113:417–422, 1974.

38. Meyers MA, Whalen JP: Radiologic aspects of intra-abdominal abscess. *In:* Ariel, TM, Kazarian, KK (Eds): Diagnosis and Treatment of Abdominal Abscesses, Baltimore, Williams and Wilkins, 1971, pp 87–127.

39. Miller WT, Talman EA: Subphrenic abscess. Am J Roentgenol 101:961–969, 1967.

40. Millett J: Solitary liver abscess. NY State J Med 66:1773–1777, 1966.

41. Molavi A, Weinstein L: Persistent perplexing pyrexia: Some comments on etiology and diagnosis. Med Clin N Amer 54:379–397, 1970.

42. Myers JA: The natural history of tuberculosis in the human body. JAMA 194:1086–1092, 1965.

43. Nomeir A-M, Watts E, Philip JR: Bacterial endocarditis: Echocardiographic and clinical evaluation during therapy. J Clin Ultrasound 4:23–27, 1976.

44. O'Brien JB: Tropical anhidrotic asthenia. Arch Intern Med 81:799–831, 1948.

45. Paton JHP: The mean temperature of healthy girls. Br Med J 2:142–144, 1932.

46. Petersdorf RG, Bennett IL Jr: Factitious fever. Ann Intern Med 46:1039–1062, 1957.

47. Petersdorf RG, Beeson PB: Fever of unexplained origin: Report on 100 cases. Medicine (Baltimore) 40:1–30, 1961.

48. Quinn RW: Health hazards associated with the welding process. Mil Surg 95:410–418, 1944.

49. Reimann HA: Habitual hyperthermia. JAMA 99:1860–1862, 1932.

50. Reimann HA: Problem of long continued low grade fever. JAMA 107:1089–1094, 1936.

51. Reimann HA: Hypothermia—Subnormal temperature and its relation to neurocirculatory asthenia (soldier's heart). JAMA 115:1606–1609, 1940.

52. Reimann HA: Periodic disease. Medicine 30:219–245, 1951.

53. Rubin RH, Weinstein L: Salmonellosis: Microbiologic, Pathologic and Clinical Features. New York, Stratton Intercontinental Medical Book, 1977.

54. Sann SA, Neff TA: Miliary tuberculosis. Am J Med 56:495–505, 1974.

55. Sheon RP, Van Ommen RA: Fever of obscure origin, diagnosis and treatment based on a series of sixty cases. Am J Med 34:486–499, 1963.

56. Simon HB, Wolff SM: Granulomatous hepatitis and prolonged fever of unknown origin: A study of 13 patients. Medicine 52:1–21, 1973.

57. Smith EH, Bartum RJ Jr, Chang YC: Ultrasonically guided percutaneous aspiration of abscesses. Am J Roentgenol 122:308–312, 1974.

58. Spink WW: The Nature of Brucellosis. Minneapolis, Univ. of Minnesota Press, 1956, pp 1–464.

59. Stiles D, Leikola J: Infectious mononucleosis. Semin Hematol 8:243–260, 1971.

60. Sunderman FW: Persons lacking sweat glands. Hereditary dysplasia of the anhidrotic type. Arch Intern Med 67:846–854, 1941.

61. Thorley JD, Jones SR, Sanford JP: Perinephric abscess. Medicine 53:441–451, 1974.

62. Tompkins P: The use of basal temperature graphs in determining the date of ovulation. JAMA 124:698–700, 1944.

63. Ulrich PC, Sanders RC: Ultrasonic characteristics of pelvic inflammatory masses. J Clin Ultrasound 4:199–204, 1976.

64. Waldvogel FA, Medoff G, Swartz MN: Osteomyelitis: a review of clinical features, therapeutic considerations and unusual aspects. N Engl J Med 282:198–206, 260–268, 316–322, 1970.

65. Weinstein EC, Geraci JE, Green LF: Hypernephroma presenting as fever of obscure origin. Proc Mayo Clin 36:12–19, 1961.

66. Weinstein L: Scarlet fever. *In:* Grulee CF, Eley RC (Eds): The Child in Health and Diseases. Baltimore, Williams and Wilkins, 1952, pp 236–247.

67. Weinstein L, Rubin RH: Infective endocarditis—1973. Prog Cardiovasc Dis 16:239–274, 1973.
68. Weinstein L, Schlesinger J: Pathoanatomic, pathophysiologic and clinical correlation in endocarditis. N Engl J Med 241:832–837, 1122–1126, 1974.
69. Weinstein L: Modern infective endocarditis. JAMA 233:260–263, 1975.
70. Williams MH: A note on the temperature of 1000 children. Lancet 1:1192–1194, 1912.
71. Wolff SM, Kimball HR, Perry S, Root R, Kappas A: Clinical Staff Conference: The biological properties of etiocholanalone. Ann Intern Med 67:1268–1295, 1967.

CHAPTER 2

GONORRHEA:
New Insights and Problems

P. Frederick Sparling, M.D. and
Terrence J. Lee, M.D.

In this review, a broad view of the epidemiology, clinical manifestations, and therapy of gonococcal infection is attempted. Because of the availability of other pertinent reviews [40,45,61,63,130,137,152] and books [120],* we have neither discussed all possible topics nor treated each in equal depth. We have tried to indicate something of the scope of present research in this field, as well as to provide information of use to physicians caring for patients with gonococcal infection.

INCIDENCE AND EPIDEMIOLOGY

Incidence

Gonorrhea is the most common reported infection in the United States, with over one million cases recorded in calendar year 1976. Although the true incidence is very difficult to estimate due to underreporting and other factors, a conservative estimate is that two to three million cases occurred in the United States in 1976.

Gonorrhea increased at an annually compounded rate of approximately 15 per cent in the late 1960s and early 1970s, but more

From the Department of Medicine, University of North Carolina School of Medicine, Chapel Hill, N.C.

Acknowledgments: We thank L. Brooks for assistance, and K. Holmes, J. Knapp, P. Perrine, M. Siegel, C. Thornsberry, and P. Wiesner, who communicated unpublished data. Work from the authors' laboratories was supported by NIH grants AI10646 and AI09574 to P.F.S., National Research Service Award AI05216 to T.J.L., and by a grant from The John A. Hartford Foundation, Inc.

* Because of limited space, citations have often been limited to only a few of the many relevant studies, or to reviews.

recent statistics show a marked slowing of the rate of increase, and in the first seven months of 1977, reported cases decreased 0.7 per cent as compared with the same period in 1976 [24]. The reasons for the apparent slowdown in the gonorrhea "epidemic" have not been defined, but one factor may be inferred from inspection of Figure 1. In 1971 a federally funded program of culture screening in asymptomatic women was instituted, and reported cases of gonorrhea in women increased abruptly thereafter. Over eight million screening cultures were performed in nonvenereal disease clinics in each of 1975 and 1976, yielding over 220,000 cases each year. As a result, the ratio of male to female cases dropped from 3:1 in 1970 to approximately 1.5:1 currently. Reduction in the pool of asymptomatic infected females is probably partly responsible for recent flattening of the incidence curve in both males and females. It is too early to be certain whether this trend will persist.

Who Has Gonorrhea?

A report by Pedersen and Bonin [102] is instructive. They found markedly different prevalence rates of asymptomatic gonorrhea in screening cultures of different populations. For instance, 5.7 per cent of cultures in a county hospital obstetrics and gynecology clinic were positive as compared with only 1.2 per cent of cultures in offices of private practicing obstetricians and gynecologists. Rates of positive cultures were higher in blacks than in whites, in patients under 30, in the nonmarried, and in patients of low socioeconomic status. Among patients seen by private physicians, 7.7 per cent of patients under 30 of low socioeconomic status had positive cervical cultures as compared with only 1.5 per cent of patients under 30 and 0.3 per cent of patients over 30 of high socioeconomic status. Similar results were reported by Pariser and Marino [99].

Anyone can acquire gonorrhea, but some are much more likely to do so than others. Studies of a prenatal clinic population at Duke University Hospital in Durham, North Carolina, in which there was a 7.5 per cent prevalence of cervical gonorrhea, showed that 30 per cent of treated patients reacquired infection prior to delivery [71]. Studies in other venereal disease clinics show similar high rates of recidivism, with approximately 15 per cent of patients showing cultural evidence of a new infection within four to six weeks of initial treatment (R. Henderson, personal communication, 1975). Therefore, it is now generally recommended that all patients should be cultured seven to 14 days after treatment (test of cure) and four to six weeks after treatment (to detect reinfection).

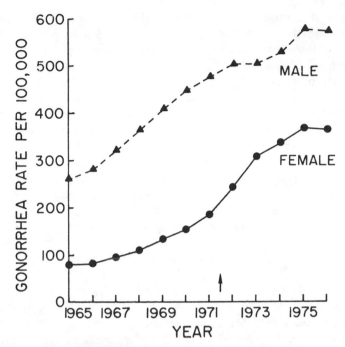

FIG. 1. Rates per 100,000 of reported gonorrhea in the United States in calendar years 1965 through 1976. The arrow indicates onset of the national program of culture screening for gonorrhea in asymptomatic women. Source: Center for Disease Control (P. Wiesner).

An analysis of behavioral and sociologic characteristics of patients with repeated venereal disease [85] showed that the repeaters had difficulty with interpersonal relationships, low self-esteem, and a negative attitude toward society, as contrasted to patients with single episodes of venereal disease. Moreover repeat patients tended to be less well educated and more mobile than non-repeat patients, and more commonly came from a broken home. Problems with alcoholism, injuries, encounters with the police, and other infections including tuberculosis and hepatitis were more common in the repeat patient, as was acquisition of gonorrhea from an infected male homosexual partner. Thus, repeated episodes of venereal disease are one of many manifestations of a disordered and unstable life, which may in turn reflect economic and social problems of the society in which these patients grew up. There will be no easy solution to this problem.

Since gonorrhea is primarily acquired by sexual contact, increased promiscuity is a seemingly obvious explanation for recent increases in gonorrhea. Although several studies of college men did not show increases in promiscuity from 1948 to 1968, college women did show a marked increase in premarital sexual activity by the late 1960s [36]. This change correlated with the advent of oral anovulatory agents ("the pill"). There is no direct evidence incriminating the pill as a causal factor in gonorrhea rates, however [36]. Juhlin and Liden found evidence of increased promiscuity but not of increased rates of gonorrhea among women who used the pill [72]. Two recent studies showed increased rates of gonorrhea in women using either the pill or intrauterine devices as compared with women using the diaphragm and/or foam for contraception [10,60], but the lower rates in women using foams could well have been due to the antigonococcal activity exhibited by certain contraceptive foams *in vitro* [127].

The Asymptomatic Male

One of the most remarkable developments in the past few years has been the rediscovery and realization of the importance of asymptomatic carriage of the gonococcus in males. Until recently, most males with infection of the urethra were thought to be symptomatic.

The concept of the asymptomatic male carrier is not a new one. The old literature is replete with anecdotal reports of individuals who were thought to have asymptomatic carriage in the prostate and elsewhere for periods up to 50 years; these reports are difficult to evaluate because of the difficulties in proving that such patients had not recently acquired asymptomatic infection. In order to circumvent this problem, Carpenter and Westphal [22] studied male inmates at the Attica prison in the late 1930s. Eleven of 1,061 tested inmates had positive genitourinary cultures for the gonococcus, and seven of these had no symptoms. Duration of the carrier state was estimated at from six weeks to over seven years, based on the time elapsed since incarceration in the prison. An assumption that no homosexual transmission took place in the prison is open to question. Despite this difficulty, their study showed that males could carry the gonococcus for considerable periods of time without obvious symptoms.

Carpenter and Westphal's paper had surprisingly little impact on the medical community. However in 1958, Landman and her associates [82] reported that over half of infected male contacts of women with gonococcal salpingitis were asymptomatic, which has since been confirmed many times (Table 1). From these studies one must conclude that approximately 50 per cent of infections found in men named as sexual contacts of women with complications of gonorrhea (salpingitis or disseminated gonococcal infection) or of women detected by screening

TABLE 1. Asymptomatic Gonorrhea in Selected Populations of Men Named as Contacts of Women with Gonorrhea

Author	Type of Contact	Infected No. Positive/No. Examined	Infection Asymptomatic
Landman et al. [82]	Women with gonococcal PID[a]	77/82 (94%)	42/77 (55%)
Pariser et al. [98]	Women in a V.D. clinic	43/115 (37%)	26/43 (60%)
Blound [14]	Women detected by prenatal or family planning clinic screening cultures	228/822 (28%)	91/228 (40%)
Handsfield et al. [56]	Women with gonococcal arthritis	21/38 (55%)	12/21 (57%)
Portnoy et al. [110]	Women in a V.D. clinic	63/133 (47%)	27/63 (43%)
Eschenbach et al. [46]	Women with gonococcal PID	22/42 (52%)	10/22 (45%)

[a] PID, pelvic inflammatory disease.

cultures in a nonvenereal disease clinic setting will be asymptomatic. The concept that most men with gonococcal urethritis are symptomatic stemmed from biased samples of men who presented to venereal disease clinics because of their symptoms.

The natural course of male asymptomatic gonococcal urethritis was studied by Hansfield et al. [56], who followed 28 untreated patients. Eighteen of them remained asymptomatic, without evidence of urethral discharge until treatment was given seven to 165 days later. Five underwent apparent spontaneous cure. The remaining five developed urethritis prior to treatment, although two of the five were subjectively asymptomatic.

Three recent studies of high-risk young men have shown prevalence rates of asymptomatic gonococcal urethritis of over 1.5 per cent [38,56,58] (Table 2). These data probably represent the upper limit of prevalence of asymptomatic urethritis in men in the United States, since the populations studied were drawn from an adolescent detention center, a venereal disease clinic, and military personnel returning from Vietnam; over 25 per cent of the latter had a history of previous gonorrhea.

Does this mean that one-half of men infected with the gonococcus will develop asymptomatic urethritis? The only pertinent data are from an unpublished study by Holmes et al. [62], who followed the course of men aboard ship after they returned from shore leave. Over 95 per cent of the men who developed gonorrhea were symptomatic. Holmes has postulated, therefore, that most men with gonococcal urethritis develop symptoms and present themselves for therapy. The minority who do not develop symptoms continue to carry the organism for prolonged periods of time and represent a disproportionate percentage of total cases in prevalence studies [56,62].

It could be argued that asymptomatic men are merely colonized and not infected. Certainly, a clear distinction is commonly drawn between colonization and infection with other pathogens, such as the meningococcus. However, since asymptomatic "colonization" with the gonococcus may lead with significant frequency to complications of the disease such as bacteremia or salpingitis [8,45,63], or to transmission to a sexual partner who may then develop serious symptomatic disease, there seems little reason to dismiss asymptomatic gonorrhea as mere colonization. This is well illustrated by a remarkable asymptomatic man who had contact with ten women over a short span. Of his eight examined sexual partners, seven were infected; three or four had bacteremia-arthritis, and six apparently had salpingitis [55].

Recently it has been suggested that asymptomatic infection may be due to infection with a particular strain of *N. gonorrhoeae*. Crawford et

TABLE 2. Prevalence of Asymptomatic Gonorrhea in Cross-Sectional Studies of High-Risk Males

Author	Population Studied	Urethral Gonococcal Carriers	No. Asymptomatic No. Infected (%)
Carpenter and Westphal [22]	Long-term inmates at Attica Prison	11 of 1061 (1.0%)[a]	7/11 (63.6%)
Thatcher et al. [140]	American military	0 of 505 (0%)	
Handsfield et al. [56]	American military ("sexually active")	59 of 2628 (2.2%)	40/59 (68%)[b]
Dexter et al. [38]	Asymptomatic venereal disease clinic population exclusive of patients with urethritis or known contact to gonorrhea	37 of 2370 (1.6%)	—[c]
Hein et al. [58]	Asymptomatic adolescents in a detention center	40 of 2064 (1.9%)	—[c]

[a] Some had prostatic focus.
[b] 15 of 40 had evidence of minimal urethritis on examination.
[c] All asymptomatic, but since the study was limited to asymptomatic patients, the proportion of carriers who were asymptomatic is unknown.

al. [29] found that strains requiring arginine, hypoxanthine, and uracil (AHU⁻) were recovered from 24 of 25 asymptomatic men with urethral gonorrhea but from only 40 per cent of symptomatic controls. In retrospect, this was perhaps predictable, since AHU⁻ strains are particularly common in patients with disseminated gonococcal infection (DGI) [41,80], and patients with DGI often have asymptomatic local infection prior to development of disseminated infection [8]. There is no direct evidence as to why AHU⁻ strains cause asymptomatic local infection, but these strains grow very slowly on most laboratory media [41,80] and are unusually sensitive to fatty acids. Their slow growth could also result from uracil starvation, since transformation to uracil prototrophy (Arg⁻ Hyx⁻ Ura⁺) results in much more vigorous growth *in vitro* (B. I. Eisenstein and P. F. Sparling, unpublished data). If growth is as poor *in vivo*, small densities of organisms on the mucosal surfaces might result, with resultant absence of host inflammatory response. Alternatively, these strains may lack specific cytoplasmic or cell surface toxins, or chemotaxins or other factors necessary for production of local polymorphonuclear inflammation.

Most interesting from an epidemiologic point of view was the preliminary observation by Crawford et al. [29] that AHU⁻ strains were more likely to be found from symptomatic white men than from symptomatic black men. These results have been extended in a large multicenter study which showed that 42 per cent of urethral isolates from white patients were AHU⁻ as compared with only 9 per cent of similar isolates from black patients (personal communication, J. Knapp, 1977). Another recent study showed that highly penicillin-sensitive (MIC ≤ 0.015 µg/ml) gonococci were more commonly isolated from white than from black patients (personal communication, C. Thornsberry, 1977); most AHU⁻ strains are very penicillin-sensitive [41,80]. The reasons for these racial differences in prevalence of AHU⁻, penicillin-sensitive strains are unclear but may arise from differences in patterns of seeking health care among different groups. Darrow [37] reported that 28 percent of black males in one clinic delayed 15 or more days after onset of symptoms before presenting for treatment, as compared with 11 percent of white males. Thus, white males may present promptly for treatment of symptomatic infection, thereby eliminating selectively strains which cause symptoms; AHU⁻ strains would tend to persist because they produce minimal or no symptoms [29]. Blacks, on the other hand, may for cultural, economic or other reasons delay significantly before seeking treatment, resulting in continued spread of strains which produce symptomatic infection. These observations, if confirmed, have important practical implications for control programs.

TABLE 3. Spectrum of Gonococcal Disease in Women at a Large Urban Hospital (adapted from McCormack et al., [88])

Diagnosis	Reason for Seeking Care					
	Routine Examination	Contact to Gonorrhea	Vaginal Discharge	Abdominal Pain	DGI[a]	Other
Gonorrhea with no or non-specific symptoms	29	52	18	2	0	3
Possible salpingitis[b]	2	20	0	27	0	14
Pelvic inflammatory disease	0	4	1	75	0	8
DGI	0	0	0	0	4	6
Other	0	1	0	2	0	9
Total	31	77	20	106	4	40

[a] DGI = disseminated gonococcal infection; patients presented with skin lesions, arthralgias.
[b] Patients labeled "anogenital gonorrhea and abdominal pain" by McCormack et al. [88] have been categorized here as possible salpingitis.

Gonorrhea in Women: Symptomatic or Not?

Symptoms are few and often nonspecific in women identified as contacts of symptomatic males in venereal disease clinics [29,39,88] or through screening cultures obtained in family planning clinics, prenatal clinics, or in private physicians' offices [28,61,102]. Thus the prevailing view has been that most gonococcal infections in women do not produce symptoms.

There is evidence, however, that if one studies different populations of patients, symptomatic gonococcal infection in women is common. McCormack et al. [88] examined the records retrospectively of the majority of women with gonorrhea seen at the Boston City Hospital over a six-month interval in 1974. Two hundred and seventy-eight episodes of infection were found in 270 women. Results were analyzed by reason for seeking medical care and type of diagnosis established (Table 3). The most common cause for presenting to hospital was abdominal pain, and the majority of these women had acute pelvic inflammatory disease. Over one-half of the women presented with symptoms. Since women with acute symptoms are likely to present to hospital, it is not yet possible to state what proportion of infected females will develop symptoms, but undoubtedly more than is indicated by studies published from venereal disease clinics.

More patients with gonococcal infection were seen over-all in the emergency room of Boston City Hospital than in the public health clinic, and more were seen in the adult walk-in or screening clinic than were found by routine culture screening in the obstetrics and gynecology clinics. These data are probably typical of experiences in most big city hospitals [28], and have led to recommendations from the Center for Disease Control for intensified follow-up on patients seen in emergency rooms. Most hospitals in the United States presently have neither organized methods for follow-up of patients seen in emergency rooms, nor systematic methods to ensure reasonable rates of examination and treatment of their sex contacts. Assignment to the emergency room of a public health nurse trained in methods of gonorrhea epidemiology would help, but interested physicians in large urban hospitals will have to be found who are willing to participate on a regular basis in management of patients with sexually transmitted disease.

Finding the Asymptomatic Carrier: Contact Tracing

Some clinics in the United States and many clinics in the United Kingdom have full-time epidemiologists assigned to this task. This is expensive, however, and epidemiologic control programs have been challenged by failure of past intensive efforts (the so-called "Speed-Zone" or "Peppy-Epi" programs) to control gonorrhea in the community. These programs were undoubtedly limited, however, by failure to recognize the importance of asymptomatic carriers in disease transmission. There is still no clear evidence that contact tracing will control gonorrhea, but from the point of view of the individual patient it is imperative to treat infected sexual contacts to prevent recurrent infections.

Limitation of funds has forced many states to encourage patients to refer their own sex partners for treatment. Patients are given a card or slip to give to their sexual contacts, which informs them that they have been exposed to an infectious disease and should be seen by a physician. A recent study [111] showed that the effectiveness of this self-referral system was equal to that of the standard method employing professional investigators. Fifty-eight per cent of the contacts of patients who were told to refer their own sex partners appeared at the clinic for examination as contrasted to 62 per cent of contacts identified through the investigator-contact tracing method. Approximately one new case of untreated gonorrhea was detected by both methods for each two patients initially treated.

Strain-Typing

In the past, the only method for strain typing gonococci was determination of antibiotic sensitivities. More recently, several improved methods have been developed, including sensitivity to bacteriocins produced by *Pseudomonas aeruginosa* [126], sensitivity to bactericidal antibodies plus complement [143], and nutritional requirements ("auxotype") on defined medium [21]. Johnston, Holmes, and Gotschlich defined 16 serotypes based on differences in antigenicity and subunit molecular weight of the major outer membrane protein [70]. Epidemiologists have already made significant use of some of these new tools [70,143], and other uses are conceivable, including better medical-legal definition of who infected whom.

COMPLICATIONS OF GONORRHEA

Pelvic Inflammatory Disease

Pelvic inflammatory disease (PID) is the most important complication of gonorrhea, since it occurs in 10 to 15 per cent of women who acquire endocervical gonorrhea [32,45,61] and frequently results in serious short- and long-term morbidity [45,113,150]. The clinical manifestations are often nonspecific and may not be severe; institutions not reporting significant incidence of PID have often found that, when more careful attention was paid to the problem, considerable cases were occurring [129]. An estimated 250,000 patients are hospitalized in the United States with PID each year (the estimate is very rough) and at least as many are treated as outpatients [137]. (The term PID is preferred for patients diagnosed by clinical findings of abdominal pain, tenderness, cervical tenderness, etc., reserving salpingitis for those cases confirmed by laparoscopy. Only 65 per cent of patients with a clinical diagnosis of PID had salpingitis by laparoscopy in one careful study [65].)

The exact role of the gonococcus in pathogenesis of PID is somewhat controversial. It can be isolated from the endocervix of 33 to over 80 per cent of patients with PID [26,30,46,113,137]; data from Seattle showed that 45 per cent of patients with their first attack of PID had gonococcal cervicitis, as compared with 25 per cent of patients with recurrent PID [45]. The lower isolation rate in recurrent disease is consistent with the suggestion that initial gonococcal infection may damage the fallopian tubes, paving the way for secondary invasion by genital streptococci, bacteroides, and aerobic gram-negative rods [90]. Such organisms have been isolated more frequently from cul-de-sac cultures of patients with nongonococcal PID than from patients with gonococcal PID in some (but not all) studies [26,30,46].

Is it reasonable to consider the gonococcus as the cause of PID, merely because it is isolated from the cervix? Other sexually transmitted organisms are frequently isolated from the cervix in association with the gonococcus, including cytomegalovirus, *Chlamydia trachomatis*, mycoplasmas, *Herpes virus hominis* [149], and one or more of them could cause PID. Indeed Mårdh et al. [87] recently reported that *C. trachomatis* was isolated from the cervix of 19 of 53 laparoscopally diagnosed cases of acute salpingitis, as compared with 11 isolates of *N. gonorrhoeae*. Moreover, *C. trachomatis* was isolated from 6 of 20 tubal specimens obtained through a laparoscope, but the gonococcus was isolated from only 2 of 14 fallopian tube cultures. They concluded that Chlamydia commonly cause acute salpingitis. Although Eschenbach et al. [46] were able to recover *C. trachomatis* from peritoneal fluid obtained by culdocentesis from only one of 54 patients with PID, their findings are not in disagreement with Mårdh et al., who also failed to recover Chlamydia from peritoneal exudate even when tubal cultures were positive [87].

Not all studies have shown such low rates of isolation of gonococci from fallopian tubes or peritoneal exudate. Eschenbach et al. [46]

recovered the gonococcus from peritoneal exudate of 8 of 21 PID patients with gonococcal cervicitis, but none of 33 with negative cervical cultures. Similarly, Cunningham et al. [30] isolated gonococci from culdocentesis fluid of 22 of 45 patients with positive cervical cultures, but none of 31 with negative cervical cultures. Curtis recovered gonococci from 19 of 64 acutely inflamed fallopian tubes in the preantibiotic era [31]. Tissue samples may yield gonococci when exudate does not; Studdiford, Casper, and Scadron [133a] isolated gonococci from 16 of 24 consecutive operative tubal samples, but not once from tubal exudate. Other evidence for a significant role of gonococci in acute PID is provided by serologic studies [32,46]. Radioimmunoassay for antigonococcal pili antibody showed significant rises or declines in 12 of 18 patients with positive cervical cultures but in only 2 of 19 with negative cultures [46].

In summary, the gonococcus is an important cause of PID, although other microorganisms, including Chlamydia, may cause the same or a similar syndrome. Clinical differentiation is difficult, but gonococcal PID is more often associated with severe illness, presence of fever, and vaginal discharge, and onset of symptoms is more closely related to onset of menses than is nongonococcal PID [137]. Pelvic abscesses are more common in nongonococcal PID [30]. There is a strong statistical association with use of an IUD and occurrence of nongonococcal PID [151].

There is no convincing evidence that strains of gonococci isolated from patients with PID are different from strains isolated from patients with uncomplicated disease, whereas strains isolated from patients with DGI appear unique (see below).

Piliated gonococci are able to attach to spermatozoa *in vitro* [68], and it is conceivable that these nonmotile organisms enter the tubes as passengers of motile spermatozoa. If this conjecture is correct, gonococcal PID should be an early complication of infection; clinical studies suggest this may be so. Eschenbach followed patients with periodic cultures after initial successful treatment, and found a mean interval of six weeks between last negative cervical culture and onset of recurrent gonococcal PID [45]. Among women with at least one previous episode of PID, the risk of developing PID again with recurrent gonococcal cervicitis was approximately 33 per cent (K. Holmes, personal communication, 1976).

The most serious long-term complication of salpingitis is infertility. Among carefully diagnosed and followed patients, Weström [150] found rates of tubal occlusion of 12.8, 35.5 and 75 per cent respectively with one, two, or three attacks of salpingitis. Approximately 20 per cent of women with one or more attacks of salpingitis became infertile [150].

With single attacks, prognosis was directly related to severity of disease (as diagnosed through a laparoscope): mild disease was followed by only 2 per cent infertility (about equal to rates in controls), but severe disease was followed by 27 per cent infertility [150].

The Fitz-Hugh-Curtis-Stajano syndrome (gonococcal perihepatitis) has classically been considered a complication of salpingitis, due to spread of gonococci upwards from the tubes to the surface of the liver. However, the syndrome sometimes occurs in men [78], and can be reproduced consistently in rabbits by induction of chronic gonococcal bacteremia [74]. There has been a recent suggestion that patients who were not relieved of right upper quadrant pain by antibiotics may benefit from lysis of adhesions through a laparoscope [112].

Therapy of PID has received little systematic study until recently. Addition of adrenal cortical steroids made no difference in a classic study by Falk [47]. Recently, Cunningham et al. [30] compared the major recommendations of the U.S. Public Health Service for outpatient therapy either tetracycline 500 mg orally four times daily for 10 days, or 4.8 million units procaine penicillin IM plus 1.0 gram probenecid by mouth, followed by ampicillin 500 mg orally four times daily for 10 days. Patients requiring initial hospitalization were excluded. Follow-up rates were excellent, although long-term results are not available yet. Results showed both regimens were quite effective, with 82 per cent of patients asymptomatic and with normal pelvic examination within three to seven days of starting treatment. Subjective responses were slightly more rapid in women with gonococcal than nongonococcal PID. Outpatient therapy was successful even in women whose follow-up physical examination was compatible with pelvic abscess, six of eight responding to a 20-day course of ampicillin or tetracycline [30]. Patients who are very ill, pregnant, or in whom there is real uncertainty as to the diagnosis should usually be hospitalized, and treatment should include high-dose penicillin or intravenous tetracycline, possibly in combination with an aminoglycoside.

Disseminated Gonococcal Infection (DGI)

Gonococcal bacteremia and its main complication, gonococcal arthritis, rank second behind salpingitis as major complications of gonorrhea. Most series report a higher incidence in women, although the ratio of female to male cases was only 56:42 in the largest series [63]. Women seem to be particularly prone to DGI during menses [63]. Barr and Danielsson [8] estimated that DGI developed in 1.2 per cent of males and 3.8 per cent of infected females, based on reported numbers of patients with uncomplicated gonorrhea in the area from which the DGI patients were drawn. The true risk of developing DGI may be less than this, since some patients with uncomplicated disease certainly are not reported, even in Sweden. Nevertheless, many centers are recognizing relatively large numbers of patients with DGI, probably secondary to increased awareness of the syndrome as well as increased incidence of uncomplicated gonorrhea in the population. Gonococcal infection is undoubtedly the leading cause of septic arthritis in adults, and accounts for one-third of all cases of acute nonrecurring arthritis at one large center [63].

Most patients have asymptomatic local disease prior to onset of bacteremia. Among Barr and Danielsson's patients, only 11 of 55 women (20 per cent) and 4 of 19 men (21 per cent) had vaginal or urethral discharge, respectively [8]. Dissemination may also occur from asymptomatic pharyngeal or rectal infection [8,63,155]. Venereal disease clinics see few patients with DGI, perhaps due to the absence of local symptoms.

Patients with gonococcal bacteremia may be acutely and severely ill, but it is striking how relatively benign the illness usually is, even when frank septic arthritis has developed. Many patients walk into screening clinics or emergency rooms with a history of several days' fever and polyarthralgias, and if skin lesions are not recognized, the diagnosis may be overlooked [8]. The subacute nature of most cases of gonococcal bacteremia is consistent with the small numbers of organisms found in blood cultures by pour-plates [63]; why gonococcal bacteremia should often behave in this fashion, in contrast to the much more severe and dramatic illness usually seen with meningococcal bacteremia, is enigmatic.

The cutaneous lesions have certain characteristic features, and when seen in a young person with fever and polyarthralgias or arthritis, with or without tenosynovitis, should make one very strongly suspicious of DGI. Lesions are usually sparse in number (10 to 15) and are located principally on the extremities. They may be petechial, maculopapular, nodular, or bullous, but most commonly are pustulate or necrotic, often on an erythematous base [8,63]. Gram stain and culture of lesions are seldom positive, although culture of skin biopsy is more frequently positive, and organisms can be seen in lesions by immunofluorescence in up to 70 per cent of cases [8,146]. Skin lesions are most common in the first week of illness [49,63], coinciding with the period of most frequent isolation of gonococci from blood cultures [63].

The arthritis also takes many forms. Early on it is migratory, often involving several joints, frequently with periarticular swelling. Later (usually after a week or more of illness) purulent arthritis of one or two joints may occur, and the gonococcus is then more easily recovered from joint fluid than from the blood [49,63]. Joints of the lower extremities are most commonly affected, and large joints are more affected than small ones [49]. We have seen one patient with acute nonrecurring arthritis of the proximal interphalangeal joints closely mimicking acute rheumatoid arthritis, from whom a joint fluid aspirate grew the gonococcus.

In addition to arthritis, other complications of gonococcal bacteremia include meningitis [63,139]; hepatitis, pericarditis, myocarditis, and endocarditis [63]; and osteomyelitis [48]. One of 43 DGI patients seen in the past three years at North Carolina Memorial Hospital was a 54 year old woman whose main manifestation of illness was purulent meningitis; *N. gonorrhoeae* was recovered from her blood. Endocarditis is now relatively rare, being seen in only 3 of over 100 DGI patients in Seattle [57,63]. Mild hepatitis and myocarditis are apparently common if one looks carefully [63], but clinically significant involvement is uncommon.

In at least 50 per cent of patients, the only positive cultures are from local sites, including the pharynx or rectum as well as genitourinary sites [8,57,63]. Culture of sexual contacts may provide useful diagnostic information on occasion.

Recently, several interesting facets of the bacteria causing DGI, as well as the host with the disease, have been elucidated. Holmes's group in Seattle showed that gonococci isolated from patients with DGI were much more antibiotic-sensitive than isolates from patients with uncomplicated disease [154], and also were more likely to require arginine, hypoxanthine, and uracil for growth in vitro (AHU$^-$) [80]. These observations have been confirmed [15,41]. In Chapel Hill, DGI isolates were more penicillin-sensitive than uncomplicated disease isolates, when analysis was limited to AHU$^+$ strains only [41]; there was less evidence for an association of AHU$^-$ with virulence independent of the penicillin sensitivity usually exhibited by AHU$^-$ strains [41]. These results suggested that some mutations to low-level (non-beta lactamase) penicillin resistance result in loss of virulence, as has been shown previously in other bacterial species [117]. The propensity of AHU$^-$, penicillin-sensitive gonococci to produce asymptomatic local infection (see above) may also be a factor, since chances of dissemination would seemingly be enhanced for strains likely to be carried long-term.

Gonococci causing bacteremia are nearly always intrinsically resistant to killing by normal human serum and complement [15,41,123], and also by homologous convalescent phase serum and complement [15,123]. (Convalescing DGI patients do produce a variety of antigonococcal antibodies [15,81], including bactericidal antibodies active against serum sensitive strains [T. Lee and P. F. Sparling, unpublished data].) Recently, Payne and Finkelstein reported that DGI isolates were particularly efficient scavengers for iron in chicken embryos [100,101]. Similar observations in other species led them to propose that ability to efficiently compete with the host for limited concentrations of free iron is an attribute of most bacteremic organisms [101].

Abnormalities of host defenses occasionally play a role in development of DGI. Patients with homozygous deficiency of complement components C5 [128], C6 [83], C7 [84], and C8 [106] have been described, who had single or recurrent bouts of either gonococcal or meningococcal bacteremia. All have been otherwise well and free of other infectious complications. Heterozygotes do not seem to be clinically affected. Homozygous complement component deficiency is rare in the general population, but study of 23 consecutive cases of Neisserian bacteremia in Chapel Hill revealed that one patient with meningococcemia was C6-deficient, and one patient with gonococcemia was C7-deficient [84; T. Lee et al, unpublished data]. The common denominator is apparently inability to mount a normal bactericidal response, since opsonization and chemotaxis were normal in several of these patients [49a,83,84,106]. There is no present evidence for other immune defects in DGI patients, including presence of IgA blocking antibodies [144], although the latter have been demonstrated in meningococcal infections [52].

Some of the clinical manifestations of DGI may be immunologically mediated. Danielsson, Norberg, and Svanbom described circulating immune complexes in one patient [33], and high levels of circulating complexes were recently detected by the Raji cell technic in a woman with unusually severe DGI and pericarditis. The level declined coincident with therapy and general clinical improvement (T. Lee, S. Sauter, P. F. Sparling, unpublished data). Further studies are necessary to define the frequency and pathogenic role of immune complexes in larger groups of patients with DGI.

Therapy of DGI is effective even if given for only three days [13], or with low doses of penicillin [145], probably because of the extreme penicillin sensitivity of DGI isolates. We prefer to hospitalize most patients, administering intravenous penicillin G 10 million units daily for three days, followed by oral ampicillin as an outpatient for another week [57]. The prognosis is excellent, although symptomatic response is slower when there is markedly purulent synovial effusion [57]. Most patients with gonococcal arthritis respond well without repeated aspiration of affected joints [8,49,57], unlike other forms of septic arthritis [51]. Patients in whom the diagnosis is clear (as, for instance, when smears or previous culture results are positive for gonococci) may be treated as outpatients with a 7- to 10-day course of ampicillin if they are not severely ill, are likely to be compliant, and do not have purulent arthritis or other serious complications.

Gonorrhea in Pregnancy

Pregnancy is apparently associated with increased risk for development of DGI [25]. Rates of post-abortion endometritis were threefold higher in women with untreated gonococcal cervicitis [19]. Women with gonococcal cervicitis near term are also at increased risk of delivering a premature or immature baby [2,54], and of prolonged or premature rupture of membranes [2,54]. Perinatal mortality was 7.6 per cent in culture-positive patients and 3.0 per cent in culture-negative patients at Strong Memorial Hospital, Rochester [2]. It is not known whether these results are due to gonococcal infection or other associated infection, or are merely a reflection of the frequency with which high-risk obstetrical patients acquire gonorrhea. Neonates with positive orogastric cultures for the gonococcus are frequently septic [54]. Infants born of infected mothers may develop gonococcal conjunctivitis, but the risk of this complication was estimated in a retrospective study at less than 2 per cent after silver nitrate prophylaxis [6].

DIAGNOSIS

Culture

A single cervical culture plated onto Thayer-Martin medium has been shown to be at least 80 to 90 per cent sensitive in detecting endocervical gonorrhea [20,34]. The yield of screening is increased only slightly by obtaining urethral or rectal cultures; approximately 5 per cent of women with anogenital gonorrhea have a positive rectal but negative cervical culture [124]. Media without antibiotics are just as good as Thayer-Martin medium for urethral samples, and are preferable for cultures of cerebrospinal or joint fluid. After plates have been streaked, they may be left at room temperature for periods of at least 12 hours without loss of sensitivity before being placed in a CO_2 incubator or candle jar [102]. Several transport media have been devised, and are used extensively outside of the United States; they are sometimes useful, but may result in fewer positive cultures as compared with direct plating [129].

Diagnosis of the asymptomatic gonococcal urethritis requires culture. Handsfield et al. [56] reported that 36 of 43 infected, asymptomatic males were positive by culture, whereas fluorescent antibody stains were positive in only 20 and gram stain was positive in only 25. Ordinary cotton-tipped swabs are too large and irritating for insertion into the male urethra. Culture is best obtained with a calcium alginate swab or a wire loop. Equally good results are obtained by having the patient urinate directly onto a cotton swab, or by culture of centrifuged urine, providing the urine is centrifuged and the sediment is plated immediately after the specimen is obtained [116].

When should cultures of the pharynx and rectum be performed? Ten to 20 per cent of patients with gonorrhea who practice orogenital sex have a positive pharyngeal culture for *N. gonorrhoeae* [97,134,155], and positive rectal cultures are common in women and in male homosexuals [39,79,124]. Infection of the pharynx or rectum is often asymptomatic [39,79,155]. Both the meningococcus and the gonococcus grow on Thayer-Martin medium, however, and proper laboratory identification is required to confirm that oxidase-positive, gram-negative colonies obtained from the pharynx or rectum are gonococci. Screening cultures from these regions are probably not indicated. Cultures of the pharynx or rectum are indicated for purposes of establishing a diagnosis in high-risk patients with symptomatic pharyngitis or proctitis; in patients who present with the clinical features of a disseminated gonococcal infection; from asymptomatic contacts who were recipients in oral or anal intercourse with an infected partner; and after treatment of known gonococcal pharyngitis or proctitis. Cultures should be obtained from the rectum as well as the cervix of all females after treatment, since addition of the rectal culture increases the likelihood of documenting treatment failure by about 70 per cent as compared with cervical culture only [124].

Blood cultures are positive in less than half of those patients whose clinical illness suggests they are undergoing gonococcal bacteremia [8,63]. In the laboratory we have consistently found that gonococci grow best in liquid media which are well aerated, or in stationary cultures with a large surface-to-volume ratio. Neither of these conditions is met by standard screw-cap flask cultures in clinical laboratories. With some strains, fastest rates of growth *in vitro* are in diphasic agar broth medium (unpublished data). There is a need for clinical trial of different methods of blood culture.

Gnarpe has shown that cell wall deficient "L-form" gonococci can be isolated on osmotically stabilized media from approximately 10 per cent of patients with genitourinary gonorrhea [50]. There is a single report of isolation of gonococci on hypertonic medium from the joint fluid of a patient with gonococcal arthritis when routine cultures were negative [64]. There is no evidence to date, however, that gonococcal L-forms are pathogenic or that they are responsible for treatment failures or relapses.

Gram Stain. Microscopic examination of exudate material is a reliable diagnostic method in men with symptomatic urethritis [34,121]. Gram stain is positive in only approximately 50 per cent of women with a positive cervical culture [20,34]. Moreover, false positive gram stains were noted in 3 to 18 per cent of women, respectively, depending on whether an experienced technician or resident physician read the smear [34]. Cultures must be used for accurate diagnosis in women.

Serology

A number of efforts have been made over the years to develop a useful serologic test for gonorrhea [35,81]. A commercial serologic test was marketed briefly in the United States recently which employed agglutination of latex particles coated with crude gonococcal antigen to detect serum antibody. Unfortunately, this test generally detected less than 50 per cent of culture-positive patients, and was positive in as many as 17 per cent of culture-negative patients [92]. It is no longer available. The most promising serologic test, if only because it uses a purified antigen, is the radioimmunoassay for antibody to gonococcal pili first developed by Buchanan et al. [18]. Approximately 85 per cent of culture-positive asymptomatic females have a positive test [18,94], but 13 per cent of culture-negative patients also had a positive test in one clinical trial [94].

In a critical review of gonococcal serology, Dans, Rothenberg and Holmes pointed out that the predictive value of a positive serologic test with 90 per cent sensitivity and 90 per cent specificity in populations with 2 per cent prevalence of gonorrhea would be only 15 per cent [35]. They urged, quite reasonably, that efforts should concentrate on improving existing clinical services and contact tracing of infected sexual partners, rather than on serology.

At present, for clinical purposes, the most useful immunologic test is probably detection of gonococcal antigens in skin lesions by immunofluorescence [146].

A novel diagnostic test is use of patient secretions to detect biologically active transforming DNA [9,69]. This test has the potential advantage of detecting minute amounts of gonococcal DNA even though cultures are negative. The test appears more sensitive than culture in populations of women [9]. Although the test is relatively simple, many laboratories may not find it practical. Moreover, the specificity of the test remains to be proved in careful clinical field trials.

TREATMENT

A recent large cooperative study in the United States compared single-dose therapy of uncomplicated gonorrhea with either 4.8 million units procaine penicillin IM or 3.5 grams ampicillin orally, each combined with 1.0 gram oral probenecid [76]. The cure rate with the ampicillin regimen (92.8 per cent) was significantly less than with procaine penicillin (96.8 per cent) [76]. In another study, use of 5 million units crystalline penicillin dissolved in lidocaine, plus oral probenecid, resulted in higher peak serum levels of penicillin and avoided potential neurotoxicity due to inadvertent I.V. administration of procaine, but was not as effective as procaine penicillin [1].

For patients who fail penicillin or ampicillin therapy, or who are penicillin-allergic, a four-to-five day course of 9.5 grams of oral tetracycline HC1 or a single injection of 2.0 grams of spectinomycin also provide approximately 95 per cent cure rates [76]. Equivalent doses of other tetracyclines are similarly effective. Presently studied single-day regimens of oral trimethoprim-sulfamethoxazole result in failure rates as high as 20 per cent, which are not acceptable [43].

Spectinomycin and single-dose ampicillin have resulted in failure rates of approximately 50 per cent in treatment of pharyngeal infection, but recommended regimens of procaine penicillin or tetracycline are probably effective [153,155]. Tetracycline should be avoided in pregnancy, and the safety of spectinomycin in pregnant patients has not been well established. More extensive analysis of treatment of uncomplicated gonorrhea may be found in a recent review [40].

Although penicillin is less effective than tetracycline in treating concomitantly acquired chlamydial or ureaplasma infections [96], suggestions that tetracyclines or other drugs might be preferable to penicillin in treating gonorrhea [73] seem premature. Syphilis also may coexist with gonorrhea, and although considerably less common than chlamydial infection, is undoubtedly much more serious. Procaine penicillin as used for gonorrhea is known to cure incubating syphilis [125], but other regimens are either of dubious efficacy (tetracycline), or none (spectinomycin) [27,125]. If Chlamydia are eventually confirmed as frequent etiologic agents in women with PID, or in other diseases more serious than nongonococcal urethritis, emphasis on therapy effective against both Chlamydia and gonococci will be warranted.

Antibiotic Resistance

Chromosomal Mutations

The success of any regimen in gonorrhea is directly related to the *in vitro* antibiotic sensitivities of the organism [66,130]. The basis of antibiotic resistance in gonococci is relatively well understood, and can be divided into two broad categories: one due to chromosomal genes, the other to plasmid-borne genes. The most prevalent type of resistance is due to chromosomal mutations, which result in either high level, single-step resistance, often due to an altered target site for the drug (examples: 30S ribosomal resistance to streptomycin or spectinomycin); or low-level resistance, often due to additive effects of several mutations (examples: common low-level penicillin or tetracycline resistance) [12,86,132].

Two of the mutations involved in low-level non-β-lactamase penicillin resistance are of particular interest, because they result in nonspecific resistance to other drugs [132]. Both alter outer membrane structure and function. The *mtr* mutation (formerly designated by the symbol *ery* [132]) markedly increases the concentration of a 50,000 dalton outer membrane protein, whereas the *penB* mutation increases the apparent subunit molecular weight of the major serotype outer membrane protein from about 35,000 daltons to 38,000 daltons on SDS-polyacrylamide gels (L. Guymon, D. Walstad, and P. F. Sparling, manuscript submitted). The *penB* locus is genetically extremely closely linked to another which determines resistance to serum antibody and complement, which also affects the apparent subunit molecular weight of the major outer membrane protein (P. F. Sparling et al, unpublished data). Thus, the major outer membrane protein is not only important antigenically [70], but may also play a key role in virulence (serum resistance) and in antibiotic resistance.

The precise mechanisms of drug resistance due to the *mtr* and *penB* mutations are unknown. Mutation at *mtr* was shown to decrease permeability to crystal violet, and probably to many other compounds, including detergents and a wide variety of antibiotics [53]. The modest increases in resistance to penicillin and tetracycline resulting from the *penB* mutation [132] could reflect alteration of a passive diffusion pore formed by the major outer membrane protein. Existence of diffusion pores formed by outer membrane proteins is now well established in the enterobacteriaceae [91,93].

In the United States, the long-term trend towards increased prevalence of low-level penicillin-resistant gonococci has abated [66], and there is recent evidence for increasing gonococcal sensitivity to penicillin and other antibiotics [114]. One factor in this turnabout may be decreased importation of resistant isolates from the Far East [56], following cessation of the Vietnam conflict. Another could be the occurrence in resistant strains of mutations which increase antibiotic sensitivity. In Chapel Hill, over 16 per cent of random isolates were recently shown by physiologic and genetic technics [122] to contain mutations (*env*) which increase the permeability of the outer envelope; 15 of 16 tested clinical *env* mutants also contained a phenotypically suppressed *mtr* mutation [156]. The explanation for this may be relatively simple. Growth *in vitro* is slowed considerably by the *mtr* mutation, but is increased after subsequent introduction of an *env* mutation. Thus there may be a balance in nature between mutations like *mtr* which increase resistance, and are favored under conditions of antibiotic pressure, and others like *env* which reduce resistance, and are biologically favorable because of restoration of more rapid growth in the absence of antibiotics.

Penicillinase Plasmids

The recent emergence [131] of penicillinase-producing gonococci (PPNG) is, without doubt, the most alarming development in years. These strains are considerably more resistant than any strains previously encountered, with minimum inhibitory concentrations (MICs) to penicillin G of over 100 μg/ml with inoculums of 10^5 to 10^6 CFU/ml [104]. By comparison, the most resistant previous isolates had MICs of two to four μg/ml penicillin G [66,130]. As would be expected, PPNG infections usually fail to respond to treatment with any penicillin or ampicillin regimen [104].

These strains were recognized nearly simultaneously in 1976 in London, Liverpool, and Southern California [7,104,107]. PPNG were isolated from patients with PID or DGI with about expected frequency in Liverpool [104], suggesting they are as virulent as other strains. Most of the initial PPNG isolates in the United States were either from individuals very recently returned from the Far East, or which could be traced epidemiologically to such individuals. Subsequently, sporadic outbreaks of infection by PPNG have occurred where no Far East connection could be made, but as of August 1977, approximately 40 per cent of new PPNG isolates in the United States could still be linked to importation (M. Siegel, personal communication, 1977). β-lactamase producing gonococci now occur throughout the world, although their prevalence is low in most areas. In the probable source cities in the Far East, however, they account for 20 to 50 per cent of all gonococcal isolates [131].

Many of the PPNG isolates exhibit low-level, chromosomal-type resistance to tetracycline, and oral tetracycline therapy has resulted in over 30 per cent failures [104]. All isolates have been sensitive *in vitro* to spectinomycin, and single injections of 2.0 or 4.0 grams of spectinomycin have been nearly 100 per cent curative [104]. Several cephalosporins, particularly cefoxitin and cefuroxime, appear effective *in vitro* [104], but as yet have not received adequate clinical trial. Oral trimethoprim-sulfamethoxazole is being investigated as alternative therapy for PPNG infections.

The basis for penicillinase production is an R plasmid of 3.2 or 4.4 megadaltons, which carries a gene for production of a typical enteric

TEM-type beta lactamase [42,44,104,107]. Most isolates from the United Kingdom contain the 3.2 megadalton plasmid, whereas most U.S. and Far East isolates contain the 4.4 megadalton plasmid [118]. Many U.S. and Far East strains also contain a larger plasmid of 23.9 megadaltons, which promotes conjugal transfer of the smaller penicillinase plasmid to gonococci, other Neisseria, or to *E. coli* [42,119]. Prior to the occurrence of PPNG, gene transfer by conjugation among gonococci was unknown. Despite the considerable problems which could result (as for instance, transfer of the penicillinase plasmid into meningococci), there is a certain fitting irony in demonstration that gonococci have their own sexuality.

The origin of the penicillinase plasmids is uncertain, but may have been from *Hemophilus influenzae* or *H. parainfluenzae*. Similar plasmids were recognized in these organisms a few years ago. There is over 90 per cent homology by DNA-DNA hybridization between the 4.4 megadalton gonococcal plasmid and a 4.1 megadalton penicillinase plasmid in *H. influenzae*, both of which apparently contain about 40 per cent of the common ampicillin-resistance transposon Tn2 [44,118]. Both the Hemophilus and gonococcal plasmids could, of course, have another ancestral origin, such as ampicillin-resistant *E. coli* in the pharynx or rectum. There is no satisfactory answer for why these plasmids have suddenly emerged in species which had heretofore been totally devoid of any R factors.

The conjugative 23.9 dalton plasmid is not new to the gonococcus. Stiffler, Lerner and Bohnhoff isolated a plasmid of similar size from two strains several years ago [133]. Recently, we found that 12 of 156 (7.7 per cent) of random (non-PPNG) strains isolated as long ago as 1971 were able to mobilize transfer of the non-self-transferable penicillinase plasmid into *E. coli*. Each of the donor strains contained a 23.9 dalton plasmid, most of which were identical to the 23.9 dalton plasmid presently found in the PPNG strains, as judged by cleavage products resulting from digestion with the restriction enzymes EcoRI, Bam I, and Hpa II (T. Sox et al., unpublished data). The observed 30 to 50 per cent prevalence of conjugative plasmids in PPNG isolated in the United States probably reflects conjugal transmission of plasmids between gonococci in nature. Further evidence for this is the large number of different strains which contain the same penicillinase plasmid, as determined by their auxotype, and chromosomal drug resistance markers.

Contrary to what many expected, PPNG isolates have so far not increased in prevalence in the United States. Only 192 PPNG isolates were confirmed by the Center for Disease Control as of August 1977. The prevalence of PPNG among all isolated gonococci is less than 0.5

per cent in Hawaii [23], and probably even less nationwide. PPNG isolates accounted for up to 9 per cent of all gonococci in Liverpool in 1976, but, surprisingly, apparently disappeared thereafter (M. Siegel, personal communication, 1977). The reason for this may be the rather marked instability of the gonococcal penicillinase plasmids in certain strains, particularly the smaller 3.2 megadalton plasmid common to Liverpool isolates [118].

Because of the low prevalence of PPNG in the United States at present, recommendations for treatment of gonorrhea remain unaltered [23,131]. Patients failing penicillin or ampicillin should be cultured and treated with spectinomycin, and their isolates should be tested for penicillinase production *in vitro*. A zone of inhibition of less than 20 mm around a 10 μg penicillin G disc is highly suggestive of penicillinase production, which can be quickly confirmed by several methods [131]. Infections by penicillinase-producing strains must be reported promptly. Because of the efficacy of spectinomycin for treatment of PPNG infections, spectinomycin should not be generally used for all gonococcal infections [131]. Only three or four high-level, single-step spectinomycin-resistant gonococci have been observed clinically [141], but more would surely occur under selective pressures of widespread spectinomycin use.

Prospects for a Vaccine

An explosive growth in knowledge of the pathogenesis and host response to gonococcal infection has occurred in the past few years [148]. Several animal models [5] as well as an organ culture system using human fallopian tubes [89] have been developed for *in vitro* study of bacterial attachment, penetration, toxicity, host response, and immunity.

Vaccination of chimpanzees with a crude formalinized preparation of whole virulent piliated gonococci resulted in partial protection to urethral or pharyngeal challenge with the homologous isolate, although the protective effect could be overcome by increasing the size of the challenge inoculum [4]. Studies in subcutaneous chambers in guinea pigs showed essentially similar results: Vaccination with purified outer membrane (containing lipopolysaccharide and several proteins, but not pili) resulted in partial, quantitative protection (approximately 1,000-fold compared with controls) to the homologous isolate, but no protection was afforded to a heterologous strain [16]. The degree and specificity of protection achieved by immunization with purified outer membrane was similar to that achieved after live infection in the same guinea pig chamber model [103]. Efforts to immunize guinea pigs with purified gonococcal pilus antigen were much less successful [147], which was disappointing in view of the clear evidence that pili are involved in attachment of gonococci to epithelial surfaces [135,136].

Studies of the host response in humans have shown significant cellular and both serum and secretory antibody responses following infection [11,18,32,75,77,138,144]. Serum responses include both opsonizing [11,15] and bactericidal [75,144] antibodies. It is not yet clear which functional antibody class is responsible for immunity [144]. Tramont recently demonstrated that vaginal and male urethral secretions of patients with gonorrhea contained relatively high titers of IgG and IgA antibody, which inhibited attachment of gonococci to epithelial cells *in vitro* [142]. The effect of local antibody was quite strain-specific [142]. Secretory antibodies did not persist long following termination of infection [95,138]. Either the brevity of the persistence of local antibody, or multiplicity of antigenic types of gonococci (or both) could explain the repeated infections which so commonly occur in some individuals.

Recent evidence shows that there is great diversity of cell surface antigens among different strains of gonococci. There are over 20 antigenically distinct types of pili [17; C. Brinton, personal communication, 1977], 16 type-specific major outer membrane proteins [70], 4 distinct polysaccharides [3], and probably at least 5 or 6 distinctive lipopolysaccharides [105]. In addition, three recent studies have provided reasonably convincing evidence for a fragile, polysaccharide surface capsule on many strains [59,67,115], which appears to have an antiphagocytic effect [115]. The precise chemical composition of the capsule, and the number of antigenically distinct capsular types, are not yet known. In the absence of definitive information as to the identity of the protective antigen(s), it is premature to speculate on the composition of a purified vaccine, but it would probably have to be polyvalent. Moreover, if one assumes that an effective vaccine would have to stimulate secretory antibody to afford protection against this primarily mucosal infection, the results of Plaut et al. are worrisome. These investigators have shown that gonococci produce an extracellular protease which specifically cleaves IgA1 into Fab and Fc fragments [108], which results in loss of functional activity of the antibodies studied so far [109]. Thus, gonococci might be able to overcome the protective effects of natural or induced immunity if protective antibodies were in the IgA1 subclass.

SUMMARY

There have been new developments in a variety of fields related to gonococcal infection. Asymptomatic males are of major importance epidemiologically, and have been largely overlooked until recently. Proper use of contact tracing, follow-up cultures of treated patients, and screening cultures in defined high-risk groups will probably help to control the incidence of gonorrhea. Present methods of diagnosis and treatment are generally adequate, although emergence of penicillinase-producing gonococci could result in major alterations in future treatment practices. Knowledge of gonococcal surface structure and function has progressed rapidly, but an effective vaccine is not likely very soon. The gonococcus is a remarkably versatile and well adapted pathogen, and most probably will continue in its intimate relationship with human behavior for some time.

REFERENCES

1. Adams HG, Turck M, Holmes KK: Comparison of aqueous sodium penicillin G in lidocaine and aqueous procaine penicillin G for the treatment of gonorrhea. *In*: Danielsson D, Juhlin L, Mårdh P-A (Eds): Genital Infections and Their Complications. Stockholm, Almqvist & Wiksell International, 1975.
2. Amstey MS, Steadman KT: Asymptomatic gonorrhea and pregnancy. J Am Vener Dis Assoc 3:14–16, 1976.
3. Apicella MA: Serogrouping of *Neisseria gonorrhoeae*: Identification of four immunologically distinct acidic polysaccharides. J Infect Dis 134:377–383, 1976.
4. Arko RJ, Duncan WP, Brown WJ et al: Immunity in infection with *Neisseria gonorrhoeae*: Duration and serological response in the chimpanzee. J Infect Dis 133:441–447, 1976.
5. Arko RJ, Wong KH: Comparative physical and immunological aspects of the chimpanzee and guinea-pig subcutaneous chamber models of *Neisseria gonorrhoeae* infection. Br J Vener Dis 53:101–105, 1977.
6. Armstrong JH, Zacarias F, Rein MF: Ophthalmia neonatorum: A chart review. Pediatrics 57: 884–892, 1976.
7. Ashford WA, Golash RG, Hemming VG: Penicillinase-producing *Neisseria gonorrhoeae*. Lancet 2: 657–658, 1976.
8. Barr J, Danielsson D: Disseminated gonococcal infections (gonococcal septicemia). *In*: Danielsson D, Juhlin L, Mårdh P-A (Eds): Genital Infections and Their Complications. Stockholm, Almqvist & Wiksell International, 1975.
9. Bawdon RE, Juni E, Britt EM: Identification of *Neisseria gonorrhoeae* by genetic transformation: A clinical laboratory evaluation. J Clin Microbiol 5:108–109, 1977.
10. Berger GS, Keith L, Moss W: Prevalence of gonorrhoea among women using various methods of contraception. Br J Vener Dis 51:307–309, 1975.
11. Bisno AL, Ofek I, Beachey EH et al: Human immunity to *Neisseria gonorrhoeae*. Acquired serum opsonic antibodies. J Lab Clin Med 86:221–229, 1975.
12. Biswas G, Comer S, Sparling PF: Chromosomal location of antibiotic resistance genes in *Neisseria gonorrhoeae*. J Bacteriol 125:1207–1210, 1976.
13. Blankenship RM, Holmes RK, Sanford JP: Treatment of disseminated gonococcal infection. A prospective evaluation of short-term antibiotic therapy. N Engl J Med 290:267–268, 1974.

14. Blount JH: A new approach for gonorrhea epidemiology. Am J Public Health 62:710–713, 1972.

15. Brooks GF, Israel KS, Petersen BH: Bactericidal and opsonic activity against *Neisseria gonorrhoeae* in sera from patients with disseminated gonococcal infection. J Infect Dis 134:450–462, 1976.

16. Buchanan TM, Arko RJ: Immunity to gonococcal infection induced by vaccination with isolated outer membranes of *Neisseria gonorrhoeae* in guinea pigs. J Infect Dis 135:879–887, 1977.

17. Buchanan TM, Pearce WA: Pili as a mediator of the attachment of gonococci to human erythrocytes. Infect Immun 13:1483–1489, 1976.

18. Buchanan TM, Swanson J, Holmes KK et al: Quantitative determination of antibody to gonococcal pili. Changes in antibody level with gonococcal infection. J Clin Invest 52:2896–2909, 1973.

19. Burkman RT, Tonascia JA, Atienza MF, King TM: Untreated endocervical gonorrhea and endometritis following elective abortion. Am J Obstet Gynecol 126:648–651, 1976.

20. Caldwell JG, Price EV, Pazin GJ et al: Sensitivity and reproducibility of Thayer-Martin culture medium in diagnosing gonorrhea in women. Am J Obstet Gynecol 109:463–468, 1971.

21. Carifo K, Catlin BW: *Neisseria gonorrhoeae* auxotyping: Differentiation of clinical isolates based on growth responses on chemically defined media. Appl Microbiol 26:223–230, 1973.

22. Carpenter CM, Westphal RS: The problem of the gonococcus carrier. Am J Public Health 30:537–541, 1940.

23. Center for Disease Control: Follow-up on penicillinase-producing *Neisseria gonorrhoeae*—worldwide. Morbidity and Mortality Weekly Report 26:153–154, 1977.

24. Center for Disease Control: Cases of specified notifiable diseases: United States. Morbidity and Mortality Weekly Report 26:253, 1977.

25. Chapman DR, Fernandez-Rocha L: Gonococcal arthritis in pregnancy: A ten-year review. South Med J 68:1333–1336, 1975.

26. Chow AW, Malkasian KL, Marshall JR, Guze LB: Acute pelvic inflammatory disease and clinical response to parenteral doxycycline. Antimicrob Agents Chemother 7:133–138, 1975.

27. Clark JW, Jr, Yobs AR: Effect of actinospectacin (Trobicin) in experimental syphilis in the rabbit. II. In subclinical incubating syphilis. Br J Vener Dis 40:53–54, 1964.

28. Cooper DL, Bernstein GS, Ivler D et al: Gonorrhea screening program in a women's hospital outpatient department: Results and analysis of risk factors. J Am Vener Dis Assoc 3:71–75, 1976.

29. Crawford G, Knapp JS, Hale J, Holmes KK: Asymptomatic gonorrhea in men: Caused by gonococci with unique nutritional requirements. Science 196:1352–1353, 1977.

30. Cunningham FG, Hauth JC, Strong JD et al: Evaluation of tetracycline or penicillin and ampicillin for treatment of acute pelvic inflammatory disease. N Engl J Med 296:1380–1383, 1977.

31. Curtis AH: Bacteriology and pathology of fallopian tubes removed at operation. Surg Gynecol Obstet 33:621–631, 1921.

32. Danielsson D, Falk V, Forslin L: Acute salpingitis and gonorrhoea on a gynaecological ward. A bacteriologic, immunofluorescent and serologic study. *In*: Danielsson D, Juhlin L, Mårdh P-A (Eds): Genital Infections and Their Complications. Stockholm, Almqvist & Wiksell International, 1975.

33. Danielsson D, Norberg R, Svanbom M: Circulating immune complexes in a patient with prolonged gonococcal septicemia. Acta Dermatovener (Stockholm) 55:301–304, 1975.

34. Dans PE, Judson F: The establishment of a venereal disease clinic. II. An appraisal of current diagnostic methods in uncomplicated urogenital and rectal gonorrhea. J Am Vener Dis Assoc 3:107–112, 1975.

35. Dans PE, Rothenberg R, Holmes KK: Gonococcal serology: How soon, how useful, and how much? J Infect Dis 135:330–334, 1977.

36. Darrow WW: Changes in sexual behavior and venereal diseases. Clin Obstet Gynecol 18:255–267, 1975.

37. Darrow WW: Venereal infections in three ethnic groups in Sacramento. Amer J Public Health 66:446–450, 1976.

38. Dexter DD, Cave VG, Faur YC et al: Asymptomatic urethral gonorrhea among men in public New York City social hygiene clinics. J Am Vener Dis Assoc 2:7–11, 1976.

39. Dunlop EMC, Lamb AM, King DM: Gonorrhoea in the asymptomatic patient: Presentation and the role of contact tracing for heterosexual men and women and for homosexual men. Infection 4:125–129, 1976.

40. Eisenstein BI: Effective treatment of gonorrhoea. Drugs 14:57–67, 1977.

41. Eisenstein BI, Lee TJ, Sparling PF: Penicillin sensitivity and serum resistance are independent attributes of strains of *Neisseria gonorrhoeae* causing disseminated gonococcal infection. Infect Immun 15:834–841, 1977.

42. Eisenstein BI, Sox T, Biswas G et al: Conjugal transfer of the gonococcal penicillinase plasmid. Science 195:998–1000, 1977.

43. Elliott WC, Reynolds G, Thornsberry C et al: Treatment of gonorrhea with trimethoprim-sulfamethoxazole. J Infect Dis 135:939–943, 1977.

44. Elwell LP, Roberts M, Mayer LW, Falkow S: Plasmid-mediated beta-lactamase production in *Neisseria gonorrhoeae*. Antimicrob Agents Chemother 11:528–533, 1977.

45. Eschenbach DA: Acute pelvic inflammatory disease: Etiology, risk factors, and pathogenesis. Clin Obstet Gynecol 19:147–169, 1976.

46. Eschenbach DA, Buchanan TM, Pollock HM et al: Polymicrobial etiology of acute pelvic inflammatory disease. N Engl J Med 293:166–171, 1975.

47. Falk V: Treatment of acute nontuberulous salpingitis with antibiotics alone and in combination with glucocorticoids. Acta Obstet Gynecol Scand 44:1–118, 1965.

48. Gantz NM, McCormack WM, Laughlin LW et al: Gonococcal osteomyelitis: An unusual complication of gonococcal arthritis. JAMA 236:2431–2432, 1976.

49. Garcia-Kutzbach A, Dismuke SE, Masi AT: Gonococcal arthritis: Clinical features and results of penicillin therapy. J Rheumatol 1:210–221, 1974.

49a. Gewurz A, Lim D, Ghaze M, Lint RF: Absence of C6 with recurrent meningococcal meningitis. Clin Res 23:532A, 1975.

50. Gnarpe H, Wallin J, Forsgren A: Studies in venereal disease. I. Isolation of L-phase organisms of *N. gonorrhoeae* from patients with gonorrhoea. Br J Vener Dis 48:496–499, 1972.

51. Goldenberg DL, Brandt KD, Cohen AS, Cathcart ES: Treatment of septic arthritis. Comparison of needle aspiration and surgery as initial modes of joint drainage. Arthritis Rheum 18:83–90, 1975.

52. Griffis JM: Bactericidal activity of meningococcal antisera: Blocking by IgA of lytic antibody in human convalescent sera. J Immunol 114:1779–1784, 1975.

53. Guymon LF, Sparling PF: Altered crystal violet permeability and lytic behavior in antibiotic-resistant and -sensitive mutants of *Neisseria gonorrhoeae*. J Bacteriol 124:757–763, 1975.

54. Handsfield HH, Hodson WA, Holmes KK: Neonatal gonococcal infection. I. Orogastric contamination with *Neisseria gonorrhoeae*. JAMA 225:697–701, 1973.

55. Handsfield HH, Holmes KK: Microepidemic of virulent gonococcal infection. J Am Vener Dis Assoc 1:20–22, 1974.

56. Handsfield HH, Lipman TO, Harnisch JP et al: Asymptomatic gonorrhea in men: Diagnosis, natural course, prevalence and significance. N Engl J Med 290:117–123, 1974.

57. Handsfield HH, Wiesner PJ, Holmes KK: Treatment of the gonococcal arthritis-dermatitis syndrome. Ann Intern Med 84:661–667, 1976.

58. Hein K, Marks A, Cohen MI: Asymptomatic gonorrhea: Prevalence in a population of urban adolescents. J Pediatrics 90:634–635, 1977.

59. Hendley JO, Powell KR, Rodewald R et al: Demonstration of a capsule on *Neisseria gonorrhoeae*. N Engl J Med 296:608–611, 1977.

60. Herson J, Crocker CL, Heshmat MY et al: A retrospective study of gonorrhea incidence in an urban family planning clinic. J Am Vener Dis Assoc 1:146–149, 1975.

61. Holmes KK: Gonococcal infection. Clinical, epidemiologic, and laboratory perspectives. Advances in Internal Med 19:259–284, 1974.

62. Holmes KK: Discussion, p. 76. *In*: Danielsson D, Juhlin L, Mårdh P-A (Eds): Genital Infections and Their Complications. Stockholm, Almqvist & Wiksell International, 1975.

63. Holmes KK, Counts GW, Beaty HN: Disseminated gonococcal infection. Ann Intern Med 74:979–993, 1971.

64. Holmes KK, Gutman LT, Belding ME, Turck M: Recovery of *Neisseria gonorrhoeae* from "sterile" synovial fluid in gonococcal arthritis. N Engl J Med 284:318–320, 1971.

65. Jacobson L, Weström L: Objectivized diagnosis of acute pelvic inflammatory disease. Am J Obstet Gynecol 105:1088–1098, 1969.

66. Jaffe HW, Biddle JW, Thornsberry C et al: National gonorrhea therapy monitoring study: In vitro antibiotic susceptibility and its correlation with treatment results. N Engl J Med 294:5–9, 1976.

67. James JF, Swanson J: The capsule of the gonococcus. J Exp Med 145:1082–1086, 1977.

68. James-Holmquest A, Swanson J, Buchanan TM et al: Differential attachment by piliated and non-piliated *Neisseria gonorrhoeae* to human sperm. Infect Immun 9:897–902, 1974.

69. Janik A, Juni E, Heym GA: Genetic transformation as a tool for detection of *Neisseria gonorrhoeae*. J Clin Microbiol 4:71–81, 1976.

70. Johnston KH, Holmes KK, Gotschlich EC: The serological classification of *Neisseria gonorrhoeae*. I. Isolation of the outer membrane complex responsible for serotypic specificity. J Exp Med 143:741–758, 1976.

71. Jones DED, Brame RG, Jones CP: Gonorrhea in obstetric patients. J Am Vener Dis Assoc 2:30–32, 1976.

72. Juhlin L, Liden S: Influence of contraceptive gestogen pills on sexual behaviour and the spread of gonorrhoea. Br J Vener Dis 45:321–324, 1969.

73. Karney WW, Pedersen AHB, Nelson M et al: Spectinomycin versus tetracycline for the treatment of gonorrhea. N Engl J Med 296:889–894, 1977.

74. Kaspar RL, Drutz DJ: Perihepatitis and hepatitis as complications of experimental endocarditis due to *Neisseria gonorrhoeae* in the rabbit. J Infect Dis 136:37–42, 1977.

75. Kasper DL, Rice PA, McCormack WM: Bactericidal antibody in genital infection due to *Neisseria gonorrhoeae*. J Infect Dis 135:243–251, 1977.

76. Kaufman RE, Johnson RE, Jaffe HW et al: National gonorrhea therapy monitoring study: Treatment results. N Engl J Med 294:1–4, 1976.

77. Kearns DH, Seibert GB, O'Reilly R et al: Paradox of the immune response to uncomplicated gonococcal urethritis. N Engl J Med 289:1170–1174, 1973.

78. Kimball MW, Knee S: Gonococcal perihepatitis in a male: The Fitz-Hugh-Curtis syndrome. N Engl J Med 282:1082–1084, 1970.

79. Klein EJ, Fisher LS, Chow AW, Guze LB: Anorectal gonococcal infection. Ann Intern Med 86:340–346, 1977.

80. Knapp JS, Holmes KK: Disseminated gonococcal infections caused by *Neisseria gonorrhoeae* with unique nutritional requirements. J Infect Dis 132:204–208, 1975.

81. Koransky JR, Jacobs NF, Jr: Serologic testing for gonorrhea. Sexually Transmitted Diseases 4:27–31, 1977.

82. Landman GS, Phillips LV, Friend L: Treatment of acute gonorrheal pelvic inflammatory disease: The use of benzathine penicillin G in the ambulatory patient. South Med J 51:899–902, 1958.

83. Leddy JP, Frank MM, Gaither T et al: Hereditary deficiency of the sixth component of complement in man. I. Immunochemical, biologic, and family studies. J Clin Invest 53:544–553, 1974.

84. Lee TJ, Utsinger PD, Yount WJ, Sparling PF: Deficiency of the seventh component of complement associated with recurrent Neisseria infections. Clin Res 25:379A, 1977.

85. Lundin RS, Wright MW, Scatliff JN: Behavioural and social characteristics of the patient with repeated venereal disease and his effect on statistics on venereal diseases. Br J Vener Dis 53:140–144, 1977.

86. Maness MJ, Foster GC, Sparling PF: Ribosomal resistance to streptomycin and spectinomycin in *Neisseria gonorrhoeae*. J Bacteriol 120:1293–1299, 1974.

87. Mårdh P-A, Ripa T, Svensson L, Weström L: *Chlamydia trachomatis* infection in patients with acute salpingitis. N Engl J Med 296:1377–1379, 1977.

88. McCormack WM, Stumacher RJ, Johnson K et al: Clinical spectrum of gonococcal infection in women. Lancet 1:1182–1185, 1977.

89. McGee ZA, Johnson AP, Taylor-Robinson D: Human fallopian tubes in organ culture: Preparation, maintenance, and quantitation of damage by pathogenic microorganisms. Infect Immun 13:608–618, 1976.

90. Monif GRG, Welkos SL, Baer H, Thompson RJ: Cul-de-sac isolates from patients with endometritis-salpingitis-peritonitis and gonococcal endocervicitis. Am J Obstet Gynecol 126:158–161, 1976.

91. Nakae T: Outer membrane of *Salmonella*: Isolation of protein complex that produces transmembrane channels. J Biol Chem 251:2176–2178, 1976.

92. Nelson M, Portoni EJ, Ishida M, Feldman MJ: Evaluation of a serologic test for gonorrhea in a low-risk female population. South Med J 70:316–319, 1977.

93. Nikaido H: Outer membrane of *Salmonella typhimurium*: Transmembrane diffusion of some hydrophobic substances. Biochim Biophys Acta 433:118–132, 1976.

94. Oates SA, Falkler WA, Jr, Joseph JM, Warfel LE: Asymptomatic females: Detection of antibody activity to gonococcal pili antigen by radioimmunoassay. J Clin Microbiol 5:26–30, 1977.

95. O'Reilly RJ, Lee L, Welch BG: Secretory IgA antibody responses to *Neisseria gonorrhoeae* in the genital secretions of infected females. J Infect Dis 133:113–125, 1976.

96. Oriel JD, Ridgeway GL, Reeve P et al: The lack of effect of ampicillin plus probenecid given for genital infections with *Neisseria gonorrhoeae* on associated infections with *Chlamydia trachomatis*. J Infect Dis 133:568–571, 1976.

97. Owen RL, Hill JL: Rectal and pharyngeal gonorrhea in homosexual men. JAMA 220:1315–1318, 1972.

98. Pariser H, Farmer AD, Marino AF: Asymptomatic gonorrhea in the male. South Med J 57:688–690, 1964.

99. Pariser H, Marino AF: Gonorrhea—frequently unrecognized reservoirs. South Med J 63:198–201, 1970.

100. Payne SM, Finkelstein RA: Pathogenesis and immunology of experimental gonococcal infection: Role of iron in virulence. Infect Immun 12:1313–1318, 1975.

101. Payne SM, Finkelstein RA: Central role of iron in experimental gonococcal and other bacterial-host interactions. Abstracts Annual Meeting Amer Soc Microbiol 1977, B95, pp 31.

102. Pedersen AHB, Bonin P: Screening females for asymptomatic gonorrhea infection. Northwest Med 70:255–261, 1971.

103. Penn CW, Parsons NJ, Sen D et al: Immunization of guinea pigs with *Neisseria gonorrhoeae*: Strain specificity and mechanisms of immunity. J Gen Microbiol 100:159–166, 1977.

104. Percival A, Rowlands J, Corkill JE, et al: Penicillinase-producing gonococci in Liverpool. Lancet 2:1379–1382, 1976.

105. Perry MB, Daoust V, Diena BB et al: The lipopolysaccharides of *Neisseria gonorrhoeae* colony types 1 and 4. Can J Biochem 53:623–629, 1975.

106. Petersen BH, Graham JA, Brooks GF: Human deficiency of the eighth component of complement: The requirement of C8 for serum *Neisseria gonorrhoeae* bactericidal activity. J Clin Invest 57:283–290, 1976.

107. Phillips I: β-lactamase-producing, penicillin-resistant gonococcus. Lancet 2:656–657, 1976.

108. Plaut AG, Gilbert JV, Artenstein MS, Capra JD: *Neisseria gonorrhoeae* and *Neisseria meningitidis*: Extracellular enzyme cleaves human immunoglobulin A. Science 190:1103–1105, 1975.

109. Plaut AG, Gilbert JV, Wistar R, Jr: Loss of antibody activity in human immunoglobulin A exposed to extracellular immunoglobulin A proteases of *Neisseria gonorrhoeae* and *Streptococcus sanguis*. Infect Immun 17:130–135, 1977.

110. Portnoy J, Mendelson J, Clecner B, Heisler L: Asymptomatic gonorrhea in the male. CMA Journal 110:169, 171, 1974.

111. Potterat JJ, Rothenberg R: The case-finding effectiveness of a self-referral system for gonorrhea: A preliminary report. Am J Public Health 67:174–176, 1977.

112. Reichert JA, Valle RF: Fitz-Hugh-Curtis syndrome: A laparoscopic approach. JAMA 236:266–268, 1976.

113. Rendtorff RC, Curran JW, Chandler RW, et al: Economic consequences of gonorrhea in women: Experience from an urban hospital. J Am Vener Dis Assoc 1:40–46, 1974.

114. Reynolds GH, Jaffe HW, Thornsberry C et al: Gonococcal resistance to antibiotics. Abstract No. 400. 16th Interscience Conference on Antimicrobial Agents and Chemotherapy, Chicago, 27–29 October 1976.

115. Richardson WP, Sadoff JC: Production of a capsule by *Neisseria gonorrhoeae*. Infect Immun 15:663–664, 1977.

116. Riggs M: Screening asymptomatic male patients for gonorrhea. JAMA 231:701–702, 1975.

117. Roantree RJ, Steward JP: Mutations to penicillin resistance in the Enterobacteriaceae that affect sensitivity to serum and virulence for the mouse. J Bacteriol 89:630–639, 1965.

118. Roberts M, Elwell LP, Falkow S: Molecular characterization of two beta-lactamase-specifying plasmids isolated from *Neisseria gonorrhoeae*. J Bacteriol 131:557–563, 1977.
119. Roberts M, Falkow S: Conjugal transfer of R plasmids in *Neisseria gonorrhoeae*. Nature 266:630–631, 1977.
120. Roberts RR (Ed): The Gonococcus. New York, John Wiley and Sons, 1977.
121. Rothenberg RB, Simon R, Chipperfield E, Catterall RD: Efficacy of selected diagnostic tests for sexually transmitted diseases. JAMA 235:49–52, 1976.
122. Sarubbi FA, Jr, Sparling PF, Blackman E, Lewis E: Loss of low-level antibiotic resistance in *Neisseria gonorrhoeae* due to *env* mutations. J Bacteriol 124:750–756, 1975.
123. Schoolnik GK, Buchanan TM, Holmes KK: Gonococci causing disseminated gonococcal infection are resistant to the bactericidal action of normal human sera. J Clin Invest 58:1163–1173, 1976.
124. Schroeter AL, Reynolds G: The rectal culture as a test of cure of gonorrhea in the female. J Infect Dis 125:499–503, 1972.
125. Schroeter AL, Turner RH, Lucas JB: Therapy of incubating syphilis: Effectiveness of gonorrhea treatment. JAMA 218:711–713, 1971.
126. Sidberry HD, Sadoff JC: Pyocin sensitivity of *Neisseria gonorrhoeae* and its feasibility as an epidemiological tool. Infect Immun 15:628–637, 1977.
127. Singh B, Cutler JC, Utidjian HMD: Studies on the development of a vaginal preparation providing both prophylaxis against venereal disease and other genital infections and contraception: II. Effect in vitro of vaginal contraceptive and noncontraceptive preparations on *Treponema pallidum* and *Neisseria gonorrhoeae*. Br J Vener Dis 48:57–64, 1972.
128. Snyderman R, Pike MC, Szatolowicz V, Meadows LM: A familial deficiency of the fifth component of complement. Clin Res 25:368A, 1977.
129. Sparks RA, Davies AJ: Gonococcal salpingitis in gynaecology—myth or missed? Br J Vener Dis 52:178–181, 1976.
130. Sparling PF: Antibiotic resistance in *Neisseria gonorrhoeae*. Med Clin North Am 56:1133–1144, 1972.
131. Sparling PF, Holmes KK, Wiesner PJ, Puziss M: Summary of the conference on the problem of penicillin-resistant gonococci. J Infect Dis 135:865–867, 1977.
132. Sparling PF, Sarubbi FA, Jr, Blackman E: Inheritance of low-level resistance to penicillin, tetracycline, and chloramphenicol in *Neisseria gonorrhoeae*. J Bacteriol 124:740–749, 1975.
133. Stiffler PW, Lerner SA, Bohnhoff M, Morello JA: Plasmid deoxyribonucleic acid in clinical isolates of *Neisseria gonorrhoeae*. J Bacteriol 122:1293–1300, 1975.
133a. Studdiford WE, Casper WA, Scadron EN: The persistence of gonococcal infection in the adnexa. Surg Gynecol Obstet 67:176–180, 1938.
134. Stutz DR, Spence MR, Duagmani C: Oropharyngeal gonorrhea during pregnancy. J Am Vener Dis Assoc 3:65–67, 1976.
135. Swanson J: Role of pili in interactions between *Neisseria gonorrhoeae* and eukaryotic cells in vitro. *In*: Schlessinger D (Ed): Microbiology—1975. Washington, D.C., American Society for Microbiology, 1975.
136. Swanson J, Sparks E, Young D, King G: Studies on gonococcus infection. X. Pili and leukocyte association factor as mediators of interactions between gonococci and eukaryotic cells in vitro. Infect Immun 11:1352–1361, 1975.
137. Sweet RL: Diagnosis and treatment of acute salpingitis. J Reproduct Med 19:21–30, 1977.

138. Tapchaisri P, Sirisinha S: Serum and secretory antibody responses to *Neisseria gonorrhoeae* in patients with gonococcal infections. Br J Vener Dis 52:374–380, 1976.
139. Taubin HL, Landsberg L: Gonococcal meningitis. N Engl J Med 285:504–505, 1971.
140. Thatcher RW, McCraney WT, Kellogg DS, Jr, Whaley WH: Asymptomatic gonorrhea. JAMA 210:315–317, 1969.
141. Thornsberry C, Jaffee H, Brown ST, et al: Spectinomycin-resistant *Neisseria gonorrhoeae*. JAMA 237:2405–2406, 1977.
142. Tramont EC: Inhibition of adherence of *Neisseria gonorrhoeae* by human genital secretions. J Clin Invest 59:117–124, 1977.
143. Tramont EC, Griffiss JM, Rose D et al: Clinical correlation of strain differentiation of *Neisseria gonorrhoeae*. J Infect Dis 134:128–134, 1976.
144. Tramont EC, Sadoff JC, Wilson C: Variability of the lytic susceptibility of *Neisseria gonorrhoeae* to human sera. J Immunol 118:1843–1851, 1977.
145. Trentham DE, McCravey JW, Masi AT: Low-dose penicillin for gonococcal arthritis: A comparative therapy trial. JAMA 236:2410–2412, 1976.
146. Tronca E, Handsfield HH, Wiesner PJ et al: Demonstration of *Neisseria gonorrhoeae* with fluorescent antibody in patients with disseminated gonococcal infection. J Infect Dis 129:583–586, 1974.
147. Turner WH, Novotny P: The inability of *Neisseria gonorrhoeae* pili antibodies to confer immunity in subcutaneous guinea-pig chambers. J Gen Microbiol 92:224–228, 1976.
148. Ward ME, Watt PJ: Studies on the cell biology of gonorrhoea. *In*: Danielsson D, Juhlin L, Mårdh P-A (Eds): Genital Infections and Their Complications. Stockholm, Almqvist & Wiksell International, 1975.
149. Wentworth BB, Bonin P, Holmes KK et al: Isolation of viruses, bacteria, and other organisms from venereal disease clinic patients: Methodology and problems associated with multiple isolations. Health Lab Sci 10:75–81, 1973.
150. Weström L: Effect of acute pelvic inflammatory disease on fertility. Am J Obstet Gynecol 121:707–713, 1975.
151. Weström L, Bengtsson LP, Mårdh P-A: The risk of pelvic inflammatory disease in women using intrauterine contraceptive devices as compared to non-users. Lancet 2:221–224, 1976.
152. Weström L, Mårdh P-A: Acute salpingitis: Aspects on aetiology, diagnosis, and prognosis. *In*: Danielsson D, Juhlin L, Mårdh P-A (Eds): Genital Infections and Their Complications. Stockholm, Almqvist & Wiksell International, 1975.
153. Wiesner PJ: Gonococcal pharyngeal infection. Clin Obstet Gynecol 18:121–129, 1975.
154. Wiesner PJ, Handsfield HH, Holmes KK: Low antibiotic resistance of gonococci causing systemic infection. N Engl J Med 288:1221–1222, 1973.
155. Wiesner PJ, Tronca E, Bonin P et al: Clinical spectrum of pharyngeal gonococcal infection. N Engl J Med 228:181–185, 1972.
156. Eisenstein BI, Sparling PF: Mutations to increased antibiotic sensitivity in naturally occurring gonococci. Nature (in press).

CHAPTER 3

BACTERIAL INFECTIONS OF
THE INTESTINE

Richard B. Hornick, M.D.

INTRODUCTION

Diarrheal diseases remain one of man's most common disabilities. In late developing areas of the world, diarrheal diseases are a leading contributor to infant mortality. However, diarrhea caused by various infectious agents is not a disease primarily of countries with poor water supplies and sewage disposal. In the United States, the incidence of infections caused by Salmonella and Shigella has not decreased in the last ten years; indeed, the annual statistics from the Center for Disease Control indicate that these infections are increasing. Yet the proportion of cases caused by these classic bacterial pathogens is small. There is no comprehensive survey as yet which identifies the infectious cause(s) of all cases of diarrhea. Host and environmental variables influence the types of organisms that may be involved during a particular time period [22,42,43,75,76]. Many new agents have been characterized in the past decade, but unknown etiologic factors remain to be identified. Unfortunately, the discovery of newer infectious causes of diarrhea has been of no diagnostic help to the clinician, as these unique microbes cannot be identified by the usual clinical microbiological laboratory. The greatest recent advance in understanding the pathogenesis of infectious diarrhea has been the knowledge gained about the presence and actions of enterotoxins. This information began with cholera toxins [8] and has rapidly spread to the identification of *E. coli* enterotoxins [17]; then various types of enterotoxins from Shigella [52], *Vibrio parahemolyticus* [97], Salmonella [56], various species of Enterobacteriaceae [54,55,57], Clostridia sp. [16,80], staphylococcus [50,51] and other bacteria [100], and recently *E. histolytica* [63] have been identified. Continuing investigations looking for other sources of enterotoxins should be rewarding.

From the Division of Infectious Diseases, University of Maryland School of Medicine, Baltimore, Md.

The role of viruses in causing the undifferentiated cases of diarrhea remains to be clarified. Newer viral agents have recently been uncovered which cause a diarrhea syndrome identical to that caused by bacterial diseases [13,65]. In the near future, many of the cases of diarrhea now undiagnosed should be identified as the etiologic role of enterotoxins and enteroviruses is exploited.

The gastrointestinal tract is a complex organ, but there are only a limited number of functions that appear to be involved in infectious diarrhea. These would include primarily fluid secretion and absorption, but also motility, immunologic defense, nonspecific nosocomial bacterial inhibition and various hormonal and biochemical reactions. The focal point in the pathogenesis of any infectious diarrhea is the epithelial cell. These cells mediate the obvious manifestations of diarrhea, i.e., liquid stools. Diarrhea is an expression of disordered fluid and electrolyte secretion and absorption in the small and/or large intestines. When secretion exceeds the absorptive capacity of the gastrointestinal tract, diarrhea will ensue. It is reasonable to assume that if the absorptive capacity of the gastrointestinal tract is impaired, loose stools may also result. Evidence for this is not as compelling as that for excessive fluid secretion. Increased peristaltic activity may be involved in some phases of bacterial infection, such as shigella dysentery, but it is not a major and universal component of the pathogenesis of infectious diarrhea. The gastrointestinal tract, infected by enteric pathogens, attempts to dilute and/or dislodge the offending organism or toxin through the outpouring of fluids. Specific immune mechanisms eventually are marshalled which contain the pathogen in the lumen of the gut and allow repairs to damaged epithelium to proceed. Thus, "diarrhea" can be viewed as a primitive defensive reaction of the host to a noxious stimulus. This discussion will focus on the pathogenic mechanisms associated with bacterial infections of the gut, the inhibitory processes which help prevent and eliminate the offending microbe, and finally treatment regimens found to be effective in the various infectious diarrhea syndromes.

I. PATHOGENESIS OF INFECTIOUS DIARRHEA

A. Intestinal Epithelial Cells

In order for any bacterial agent to cause diarrhea, it must interact directly or indirectly with epithelial cells. They appear to be the final common pathway in the production of a diarrheal stool. Epithelial cells are born in the crypts of Lieberkühn, migrate along the sides of the villi, and are sloughed off into the lumen of the gut from the tips of the villi. Their half life appears to be about two days. It has been estimated by Croft and his colleagues [9,10] that the shedding rates of intestinal cells in adult man are (a) stomach, 0.5×10^6 cells per minute, (b) small intestine, $20–50 \times 10^6$ cells per minute, and (c) colon, $2–5 \times 10^6$ cells per minute. It is interesting to speculate on the influence this shedding might have on the infectious process. Could the self-limited nature of several bacterial diarrheal states be a reflection of the rapid turnover of cells in the small intestine? As these cells are sloughed into the lumen of the intestine, they may carry the bacteria or enterotoxin with them and prevent them from attaching to other cells in other parts of the small intestinal tract, thereby aborting the infection. During the short life span of these cells they perform many functions, which, when disturbed by infection, may contribute to the diarrhea. They contain digestive enzymes, and are responsible for absorption and secretion of fluid and absorption of foods. Children with diarrhea may have the added complicating problem of being unable to digest carbohydrates due to acquired disaccharide or monosaccharide deficiencies [4]. Undigested sugar can induce an osmotic effect to prolong the diarrhea. Viral diarrhea induced in adult volunteers induced not only disaccharide deficiency but also steatorrhea [84]. The mechanisms involved in fluid production will be discussed below.

The goblet cells interspersed between epithelial cells on the sides of the villi release a mucin which may be a protective coating. This thin, undifferentiated layer appears to be a barrier to several enteric pathogens. Thus, organisms attempting to attach to epithelial cells or invade them must penetrate this mucous layer. Some pathogens such as *Vibrio cholerae,* contain a mucinase which facilitates their ability to penetrate through this layer to adhere to the epithelial cells. Organisms which lack motility because of induced mutations and resulting absence of flagella have much less virulence than fully motile strains [40]. This motility apparently permits the organisms to swim through the mucin layer and approach the surface of the epithelial cells. Antibodies which clump flagella would inhibit the motile bacteria in the mucin layer.

Epithelial cells contain gangliosides in their cellular membranes which act as receptors for cholera and *E. coli* enterotoxins [48,98]. This is the primary step in the pathogenesis of enterotoxic induced diarrhea. In addition, *E. coli* have a protein colonization factor which can be shown to enhance attachment to epithelial cells in a tissue culture system [24]. Bacteria lacking the colonization factor are relatively nonvirulent for volunteers and do not attach readily to the cells [82]. The covering of these receptor sites by other substances, such as toxoids or mucin, may prevent diarrhea. Epithelial cells will also be invaded by certain entero-pathogens; since intracellular killing apparently does not occur, these bacteria will multiply and either destroy the epithelial cells or else extend through the cells into the lamina propria. Both of these processes have been identified with shigella and salmonella infections (see below). The lamina propria contains significant defense mechanisms; it is in this area where physiologic inflammation is rapidly developed during the first few hours and days of life. The cells in this area (consisting primarily of plasma cells, lymphocytes, and some neutrophils) appear to assist in pre-venting nosocomial flora as well as enteric pathogens which may penetrate epithelial cells from entry into the lymphatics or the capillary circulation in the villus. This region, with its ability to evoke an intense inflammatory response, may contribute to the production of diarrhea by indirectly stimulating fluid production, by impairing fluid absorption and perhaps by stimulating peristalsis. The interaction of bacteria with the epithelial cells is necessary to cause diarrhea.

B. Interaction between Epithelial Cells and Enteric Pathogens

Table 1 outlines the various bacterial agents that are known to cause bacterial diarrhea and lists the mechanism by which these organisms are thought to cause disease and the location in the gastrointestinal tract where they exert their primary effect which results in diarrhea. In general, there are two main mechanisms by which bacterial pathogens can cause diarrhea. The first is by eliciting an enterotoxin which attaches to the epithelial cells and results in the enhancement of fluid secretion. The second is by invasion of the epithelial cell and initiating diarrhea by either interfering with absorption or by indirectly stimulating fluid secre-tion. In some instances both mechanisms may be involved.

1. Enterotoxigenic Induced Diarrhea

(a) Cholera
Enterotoxin-induced diarrheal disease had its beginning in the studies conducted with *Vibrio cholerae* [8]. The observation was made that stools from patients suffering from cholera contained an enterotoxin which would cause fluid accumulation in ligated intestinal segments of various animal models as well as bring about permeability changes in skin blood vessels. Additional experiments in animals and *in vitro* have demonstrated the steps necessary for this enterotoxin to induce fluid production. The *Vibrio cholerae* must be able to approach and attach to

TABLE 1. Bacterial Enteropathogens

Organism	Site of Infection	Pathogenic Mechanism	Remarks
Cholera vibrio	Small intestine	Enterotoxin	Very potent enterotoxin
E. coli (ETEC)	Small intestine	Heat-labile and heat-stable enterotoxin	Some strains produce both types of enterotoxins. Toxins plasmid controlled.
Vibrio parahemolyticus	Small intestine	Probably enterotoxin and invasion	Invades epithelial cells in experimental animals. Toxin less potent than cholera toxin.
Bacillus cereus	Small intestine	Probable enterotoxin and invasion	Cause uncertain. Perhaps toxin or bacterial
Clostridia perfringens Type A	Small intestine	Probable enterotoxin plus	Type F organisms cause necrotizing enteritis. mucosal damage
Staphylococci	Stomach and small bowel	Several enterotoxins	Delta toxin—cytotoxic and increases cAMP levels. May be important in staph enterocolitis.
Miscellaneous	Small bowel	Probable enterotoxin	*Aeromonas shigelloides, Klebsiella pneumoniae, Pseudomonas aeruginosa, Enterobacter cloacae*
Shigella	Colon	Invasion and multiplication	Probable role for cytotoxin. Ill defined at present. Prostaglandins implicated?
Salmonella	Ileum	Invasion and multiplication	? enterotoxin. Prostaglandins implicated?
E. coli (InvEC)	Colon	Invasion and multiplication	No toxin isolated at present
Yersinia enterocolitica	Small bowel and colon	Invasion	Unique enteric syndromes—mesenteric adenitis, terminal ileitis.

the microvilli on the epithelial cells. Cholera toxin is an exotoxin released, and which also must adhere to a membrane receptor to cause disease. The toxin attaches to the GM_1 ganglioside in the cell membrane [98]. This attachment initiates a series of events which culminates in stimulation of membrane-bound adenylate cyclase activity which activates cyclic AMP [29]. This energy system, then, is responsible for an active secretion of chloride ion and the inhibition of absorption of sodium. This ion flux results in an outpouring of a protein-free isotonic fluid containing, in addition to sodium and chloride, potassium and bicarbonate ion. There is no histologic change which occurs in the epithelial cells as a result of the attachment of the cholera vibrio or its toxin. Thus, the epithelial cells retain their ability to absorb fluid, but an exogenous energy source, like glucose, is needed for absorption to occur. Fluid appears to come primarily from the area rich in capillaries around the base of the villi [83,85]. The outpouring of fluid from the stimulated cells of this segment of the small intestine may be of such a volume or rate as to preclude significant absorption distally. As a result, large volume liquid stools occur. Much of this fluid production occurs in the upper small intestine.

The cholera toxin consists of two subunits, A and B [98,99]. Only one fragment of the cholera enterotoxin, fragment B, appears to contain a site that binds to the membrane receptor, whereas the other fragment, fragment A, is concerned with toxogenicity. *In vitro* studies indicate that once the attachment has occurred and is allowed to progress for a period of 10–30 minutes [68], the process will continue despite the fact that the toxin is now washed away from the binding sites. The vibrios and the toxin itself appear somehow to enter the systemic circulation either as a consequence of phagocytosis by leukocytes or by absorption through the epithelial cells into the lamina propria, because patients recovering from cholera develop serum antitoxin and vibriocidal antibodies.

The clinical consequences of infection with cholera vibrios are predictable, considering the altered physiologic process involved. Patients lose large volumes of isotonic fluid, reducing their intravascular volume [29]. Therefore, a dehydrating diarrhea leading to hypovolemic shock rapidly ensues in patients with cholera. There are patients with mild cases of cholera, and in endemic areas of the world, such cases are the rule rather than the exception. They will lose much smaller volumes of fluid and not go into shock. Isotonic fluid replacement either by the oral or parenteral routes [31,69] is indicated in all forms of cholera disease. Restoration of fluid and electrolyte balance will not shorten the course of the disease but will maintain a sense of well being. Patients do not develop fever with cholera presumably because no inflammatory response occurs in the gastrointestinal tract and bacteremia is not present. They rarely have cramps (produced by an irritated segment of the gut) other than those that are mediated by a large bolus of fluid. The retention of large amounts of fluid in the gut may occur and should be recognized. The fluid balance charts will be misleading, and additional fluid will be needed to maintain blood pressure, and normal serum specific gravity measurements.

(b) Enterotoxigenic E. coli (ETEC)

The knowledge obtained from the study of cholera has led to the search for enterotoxins in other bacterial species. There are E. coli which are enterotoxigenic and are responsible for diarrheal disease among infants and adults of many animal species, including man [17]. They have caused large scale epidemics [74] and have been associated with varying numbers of cases of traveler's diarrhea [36,78,88]. The disease is associated with the temporary colonization of the proximal small bowel with ETEC. Once they have been cleared from this area, the disease is finished despite the carriage of the organisms in the large bowel. For these organisms to cause disease, two virulence properties are necessary. The first is the ability of the strain to produce an enterotoxin [17], and the second is the possession of a colonization factor(s) [24] which enables it to attach to selected sites in the host's upper gastrointestinal tract.

E. coli can elaborate two types of enterotoxin—heat labile (LT) and heat stable (ST) [44]. The LT toxin has been more extensively studied and characterized. Genes for the synthesis of LT are found in transferable plasmids (Ent +) [90]. LT resembles cholera toxin physiologically as well as immunologically; however, the disease initiated by LT is usually much less severe than that produced by the cholera toxin. The initiation of fluid secretion in the small intestine by LT is mediated by the stimulation of an adenylate cyclase-cyclic AMP system identical to the mechanisms activated by cholera toxin. The receptor site on the epithelial cells for both E. coli enterotoxins appears to be the same as cholera, i.e., GM_1 gangliosides [15,48,98].

Isolation of LT-producing E. coli requires special laboratory technics. LT and cholera toxin can be identified in the intestinal loop model of such animals as rabbits or dogs. The organism or its toxin will cause an increase in fluid secretion in these test loops, as compared with controls. In addition, there are tissue culture systems which can be utilized to assay for these enterotoxins. The principle involved in the tissue culture system is similar to that occurring in the gastrointestinal tract; that is, the toxins attach to the cells, trigger the adenylate cyclase-cyclic AMP system, and in the Y_1 adrenal cell system the energized cells will produce steroid hormones [14]. Presumably for the same reason, the stimulated Chinese hamster ovary [41] tissue culture system will undergo overt morphologic alterations. There is a similar cell shape alteration that occurs with the adrenal cells, so that measurement of the steroid hormones is not necessary. Recently a microtiter solid phase radioimmunoassay (RIA) system has been developed for the detection of E. coli LT enterotoxin [39]. This system has several advantages: first, because it is a microtiter system, it is easily performed; secondly, it appears to be as sensitive as or even more sensitive than the adrenal cell system. It also can be used for detection of cholera enterotoxin. A widespread availability of this technic could simplify the diagnosis of ETEC-induced disease. At the present time there are no recognized distinguishing biochemical or bacteriologic characteristics which permit isolation of the E. coli from stool cultures of infected patients. One of the aforementioned procedures is required to select enterotoxin-producing strains from pooled E. coli isolated from a diarrhea stool specimen. There is increasing evidence that certain O:H (cell wall lypopolysaccharide antigen) serotypes are more prone to contain the enterotoxin [78]. O6:H16, O8:H9, O25:H42, O15:H11, O78:H11, and O78:H12 have been repeatedly found among several geographic locations. This suggests that certain serotypes of E. coli have a propensity to be enterotoxigenic pathogens. However, serologic typing is not a reliable means for selecting strains thought to be ETEC. The enterotoxin production is plasmid-mediated, and it is conceivable that some strains could lose this plasmid during in vitro passages and fail in the various tests designed to measure enterotoxin activity.

E. coli also produce a heat-stable (ST) enterotoxin. Some E. coli strains will produce both heat-stable and heat-labile enterotoxins. ST-producing strains have been associated with traveler's diarrhea [79]; recent studies in volunteers have clarified the clinical characteristics of ST-induced diarrhea [59]. There are significant differences in these toxins; the LT is of high molecular weight as compared with low molecular weight for ST [25]. The LT toxin is immunogenic and is immunologically closely related to cholera toxin. The ST toxin is nonimmunogenic and it evokes fluid secretion immediately after exposure to intestinal mucosa, whereas the LT toxin has a delay in initiating fluid depending upon the quantity of LT that is utilized [25]. ST is resistant to boiling, whereas LT is not. The genes for ST production appear also to be found in transferable plasmids. The ST toxin has a different diarrheogenic action than LT; it has not been precisely defined as yet. In order to analyze for ST toxin, the infant mouse model must be used [12]. This consists of injecting the suspected organisms into the stomach of infant mice and looking for the accumulation of fluid. LT will not induce fluid in this model, nor will ST induce fluid in the adult rabbit ileal loop model. ST is not capable of effecting morphologic changes in the Y1 adrenal cell system or Chinese hamster ovaries. Therefore, it does not appear to have the same mechanism for turning on the adenylate cyclase-cyclic AMP system as the LT does.

In addition to the enterotoxin production, ETEC must possess appendages on the cell surface that enable the organisms to absorb to intestinal mucosal epithelial cells. Bacterial organelles with this property, such as adhesion pili, represent a colonization virulence factor. Pili associated with enterotoxigenic strains pathogenic for piglets and calves have been well described [67]. Genetic information for pili production is coded in plasmids, as is enterotoxin production [26]. Animal and human studies indicate that both enterotoxin and adhesion pili are necessary for many *E. coli* to be fully pathogenic [67,82]. The adhesion pili appear to be species-specific; the pig pili antigen which allows *E. coli* to adhere to porcine intestinal cells will not adhere to bovine cells. Presumably, similar colonization factors, i.e., pili, are also necessary for a human enterotoxigenic *E. coli* to be pathogenic [82]. A non-piliated *E. coli* strain derived from normal human flora was the recipient in a genetic cross of an enterotoxin plasmid from an *E. coli* strain virulent for pigs [18]. When large numbers ($10^8 - 10^9$) of the resultant enterotoxigenic HS strain were fed to adult volunteers, no disease occurred. This established that other virulence properties (i.e., colonization factor) in addition to enterotoxin production were necessary for human virulence of *E. coli* strains. Recent investigations indicate that colonization for humans is distinct from the common *E. coli* pili [24].

The clinical manifestations of ETEC are similar to those of cholera but differ quantitatively in enterotoxigenicity. Only an exceptional strain will induce a dehydrating diarrhea, despite the fact that the toxins from *E. coli* and cholera vibrios are immunologically and physiologically look-alikes. The vast majority of patients infected with ETEC have a mild self-limited, afebrile diarrheal disease. It persists for usually 2–3 days. No epithelial cell damage occurs, and oral fluid replacement therapy is effective in relieving symptoms.

In several areas of the world, ETEC have been isolated from children with diarrhea who have evidence of enteric virus infections [43,76]. Some of these children will have serologic evidence of recent infection with ETEC; they have developed antitoxin titers to LT. Do these represent coincidental or mixed infections or is there possibly synergism between the viruses and ETEC?

The search for enterotoxin activity in other species of coliform bacteria has identified LT and/or ST from *Aeromonas shigelloides, Enterobacter cloacae* and *Klebsiella pneumoniae* [43,54,55]. These strains have been isolated from the jejunum of patients with diarrhea or tropical sprue. Additional studies are needed to identify the importance such enterotoxigenic enterobacteriaceae have in the production of human disease.

The enteropathogenic *E. coli* (EPEC) have long been associated with outbreaks of diarrhea in newborn nurseries. These strains are identified by their serotype, which belong to one of the 12 of the approximately 150 O antigen groups (O groups 26, 55, 111, 127, etc) [27]. The mechanism(s) by which they cause disease is unknown. They do not produce the classic LT or ST enterotoxins. Recent studies in volunteers have confirmed earlier feeding experiments demonstrating that these strains will produce diarrhea in adults or babies [62].

2. Diarrhea Caused by Invasive Enteric Pathogens

The classic examples of invasive bacterial pathogens are Shigellae, Salmonellae, and invasive *E. coli*. Each of these species must invade the epithelial cells in order to cause disease. In addition, they must be able to multiply either in the epithelial cells or in the lamina propria for expression of their virulence. Most of the disease process occurs in the distal ileum or in the large bowel; however, there is suggestive evidence indicating involvement of the secretory cells of the upper small intestine which may be stimulated by novel toxins or messenger substances released from the inflammatory cells. Fever, abdominal cramps, and malaise that accompany infections caused by shigella or salmonella and invasive *E. coli* may be caused in part by the inflammatory response stimulated by the invasion of these enteric pathogens. Indeed, with the invasive *E. coli* and shigella species, there is marked destruction of epithelial cells and formation of multiple small abscesses. These pathologic changes can be expected to precipitate a febrile response and alterations in the metabolic and physiologic activities of the host resulting in malaise. The pathogenesis of diarrhea caused by these species varies and will be dealt with separately.

(a) Shigella
Of all the enteric pathogens, Shigella species appear to be the most virulent in terms of the small numbers of organisms that are required to cause disease. As few as 10 organisms of *Shigella dysenteriae* are suffi-

cient to cause disease in about 10–20% [60], and 200 organisms of *Shigella flexneri* will cause disease in about 40–50% of healthy volunteers [21]. None of the other enteric pathogens appears to be able to initiate disease with such a small inoculum (see Table 2). Shigella transverse the stomach without causing apparent disease. In experimental infections in monkeys, gastritis has been described. This must be a very unusual occurrence in man. However, it could account for some of the nausea and vomiting that is sometimes seen early in this infectious process. Once the organisms reach the small bowel, they may multiply and release a toxin which will initiate active secretion of water and electrolytes from the jejunal area (see below). Many patients have liquid stools prior to the onset of bacillary dysentery [20]. There does not appear to be any penetration of the epithelial cells in the small intestine. Invasion is thought to occur in the distal ileum and colon, and without penetration shigella dysentery does not occur [58]. Virulent shigella will invade the epithelial cells, where they multiply, spread to adjacent cells, and cause destruction of these cells. This is a diffuse inflammatory process associated with ulceration and small abscess formation [58]. An analscopic examination would reveal uniform erythema of the friable rectal mucosa. These destructive changes elicit a profuse outpouring of polymorphonuclear leukocytes. Apparently the neutrophils prevent further spread of the shigella and the infection is limited to the superficial layers of the gastrointestinal tract. Rarely does bacteremia with shigella species occur in man. On occasion, children suffering from shigella infection will have *E. coli* bacteremia [45]. It is strong testimony to man's cellular defenses that despite the marked destruction of the epithelial surface, members of the nosocomial flora of the colon do not

TABLE 2.   Dose of Certain Enteric Pathogens for Man*

Organism	Number of Organisms	Attack Rate (%)
Shigella dysenteriae (Shiga bacillus)	10	10
Shigella flexneri and *sonnei*	200	20–30
Salmonella typhosa	100,000	30–40
Clostridia perfringens (type A)	10^9–10^{10}	45
E. coli (ETEC)	10^{6-8}	50–60
E. coli (ST only)	10^{9-10}	80
V. cholerae	10^6†	40–50

* Based on various volunteer studies.
† Inoculum administered with bicarbonate.

penetrate and establish bacteremia. Apparently the leukocyte barrier also prevents these organisms from entering the blood stream.

There are 39 shigella serotypes, which are divided into four grous: (a) *Shigella dysenteriae,* (b) *Shigella flexneri,* (c) *Shigella boydii,* and (d) *Shigella sonnei. Shigella sonnei* is the most common serotype isolated in the industrial countries, while *Shigella flexneri* serotypes predominate in the less developed world. There is a spectrum of clinical illness caused by the various serotypes, although any particular serotype can cause either mild diarrhea or fulminating dysentery. *Shigella sonnei* tends to be associated with milder disease than flexneri serotypes. *Shigella dysenteriae* 1, or Shiga's bacillus, was the first serotype isolated, and has always stood apart from other shigellae because of its clinical virulence, its pandemic potential and elaboration of an exotoxin *in vitro.* This toxin was initially demonstrated to have neurotoxicity. Subsequently, Keusch and co-workers [52,53] were able to show that it caused transudation of fluid in the isolated rabbit ileal loop, was cytotoxic for cells in tissue culture and would cause death when injected intraperitoneally into mice. The role of this enterotoxin in causing the diarrhea associated with shigella infection remains to be defined. In addition, the demonstration recently [72] that *Shigella flexneri* 2a produces a toxin which is serologically related to *Shigella dysenteriae* 1 toxin now expands the unknown relationship of these enterotoxins to the pathogenesis of shigella diarrheal disease. The toxin produced by *Shigella flexneri* 2a is about 1000-fold less active than that produced by Shiga extracts [72]. The reasons for this might be that *Shigella flexneri* have regulatory mechanisms for the synthesis of the toxin which are different than those of *Shigella dysenteriae* and the toxin production is repressed in these species. Second, it is possible that the *Shigella flexneri* produces a protoxin which must be activated in order to express its toxin activity. Third, the low levels of toxin activity in *Shigella flexneri* could reflect the presence of some inhibitory substance that dramatically alters its activity. The enterotoxin produced by *Shigella dysenteriae* was initially thought to be unable to stimulate the production of adenylate cyclase. However, new evidence indicates that if the concentrations of some of the substrates utilized in the determination of adenylate cyclase are increased, then it is possible to demonstrate that *Shigella dysenteriae* toxin will stimulate the production of adenylate cyclase [7]. How these *in vitro* manipulations impact on the environment *in vivo* remains to be determined. It is conceivable that the Shigella enterotoxins may be important in some of the cytopathic changes that occur during these infections. Indeed, the *Shigella dysenteriae* enterotoxin has been shown to have an ability to inhibit protein synthesis, which may be responsible for its cytotoxicity in tissue culture systems [95]. Limited studies in volunteers indicated that strains of shigella which produced a toxin would not initiate disease unless they were able to penetrate and multiply in the epithelial cells [60]. Thus, the primary virulence factor of shigella species is associated with the ability to penetrate and multiply. Assistance in penetrating cells could be provided by these cytotoxic enterotoxins as well as causing the subsequent destruction of the epithelial surface. Under appropriate conditions, the toxins could also stimulate the epithelium of the small intestine or colon to actively secrete water and electrolytes. This fluid then may be unable to be absorbed in the colon, where a diffuse inflammatory response has occurred along with disruption of the epithelial surface.

There is another explanation for the activation of secretory activity of the bowel during shigella infection. It has been shown by Gianelli and co-workers that the intense inflammatory response associated with the invasive pathogens is associated with high concentrations of prostaglandins [38]. Prostglandins can stimulate the cyclic AMP energy system and thereby turn on the secretory process. In their beautiful animal experimentations, they were able to demonstrate that indomethacin given prophylactically would inhibit intestinal loop fluid accumulation presumably by its direct anti-prostaglandin activity.

The ability of shigella to penetrate the epithelial surface may be related to the constituents in the cell wall. The side chains that make up the "O" antigen appear to be a determinant of invasiveness of shigella [32]. Smooth colonies of *Shigella sonnei* contain bacteria which are fully virulent, i.e., able to multiply within the gut mucosa after invasion. Rough derivatives from the same strain do not have the capacity to penetrate epithelial cells and are avirulent. Chemical composition of the lipopolysaccharide structure may be a characteristic which is necessary for invasiveness of shigella strains. Hybrids which are created between *Shigella flexneri* and *E. coli* demonstrate that the *E. coli* antigenic structures, O25 and O8, differ in their invasive capabilities. They hybrids which express the *E. coli* O25 factor will conserve virulence, whereas the hybrids with the O8 antigen fail to penetrate. There is a distinct chemical composition difference between the O repeat units in the O8 and O25 serotypes. There is evidence to suggest that rhamnose is present in the O25 lipopolysaccharide repeat O units, and perhaps this chemical is associated with the ability to invade [32].

The pathophysiologic alterations secondary to shigella invasion, characterized by marked destruction of epithelial cells, empty goblet cells, proliferation of leukocytes, and dilatation and leaking of capillaries, are responsible for the classic bacillary dysentery signs and symptoms. The diarrhea consists of small-volume stools composed largely of blood and mucus. A smear of such a stool stained with methylene blue will show sheets of polymorphonuclear leukocytes [46]. This type of a reaction is specific for invasive enteric pathogens involving disease of the large intestine. Similar stool specimen smears will be seen in patients with ulcerative colitis or amebic colitis. The classic bacillary dysentery syndrome associated with sheets of leukocytes in the stools may not occur in many patients infected with shigella. More common is a presentation of undifferentiated diarrhea, which would suggest small bowel disease without any dysenteric signs at all. A few of these patients progress to bacillatory dysentery after 1 or 2 days of watery diarrhea [20]. Careful collection and handling of stool specimens is necessary to enhance the chances for isolation of shigella. Fresh stools are most likely to yield the pathogen.

The association of shigella disease and subsequent development of Reiter's syndrome in significant numbers of patients who have HLA-B27 serotype is a cause for concern [5]. It suggests that early diagnosis and prompt eradication of the shigella antigens be carried out.

(b) Invasive *E. coli* (InvEC)

The invasive *E. coli* (InvEC) represent a species of organisms that have been isolated from Camembert cheese imported from France [96]; although not responsible for endemic disease, they are of interest because of their resemblance to shigella and have been responsible for several mini-epidemics of diarrheal disease in this country. The clinical picture mimics that of shigellosis. These organisms must penetrate epithelial cells in order to cause disease. There are at least nine O serotypes of invasive *E. coli* which have been associated with outbreaks of diarrhea. These strains produce a keratoconjunctivitis in eyes of guinea pigs (positive Sereny test) [86] which is identical to that of shigella. This test detects the invasiveness of such bacteria. Similarly, InvEC will penetrate monolayers of HeLa cells. The *E. coli* that do invade closely resemble shigella in that they may be aerogenic, nonmotile and unable to ferment lactose. In addition, they may share antigens or have an antigenic structure identical with one or another shigella serotype. It appears that the mechanism(s) for producing diarrhea is/are probably quite similar to that of shigella strains. However, as yet no enterotoxin has been found in the invasive *E. coli* strains. Patients infected with these organisms will produce small-volume stools which consist of blood and mucus and will demonstrate sheets of white cells when stained with methylene blue. There are no characteristic morphologic or biochemical features of these *E. coli,* so that their isolation from a stool specimen is difficult and would involve screening by the Sereny test or testing in HeLa cell monolayers.

(c) Salmonella

The genus, Salmonella, is exceedingly large, comprising approximately 1400 serotypes, most of which are widely distributed in nature as enterobacteria of animals. Human disease caused by salmonella may be divided into three clinical pathologic classifications: (1) self-limiting gastroenteritis, (2) enteric fever, and (3) septicemia and metastatic infections. A fourth clinical type would be the chronic carrier state, usually seen with patients having had previous typhoid fever. Many serotypes are responsible for the self-limited cases of gastroenteritis. Some of these strains may cause bacteremic enteric fever in infants; they include *Salmonella typhimurium, S. heidelberg,* and *S. st. paul* [74a].

The pathogenesis of salmonella infection requires that the organisms must penetrate the epithelial surface in order to cause disease [33]. This penetration apparently occurs in the terminal portions of the small intestine and colon. The bacteria first are absorbed to the brush border of the cells and then are engulfed into the cell and into vacuoles (pinocytosis). They migrate through the epithelial cell into the lamina propria region [93,94]. Some bacteria may also reach the lamina propria by migrating between cells after passing the tight junction. The presence of salmonella in the lamina propria stimulates an inflammatory response [33]. Those organisms responsible for self-limited gastroenteritis induce a polymorphonuclear response, while *Salmonella typhosa* invasion is associated with a monocytic response [91]. The former serotypes ordinarily remain confined to the intestinal wall. *S. typhi,* on the other hand, remain viable in the macrophages and are carried to cells of the reticuloendothelial system, where intracellular multiplication occurs. There is *in vitro* evidence to indicate that *S. typhi* once ingested by leukocytes are able to inhibit the increased oxygen utilization associated with the digestive processes of phagocytosis [66]. Therefore, *S. typhi* are not killed by polymorphonuclear cells (the cells remain capable of phagocytizing other non-typhoid bacteria), whereas those salmonella responsible for gastroenteritis are readily killed in the neutrophil following phagocytosis.

The factors involved in penetration by salmonella species are not known. It is definite, however, that they must invade in order to cause disease [33]. The studies by Got et al. [38] have demonstrated that the inflammatory response that occurs following salmonella penetration will release sufficient amounts of prostaglandins to stimulate the production of cyclic AMP and this energy source stimulates active fluid secretion. Prophylactic administration of indomethacin almost completely abolished the accumulation of fluid in salmonella-infected rabbit loops. This inhibition occurred without any improvement in the expected histologic changes in the affected villi. Control and treated animals had identical inflammatory responses. Thus the penetration and stimulated inflammation were not solely responsible for the fluid production. Those animals which received indomethacin had little fluid production, suggesting that prostaglandins were suppressed by this drug.

Attempts have been made to demonstrate an enterotoxin produced by salmonella such as has been demonstrated in *E. coli,* cholera and shigella. At least three types of toxins have been studied. One toxin (SE) was isolated from the outer-membrane fraction of *Salmonella enteritidis* [56]. When assayed in suckling mice, positive fluid secretion was demonstrated. ST of *E. coli* is also assayed in this system, and while the SE shows this property, there are differences between the two toxins, i.e., SE is heat-labile. The other salmonella toxins have been tested for their skin permeability properties and ability to alter the morphology of the Chinese hamster ovary (CHO) tissue culture cells [81]. Skin permeability activity requires less cholera toxin for a positive test than a rabbit ileal loop system, hence is a more sensitive screening procedure. The Salmonella toxins isolated from *S. typhimurium* culture filtrates (PFs) demonstrated rapid and delayed skin induration reactions and also positive CHO cell assay. These factors have not been compared with the SE isolated from *S. enteritidis.* One of the two PFs is heat-stable and the other heat-labile. The latter is the delayed PF and produces skin changes identical to cholera and *E. coli* toxins. There is evidence, therefore, that salmonella produce toxins which have properties similar to the enterotoxins of *E. coli* and *V. cholerae.* It is reasonable to assume that they may be involved in the pathogenesis of salmonella-induced diarrhea. Further evidence is needed to confirm and elucidate their roles.

Studies have been conducted in animals infected with both shigella and salmonella to determine whether there is a transudation of fluid through the damaged epithelial surface which would contribute to the diarrhea [35]. These studies have involved both large and small sized particles, albumin and mannitol. No evidence was accumulated which indicate a leak of these particles from the vascular space into the lumen of the bowel through the damaged villus structures. Similar studies have been conducted in animal and man following cholera infection [37]. The same results were obtained: no increase in the filtration capabilities of the epithelial lining as a result of cholera enterotoxin activity. Fluid secretion occurs by active secretory mechanisms powered by cyclic AMP energy systems.

Diarrheas caused by salmonella are usually short-lived episodes in an otherwise healthy adult. Infants and geriatric patients may get life threatening disease probably due to the fluid loss and the associated metabolic stress of an invasive pathogen. Fever, abdominal cramps and liquid to pasty stools are common. The inflammatory response induced by salmonella is primarily in the lamina propria area and located in the terminal ileum. For these reasons, the methylene blue smear of the stool will not reflect a striking picture as seen with shigella infections. A few to moderate number of white blood cells will be seen in salmonella stool smears, as compared with the sheets and clumps shed from the inflamed colon in shigella infections [46].

Salmonella are readily isolated from stool cultures. All isolates should be typed, since unusual or new strains will be of epidemiologic significance in tracing the origin of the organism.

(d) *Yersinia enterocolitica*

This organism can cause severe, life-threatening enteric infections in addition to cases of undifferentiated diarrhea. The spectrum of disease ranges from a severe terminal ileitis mimicking bacillary dysentery to mesenteric adenitis presenting as an acute appendicitis and to a watery diarrhea of brief duration. Associated clinical syndromes include erythema nodosum and arthritis [71,101]. The organism is not well known as yet in this country because it requires special growth conditions and media. It is becoming increasingly important to the food industry, however, as surveys conducted by the Department of Agriculture uncover Yersinia in significant numbers of meat products. A survey of elevated antibody titers in normal subjects, patients with non-thyroid disease and patients with thyroid disease revealed a prevalence of 8% of titers in normals [87]. The association of elevated titers ($>1:8$) in patients with thyroid disease (75% with titers) is surprising and unexplained. It may represent a cross-reaction between thyroid antigen(s) and the microorganism. Whether this organism is responsible for a proportion of undiagnosed diarrheal cases needs to be ascertained. Several outbreaks have been reported [1,102], with one epidemic caused by contaminated chocolate milk resulting in 13 of 213 sick school children undergoing appendectomies [102]. The illness was characterized by abdominal pain, fever and, in some, diarrhea. There was no evidence of acute appendicitis in the children submitted to surgery. Mesenteric adenopathy and inflammation of the terminal ileum were observed.

Little is known of the histologic changes or pathogenesis of the acute diarrheal syndrome in man. The earliest lesion noted in mice infected by the intragastric route occurs in Peyer's patches of the distal ileum [6]. The initial reaction consists of a collection of neutrophils within the lymphoid nodules in the submucosal region. Spread of the infection ensues into mesenteric nodes and then systemically. This model may be a useful tool for further investigations into the pathogenesis and treatment of this infection.

(e)   *Vibrio parahemolyticus*

American physicians were first introduced to this enteric pathogen in 1970, when the first case report was published [11]. This is a unique microorganism because it is halophilic and can be isolated in media containing 3% of sodium chloride. Patients usually develop disease from ingesting contaminated seafood. Much of the knowledge of this illness and the organism comes from Japan, where infections have been common and recognized since the 1950s [30]. The disease resembles that produced by Salmonella or Shigella. Diarrhea with abdominal pain are nearly universal symptoms. Diarrhea may be profuse, but dehydration is unlikely. Blood and mucus in stools is common, attesting to the destructive nature of the infection in the distal portions of the gut. Sigmoidoscopy may reveal small superficial ulcerations. Leukocytosis of 20,000 cells/mm^3 or more is a unique and frequent laboratory clue to the diagnosis. The incubation period is around 15–20 hours, and the illness wanes over a 2–3 day period.

A thermostable hemolysin toxin can be isolated from virulent *V. parahemolyticus* [46,97]. This toxin is lethal in mice when injected parenterally or given orally. In rabbits, the toxin has produced positive ileal loops and has been called an enteropathogenic toxin. The dose required to produce a positive ileal loop test was 100 times that of cholera toxin. It is unclear whether this toxin is involved in the diarrheal syndrome produced by *V. parahemolyticus*.

(f)   *Clostridia perfringens*

The type A organism of this species is a relatively common cause of food-borne disease in the United States. The illness is acquired from ingesting large numbers of organisms from such foods as meats, or gravy that has been reheated. This process encourages germination of heat-resistant spores. Crampy abdominal pain and diarrhea appear after an overnight incubation period, and these symptoms usually disappear within 24 hours [92]. The diagnosis is established by detecting large numbers of this anaerobe in the incriminated food.

In the rabbit ileal loop system, type A cells or culture filtrates will induce fluid secretion but there are also variable histologic changes [16]. Some strains caused no change, while others destroyed much of the epithelial cell lining. Strains selected for their rabbit virulence were likely to cause diarrhea in volunteers ingesting large numbers of the bacteria and spores. The enteropathogenic factor appears to be a toxin with parasympathomimetic activity [70]. Many of its actions in sheep were alleviated with atropine.

Type F organisms and some type C produce several toxins; beta toxin is thought to be closely correlated with necrotic enteritis of animals and man [89]. Although rare, it is a severe illness characterized in man by acute onset of severe abdominal pain, vomiting, diarrhea, prostation and shock; it may be rapidly fatal. The necrotizing enteritis may extend from the jejunum to the colon.

II. THERAPY

A. Fluid and Electrolyte Therapy

The keystone to the treatment of diarrheal diseases is replacement of fluid and electrolyte losses. In the diseases mediated by enterotoxins without cellular damage, the fluid lost is isotonic, protein-free. Oral fluid replacement therapy is practical and effective in treating patients with cholera [69] or ETEC disease. The formula for an acceptable solution for adults and children has been modified slightly in recent years. The following is the solution used in the treatment of mildly and moderately dehydrated children with summer diarrhea on an Apache Indian reservation [47]. This formula (which has been adopted by the World Health Organization and Pan American Health Organization) contains per liter of water: 3.5 grams of sodium chloride, 2.5 grams of sodium bicarbonate, 1.5 grams of potassium chloride and 20 grams of glucose, which gives the following approximate concentrations: Na^+, 90 mEq; K^+, 20 mEq; Cl^-, 80 mEq; HCO_3^-, 30 mEq; and 110 Mm glucose [23]. This solution contains less sodium than earlier formulations, so that the risk of producing hypernatremia in children is reduced. In severe cases of cholera there may be a need for additional sodium. In acute onset mild diarrheal disease, the patient should be encouraged to ingest larger than usual amounts of nonalcoholic liquids. Fruit juices, broths, soft drinks, and water are useful. Milk should be used with caution in the elderly because of the risk of lactase deficiency in this population aggravating the diarrhea [3]. The risk of dehydration in the elderly, who frequently are world travelers, needs to be emphasized. Significant fluid loss can lead to postural hypotension and possibly lead to a coronary or cerebral artery occlusion. Encouragement to maintain fluid intake despite nausea and diarrhea is an important educational measure. Unfortunately, no readily available commercial source of the electrolyte-glucose mixture is available, so that less desirable but available fluids and salt should be utilized. Patients infected with invasive pathogens will have varying amounts of protein in the stools, which represents the release of intracellular protein from the destroyed cells [68]. This loss of protein is not clinically significant in the usual case of shigellosis or salmonellosis and requires no attempt at replacement. Children with these infections have been rehydrated with isotonic oral fluid replacement.

Rapid infusion of parenteral fluids is indicated for diarrheal diseases associated with shock. Intravenous lactated Ringer solution with supplemental oral doses of potassium chloride should be used [31]. Alternatively, isotonic saline solution and isotonic sodium lactate (or bicarbonate) administered in a 2:1 ratio may be given.

B. Antimicrobial Therapy

1. *Vibrio cholerae* and *E. coli* Syndromes

Enterotoxigenic diarrheal syndromes produced by *Vibrio cholerae* and *E. coli* present unusual therapeutic considerations. Of prime importance in each case is appropriate fluid replacement; however, antibiotics do have an effect. Broad spectrum antibiotics, especially tetracycline, will shorten the period of diarrhea and excretion of cholera vibrios in the stool. Presumably, the antibiotics are reaching the vibrios in the lumen of the gut and perhaps are also being actively secreted during the diarrheal phase. The evidence that antibiotics are useful for treating ETEC disease is meager. In Bangladesh, where many patients with ETEC have diseases resembling cholera and require hospitalization for rehydration, tetracycline therapy was found to be effective in those patients with infections caused by LT-ST strains [64]. Duration of illness was shortened, as was excretion of the etiologic agent. ST-only strains produced a milder illness and did not respond to tetracycline. No comparable study has been performed in U.S. citizens who have mild self-limiting illnesses; a strong recommendation for antibiotic treatment in these patients cannot be made.

The prophylactic use of antimicrobial agents to prevent that portion of traveler's diarrhea caused by ETEC has been recently studied in a well controlled investigation. Earlier studies had suggested less disease in students traveling to Mexico while on sulfa drugs or tetracycline but the causative agents of the diarrhea were not identified. Sack et al. have reported a study conducted on Peace Corps volunteers going to Kenya [77]. Those taking 100 mg of doxycycline each day for the first 3 weeks had significantly less ETEC disease than placebo and, in fact, less diarrhea (6% versus 62%). Judicious prescribing of this drug in selected high risk patients traveling to endemic areas might be indicated until additional information is obtained. One must weigh the risk of antibiotic reactions (gastrointestinal upset, allergic reactions, etc.) to the discomfort associated with diarrhea if acquired.

2.   Shigella Infections

The use of antibiotics in treating patients with shigellosis is clearly indicated during the acute stage of the dysenteric phase (bloody mucoid stools). These individuals will have shortening of the febrile course and prompt elimination of shigella organisms from the feces. In those patients whose diagnosis becomes apparent only after identification of the pathogen in stool cultures, since the clinical picture was not distinctive antibiotic treatment is probably not needed. The illness may have already run its course and there is no indication for antibiotics to eradicate the organism from the colon; a chronic carrier state is very unusual. Information gathered at the Center for Disease Control suggests that only a small percentage of patients with shigellosis are cultured, and this is usually on the seventh day of illness. The results of the culture are then reported on day ten. Very few cases of shigellosis in children or adults will persist through this stage unless inappropriate antidiarrheal treatment is given. In those rare instances of chronic carriers, antibiotics have not been effective, but promising results were obtained with lactulose, a nonabsorbable disaccharide [61]. As this sugar is metabolized in the colon, short-chain fatty acids are produced and a lower pH results. This environment is inhibitory to shigella as well as to salmonella.

Ampicillin is an effective antibiotic but resistant strains are common in some localities, especially sonnei strains. Most of the flexneri strains at present are susceptible. The likelihood of infection with shigella in the United States is greatest with sonnei strains, since they represent 65–75% of isolations in the past several years. Alternative drugs for ampicillin-resistant strains include trimethoprim-sulfamethoxazole, tetracycline (may be given as a single bolus of 3 grams to adults) and nalidixic or oxolinic acid.

3.   Salmonella Infections

Unlike shigellosis, patients with salmonellosis have not had a beneficial effect from antibiotic therapy. There is no shortening of the diarrheal stage, and of great interest is the paradoxic consequence of a prolongation of the convalescent carrier state. The expected duration of positive stool cultures after a bout of salmonella gastroenteritis is several weeks and occasionally as long as a month. About 10% of individuals will be in the latter group. However, of patients treated with an antibiotic, those who will have positive cultures for a month increase to 25% [2]. This carrier state need not be treated and usually will subside spontaneously within several months.

The use of antibiotics is indicated in the very old and probably in infants, but the course should be brief, 3–5 days. Ampicillin would be the drug of choice but it is not a substitute for appropriate fluid replacement.

C. Symptomatic Treatment of Diarrhea

There are four mechanisms by which antidiarrheal drugs may interfere with the pathogenesis of diarrhea: (a) alter intestinal motility, (b) absorb toxins or bacteria present in the lumen of the gastrointestinal tract, (c) influence the milieu of the gut fluid so as to inhibit growth of enteric pathogens, and (d) block secretion of fluid in the small bowel. Each of these mechanisms has theoretical possibilities for being effective treatment of diarrhea. However, actual practice has indicated that adverse results may be attained.

First, antimotility drugs: Examples of this class of agents include paregoric, opium, anticholinergic drugs, and combinations such as Lomotil. These drugs are dangerous in infants, the population most susceptible to diarrheal disease. Their effectiveness in lessening motility in adults has been shown to be counterproductive in patients with shigellosis [19], salmonellosis and in children with ETEC infections [100]. Patients with shigellosis treated with such drugs have a worsening of their clinical state, with increased fever and prolongation of diarrhea and excretion of the pathogen. This has occurred despite effective antibiotic treatment [19]. Slowing of the peristaltic activity appears to allow extension of the infection by interfering with an effective cleansing mechanism. For relief of severe cramps, Lomotil is of benefit but should be used only infrequently and not prolonged beyond two or three doses. It is difficult for most travelers and many physicians to accept the fact that antiperistaltic drugs may be counterproductive, and thus their ill advised utilization continues. Physicians should emphasize fluid therapy, not antidiarrheal drugs, for their patients.

The second group includes those medications that can absorb toxins in the intestinal lumen prior to their attachment to receptor sites on the epithelial cell membranes. In experimental animals it is possible to bind cholera or *E. coli* toxin to gangliosides therefore preventing them from reaching gangliosides in the cell membrane. This approach has not been tested in man. The popular over-the-counter medicines containing kaolin, pectin, bismuth, etc., are compounded for the purposes of absorbing and detoxifying toxins. In recent studies conducted in Central America, these agents failed to alter the diarrhea syndrome in tested children. One compound, Pepto Bismol, did have an effect, but as will be discussed later it was not due to the bismuth [100]. There is very little evidence at present to justify strong recommendations for the general utilization of these drugs in the control of diarrhea.

Included in the third group of agents which may change the intestinal milieu so as to inhibit enteric pathogens are lactulose, *Lactobacillus acidophilus* and yogurt. Lactulose is nonabsorbable and not metabolized in the upper small intestine [61]. However, this disaccharide will promote acidification of the lower intestinal contents because of degradation by the intestinal flora. While this may be effective in salmonella or shigella infections, it is not useful in treating ETEC infection, where the disease is primarily proximal small intestinal. In addition, a large dose of lactulose will cause diarrhea. The use of lactobacilli or yogurt to combat diarrhea has not been widely accepted. These organisms are not normal inhabitants of the upper small intestine and do not seem to be important in the nonspecific defenses established by bacterial interference phenomena.

The fourth group of drugs included in this discussion offers exciting prospects for future use. As additional studies demonstrate the mechanisms involved in fluid secretion, efforts have been made to interfere with one of the many steps involved. Studies in rabbits have suggested that prostaglandins may play a role in the production of fluid by salmonella, shigella and perhaps cholera in experimental models [38] (see above). By employing a prostaglandin inhibitor (indomethacin) prophylactically, most of the fluid produced by salmonella and cholera and about half of that induced by shigella infection could be inhibited. After further animal studies, similar inhibitors may be investigated in man. Salicylates are inhibitors of prostaglandins, but, in addition, they and indomethacin have also been shown to have a direct absorptive effect on intestinal epithelial cells [28,34]. Thus, the beneficial effects noted with Pepto Bismol in the amelioration of diarrhea in children may be due to the subsalicylate contained in the product. These results need to be expanded and confirmed.

Finally, future studies in animals will be directed at "turning off" the secretory stimulus in the epithelial cells. Currently, various binding nucleotides are being studied to determine if they can not only block the action of enterotoxins but also not activate the adenyl cyclase in intestinal epithelial cells. The results of these studies may be significant indicators in directing the development of future effective and indicated antidiarrheal drugs.

CONCLUSIONS

The great advances in our knowledge of the pathogenesis of bacterial diarrheas have evolved around the defining of the mechanisms involved in fluid secretion. The numerous enterotoxins that have been identified help to explain how various pathogens cause diarrhea. It remains for future studies to identify all the microbes which are responsible for the mass of undiagnosed infectious diarrheas. The therapy of diarrheal diseases is based on fluid and electrolyte replacement. Antibiotics are of some value in selected types of infectious diarrhea. Antidiarrheal drugs that inhibit motility should be avoided in the management of patients with infectious diarrhea.

REFERENCES

1. Asakawa Y, Akahane S, Kagata N, Noguchi M: Two community outbreaks of human infections with *Yersinia enterocolitica*. J Hyg (Camb) 71:715–723, 1973.
2. Aserkoff B, Bennett JV: Effect of antibiotic therapy in acute salmonellosis on the fecal excretion of Salmonellae. N Engl J Med 281:636, 1969.
3. Bayless TM, Rosensweig N, Christopher N, Huang S-S: Milk intolerance and lactose tolerance tests. Gastroenterology 54:475, 1968.
4. Burke V, Kerry KR, Anderson CM: The relationship of dietary lactose to refractory diarrhoea in infancy. Aust Pediat J 1:147, 1965.
5. Calin A, Fries JF: An "experimental" epidemic of Reiter's syndrome revisited. Follow-up evidence on genetic and environmental factors. Ann Intern Med 84:564–566, 1976.
6. Carter PB: Pathogenicity of *Yersinia enterocolitica* for mice. Infect Immun 11:164–170, 1975.
7. Charney AN, Gots RE, Formal SB, Gianella RA: Activation of intestinal mucosal adenylate cyclase by *Shigella dysenteriae* 1 enterotoxin. Gastroenterology 70:1085–1090, 1976.
8. Craig JP: A permeability factor (toxin) found in cholera stools and culture filtrates and its neutralization by convalescent cholera sera. Nature (London) 207:614–616, 1965.
9. Croft DN, Cotton PB: Gastro-intestinal cell loss in man: its measurement and significance. Digestion 8:144–160, 1973.
10. Croft ND, Loehry CA, Taylor JFN, Cole J: D.N.A. and cell loss from normal small-intestinal mucosa. Lancet 2:70–73, 1968.
11. Dadisman TA, Nelson R, Molenda JR, Garber HJ: *Vibrio parahaemolyticus* gastroenteritis in Maryland. I. Clinical and epidemiologic aspects. Am J Epidemiol 96:414, 1972.
12. Dean AG, Ching Y-C, Williams RG, Harden LB: Test for *Escherichia coli* enterotoxin using infant mice: application in a study of diarrhea in children in Honolulu. J Infect Dis 125:407–411, 1972.
13. Dolin R, Blacklow NR, DuPont H, et al: Transmission of acute infectious nonbacterial gastroenteritis to volunteers by oral administration of stool filtrates. J Infect Dis 123:307–312, 1971.

14. Donta ST, King M, Sloper K: Induction of steroidogenesis in tissue culture by cholera enterotoxin. Nature (New Biol) 243:246–247, 1973.

15. Donta ST, Viner JP: Inhibition of the steroidogenic effects of cholera and heat-labile *Escherichia coli* enterotoxins by G_{M1} gangliosides: evidence for a similar receptor site for the two toxins. Infect Immun 11:982–985, 1975.

16. Duncan CL, Sugiyama H, Strong DH: Rabbit ileal loop response to strains of *Clostridium perfringens*. J Bacteriol 95:1560–1566, 1968.

17. DuPont HL, Formal SB, Hornick RB, et al: Pathogenesis of *Escherichia coli* diarrhea. N Engl J Med 285:1–9, 1971.

18. DuPont HL, Hornick RB: Unpublished data.

19. DuPont HL, Hornick RB: Adverse effect of Lomotil therapy in shigellosis. JAMA 226:1525, 1973.

20. DuPont HL, Hornick RB, Dawkins AT, et al: The response of man to virulent *Shigella flexneri* 2a. J Infect Dis 119:296–299, 1969.

21. DuPont HL, Hornick RB, Snyder MJ, et al: Immunity in Shigellosis. II. Protection induced by oral live vaccine or primary infection. J Infect Dis 125:12–16, 1972.

22. Echeverria P, Ho MT, Blacklow NR, et al: Relative importance of viruses and bacteria in the etiology of pediatric diarrhea in Taiwan. J Infect Dis 136:383–390, 1977.

23. Editorial: Oral glucose/electrolyte therapy for acute diarrhoea. Lancet 1:79, 1975.

24. Evans DG, Evans DJ Jr, DuPont HL: Virulence factors of enterotoxigenic *Escherichia coli*. J Infect Dis 136:S118–123, 1977.

25. Evans DG, Evans DJ Jr, Pierce NF: Differences in the response of rabbit small intestine to heat-labile and heat-stable enterotoxins of *Escherichia coli*. Infect Immun 7:873–880, 1973.

26. Evans DG, Silver RP, Evans DJ Jr, et al: Plasmid-controlled colonization factor associated with virulence in *Escherichia coli* enterotoxigenic for humans. Infect Immun 12:656–667, 1975.

27. Ewing WH: Sources of *Escherichia coli* cultures that belonged to O antigen groups associated with infantile diarrheal disease. J Infect Dis 110:114–120, 1962.

28. Farris RK, Tapper EJ, Powell DW, Morris SM: Effect of aspirin on normal and cholera toxin-stimulated intestinal electrolyte transport. J Clin Invest 57:916–924, 1976.

29. Field M: Intestinal secretion: Effect of cyclic AMP and its role in cholera. N Engl J Med 284:1137–1144, 1971.

30. Fujino T: On the bacteriological examination of Shirasu food poisoning. Med J Osaka Univ 4:299, 1953.

31. Gangarosa EJ, Barker WH: Cholera: Implications for the United States. JAMA 227:170–171, 1974.

32. Gemski P Jr, Formal SB: Shigellosis: an invasive infection of the gastrointestinal tract. Microbiology 165–169, 1975.

33. Giannella RA, Formal SB, Dammin GJ: Pathogenesis of salmonellosis: studies of fluid secretion, mucosal invasion, and morphologic reaction in the rabbit ileum. J Clin Invest 52:441–453, 1973.

34. Giannella RA, Gots RE, Charney AN, et al: Pathogenesis of salmonella-mediated intestinal fluid secretion. Gastroenterology 69:1238–1245, 1975.

35. Giannella RA, Rout WR, Formal SB, Collins H: Role of plasma filtration in the intestinal fluid secretion mediated by infection with Salmonella typhimurium. Infect Immun 13:470–474, 1976.

36. Gorbach SL, Kean BH, Evans DG, et al: Travelers' diarrhea and toxigenic *Escherichia coli*. N Engl J Med 292:933–936, 1975.

37. Gordon RS, Gardner JD, Kinzie JL: Low mannitol clearance into cholera stool as evidence against filtration as a source of stool fluid. Gastroenterology 63:407–412, 1972.

38. Gots RE, Formal SB, Giannella RA: Indomethacin inhibition of *Salmonella typhimurium, Shigella flexneri,* and cholera-mediated rabbit ileal secretion. J Infect Dis 130:280–284, 1974.

39. Greenberg HB, Sack DA, Rodriguez W, et al: Microtiter solid-phase radioimmunoassay for detection of *Escherichia coli* heat-labile enterotoxin. Infect Immun 17:541–545, 1977.

40. Guentzel MN, Berry LJ: Motility as a virulence factor for *Vibrio cholerae.* Infect Immun 11:890–897, 1975.

41. Guerrant RL, Bruton LL, Schnaitman TC, et al: Cyclic adenosine monophosphate and alteration of Chinese hamster ovary cell morphology: a rapid, sensitive *in vitro* assay for the enterotoxins of *Vibrio cholerae* and *Escherichia coli.* Infect Immun 10:320–327, 1974.

42. Guerrant RL, Moore RA, Kirschenfeld PM, Sande MA: Role of toxigenic and invasive bacteria in acute diarrhea of childhood. N Engl J Med 293:567–573, 1975.

43. Gurwith MC, Williams, TW: Gastroenteritis in children: A two-year review in Manitoba. I. Etiology. J. Infect Dis 136:239–247, 1977.

44. Gyles CL: Heat-labile and heat-stable forms of the enterotoxin from *E. coli* strains enteropathogenic for pigs. Ann NY Acad Sci 196:314–322, 1971.

45. Haltalin KC, Nelson JD: Coliform septicemia complicating shigellosis in children. JAMA 129:441, 1965.

46. Harris JC, DuPont HL, Hornick RB: Fecal leukocytes in diarrheal illness. Ann Intern Med 76:697, 1972.

47. Hirschhorn N, McCarthy BJ, Ranney B, et al: Ad libitum oral glucose-electrolyte therapy for acute diarrhea in Apache children. J Pediatr 83:562–571, 1973.

48. Holmgren J: Comparison of the tissue receptors for *Vibrio cholerae* and *Escherichia coli* enterotoxins by means of gangliosides and natural cholera toxoid. Infect Immun 8:851–859, 1973.

49. Honda T, Taga S, Takeda T, et al: Identification of lethal toxin with the thermostable direct hemolysin produced by *Vibrio parahaemolyticus,* and some physicochemical properties of the purified toxin. Infect Immun 13:133–139, 1976.

50. Huang KC, Chen TST, Rout WR: Effect of staphylococcal enterotoxins A, B, and C on transport and permeability across the flounder intestine. Proc Soc Exp Biol Med 147:250–254, 1974.

51. Kapral FA, O'Brien AD, Russ PD, Drugan WJ Jr: Inhibition of water absorption in the intestine by *Staphylococcus aureus* delta-toxin. Infect Immun 13:140–145, 1976.

52. Keusch GT, Grady GF, Mata LJ: The pathogenesis of *Shigella dysenteriae.* J Clin Invest 51:1212–1218, 1972.

53. Keusch GT, Jacewicz M: The pathogenesis of Shigella diarrhea. V. Relationship of Shiga enterotoxin, neurotoxin and cytotoxin. J Infect Dis 131:S33–39, 1975.

54. Klipstein FA, Engert RF: Partial purification and properties of *Enterobacter cloacae* heat-stable enterotoxin. Infect Immun 13:1307–1314, 1976.

55. Klipstein FA, Engert RF: Enterotoxigenic intestinal bacteria in tropical sprue. III. Preliminary characterization of *Klebsiella pneumoniae* enterotoxin. J Infect Dis 132:200–203, 1975.

56. Koupal LR, Deibel RH: Assay, characterization, and localization of an enterotoxin produced by *Salmonella.* Infect Immun 11:14–22, 1975.

57. Kubota Y, Liu PV: An enterotoxin of *Pseudomonas aeruginosa*. J Infect Dis 123:97–98, 1971.
58. LaBrec EH, Schneider H, Magnani TJ, Formal SB: Epithelial cell penetration as an essential step in the pathogenesis of bacillary dysentery. J Bacteriol 88:1503–1518, 1964.
59. Levine MM, Caplan ES, Waterman D, et al: Diarrhea caused by *Escherichia coli* that produce only heat-stable enterotoxin. Infect Immun 17:78–82, 1977.
60. Levine MM, DuPont HL, Formal SB, et al: Pathogenesis of *Shigella dysenteriae* 1 (Shiga) dysentery. J Infect Dis 127:261–270, 1973.
61. Levine MM, DuPont HL, Khodabandelou M, Hornick RB: Long-term shigella carrier state. N Engl J Med 288:1169–1171, 1973.
62. Levine MM, Nalin DR: Unpublished data.
63. Lushbaugh WB, Karialla AB, Cantey JR, Pittman FE: Isolation of an enterotoxin from axenically cultivated *Entamoeba histolytica*. Clin Res 26:58A, 1978.
64. Merson MH, Sack RB, Islam S, et al: Tetracycline therapy of enterotoxigenic *Escherichia coli* (ETEC) diarrhea. (Abstract #401) 17th Interscience Conference on Antimicrobial Agents and Chemotherapy, 12–14 October 1977.
65. Middleton PJ, Abbott GD, Szymanski MT, Hamilton JR: Oribvirus acute gastroenteritis in infancy. Lancet 1:1241–1244, 1974.
66. Miller RM, Garbus J, Hornick RB: Lack of enhanced oxygen consumption by polymorphonuclear leukocytes on phagocytosis of virulent *Salmonella typhi*. Science 175:1010–1011, 1972.
67. Moon HW, Nagy B, Isaacson RE: Intestinal colonization and adhesion by enterotoxigenic *Escherichia coli:* ultrastructural observations on adherence to ileal epithelium of the pig. J Infect Dis 136:S124–129, 1977.
68. Nalin DR, Bhattacharjee AK, Richardson SH: Cholera-like toxic effect of culture filtrates of *Escherichia coli*. J Infect Dis 130:595–601, 1974.
69. Nalin DR, Cash RA: Oral maintenance for cholera and other severe diarrhea in children. J Pediatr 78:355, 1971.
70. Niilo L: Mechanism of action of the enteropathogenic factor of *Clostridium perfringens* type A. Infect Immun 3:100–106, 1971.
71. Nilehn B: Studies on *Yersinia enterocolitica* with special reference to bacterial diagnosis and occurrence in human acute enteric disease. Acta Pathol Microbiol Scand (Suppl) 206:S1–48, 1969.
72. O'Brien AD, Thompson MR, Gemski P, et al: Biological properties of *Shigella flexneri* 2a toxin and its serological relationship to *Shigella dysenteriae* 1 toxin. Infect Immun 15:796–798, 1977.
73. Portnoy BL, DuPont HL, Pruitt D, et al: Antidiarrheal agents in the treatment of acute diarrhea in children. JAMA 236:844–846, 1976.
74. Rosenberg ML, Koplan JP, Wachsmuth IK, et al: Epidemic diarrhea at Crater Lake from enterotoxigenic *Escherichia coli*. Ann Intern Med 86:714–718, 1977.
74a. Rubin RH, Weinstein L: Salmonellosis: Microbiologic, Pathologic and Clinical Features. New York, Stratton Intercontinental, 1977.
75. Rudoy RC, Nelson JD: Enteroinvasive and enterotoxigenic *Escherichia coli* occurrence in acute diarrhea of infants and children. Am J Dis Child 129:668–672, 1975.
76. Ryder RW, Sack DA, Kapikian AZ, et al: Enterotoxigenic *Escherichia coli* and reovirus-like agent in rural Bangladesh. Lancet 1:659–662, 1976.
77. Sack DA, Kaminsky DC, Sack RB, Arthur R: Prophylactic doxycycline for travelers' diarrhea. (Abstract #402) 17th Interscience Conference on Antimicrobial Agents and Chemotherapy, 12–14 October 1977.

78. Sack DA, Kaminsky DC, Sack RB, et al: Enterotoxigenic *Escherichia coli* diarrhea of travelers: a prospective study of American Peace Corps volunteers. Johns Hopkins Med J 141:63–70, 1977.
79. Sack DA, Merson MH, Wells JG, et al: Diarrhea associated with heat-stable enterotoxin-producing strains of *Escherichia coli*. Lancet 2:239–241, 1975.
80. Sakurai J, Duncan CL: Purification of beta-toxin from *Clostridium perfringens* type C. Infect Immun 18:741–745, 1977.
81. Sandefur PD, Peterson JW: Isolation of skin permeability factors from culture filtrates of *Salmonella typhimurium*. Infect Immun 14:671–679, 1976.
82. Satterwhite TK, Evans DG, DuPont HL, Evans DJ Jr: Volunteer studies on the role of *Escherichia coli* H-10407 colonization factor antigen (CFA) in acute diarrhea. Clin Res 26:29A, 1978.
83. Schrank GD, Verwey WF: Distribution of cholera organisms in experimental *Vibrio cholerae* infections: Proposed mechanisms of pathogenesis and antibacterial immunity. Infect Immun 13:195–203, 1976.
84. Schreiber DS, Blacklow NR, Trier JS: The mucosal lesion of the proximal small intestine in acute infectious nonbacterial gastroenteritis. N Engl J Med 288:1318–1323, 1973.
85. Serebro HA, Iber FL, Yardley JH, Hendrix TH: Inhibition of cholera toxin action in the rabbit by cycloheximide. Gastroenterology 56:506, 1969.
86. Sereny B: Experimental keratoconjunctivitis Shigellosa. Acta Microbiol Hung 4:368–376.
87. Shenkman L, Bottone EJ: Antibodies to *Yersinia enterocolitica* in thyroid disease. Ann Intern Med 85:735–739, 1976.
88. Shore EG, Dean AG, Holik KJ, Davis BR: Enterotoxin-producing *Escherichia coli* and diarrheal disease in adult travelers: a prospective study. J Infect Dis 129:577–582, 1974.
89. Skjelkvale R, Duncan CL: Characterization of enterotoxin purified from *Clostridium perfringens* type C. Infect Immun 11:1061–1068, 1975.
90. Smith HW, Halls S: The transmissible nature of the genetic factor in *Escherichia coli* that controls enterotoxin production. J Gen Microbiol 52:319–334, 1968.
91. Sprinz H: Pathogenesis of intestinal infections. Arch Pathol 87:556–562, 1969.
92. Strong DH, Duncan CL, Perna G: *Clostridium perfringens* type A food poisoning. II. Response of the rabbit ileum as an indication of enteropathogenicity of strains of *Clostridium perfringens* in human beings. Infect Immun 3:171–178, 1971.
93. Takeuchi A: Electron microscope studies of experimental Salmonella infections: I. Penetration into the intestinal epithelium by *Salmonella typhimurium*. Am J Pathol 50:109–136, 1967.
94. Takeuchi A, Sprinz H: Electron microscope studies of experimental Salmonella infection in the preconditioned guinea pig. II. Response of the intestinal mucosa to the invasion by *Salmonella typhimurium*. Am J Pathol 51:137–167, 1967.
95. Thompson MR, Steinberg MS, Gemski P, et al: Inhibition of *in vitro* protein synthesis by *Shigella dysenteriae* 1 toxin. Biochem Biophys Res Commun 71:873–788, 1976.
96. Tullock EF, Ryan KJ, Formal SB, Franklin FA: Invasive enteropathogenic *Escherichia coli* dysentery: Outbreak in 28 adults. Ann Intern Med 79:13, 1973.
97. Ueyama T, Baba T, Bito Y: Studies on the toxic substance of *Vibrio parahaemolyticus*. Jpn J Bacteriol 19:480–482, 1964.
98. van Heyningen S: Cholera toxin: interaction of subunits with ganglioside G_{M1}. Science 183:656–657, 1974.

99. van Heyningen S, King CA: Subunit A from cholera toxin is an activator of adenylate cyclase in pigeon erythrocytes. Biochem J 146:269–271, 1975.
100. Wadstrom T, Ljungh A, Wretland B: Enterotoxin, haemolysin and cytotoxic protein in *Aeromonas hydrophilia* from human infections. Acta Pathol Microbiol Scand (B) 84:112–114, 1976.
101. Worldwide spread of infections with *Yersinia enterocolitica*. WHO Chronicle 30:494–496, 1976.
102. *Yersinia enterocolitica* outbreak—New York. Morbidity and Mortality Weekly Report, Center for Disease Control 26:53–54, 1977.

CHAPTER 4

PERSPECTIVES ON ANTIBIOTICS

Harold C. Neu, M.D.

Antimicrobial agents have been a significant factor in man's progress in health sciences since the discovery of the antibacterial effect of sulfonamides by Domagk in the late 1930's. Penicillin in 1940 truly opened up an era which has seen the development of agents which can attack most parts of the bacterial cell. In the three and a half decades since penicillin was first used clinically in World War II, bacteria have developed resistance to many of the standard agents. Indeed, *Neisseria gonorrhoeae*, for which much of the early penicillin was used, recently has acquired the ability to destroy penicillin via a plasmid mediated β-lactamase[4]. Many other bacteria have also become resistant to agents once highly effective in the therapy of diseases caused by these bacteria. Pneumococci thought to be always susceptible to penicillin have been shown to be resistant[3]. In addition to this acquired resistance, there has been the increased appearance of microorganisms which are intrinsically resistant to many agents. This is due to progress in the chemotherapy of hematologic and other malignancies as well as increased use of technics which violate the body's natural defenses and permit entry of organisms of low invasiveness but high antibacterial resistance. As "bigger and better" antibiotics have come along to meet these demands, they have introduced undesirable side effects of the antimicrobial agents on human cells and tissues. Molecular modifications of antibiotics to overcome the problems of bacterial resistance and human toxicity have been extensive[51]. This review will look at progress which may occur in the next few years to overcome some of these problems.

PENICILLINS

In the past it has been common to state that the action of penicillin upon bacterial cells was to interfere with the peptidoglycan structure by

From the Departments of Medicine and Pharmacology, College of Physicians and Surgeons, Columbia University, New York, N.Y.

preventing linkage between peptide chains, hence causing an unstable cell wall and lysis of the bacterium. Although early experiments, primarily with gram-positive species, supported this concept, the increased use of penicillin compounds against gram-negative species resulted in a reevaluation of the relevance of this model to gram-negative species. Spratt [83] demonstrated that there are a number of penicillin binding proteins in *E. coli*. Other laboratories have shown that these penicillin binding proteins are also present in other members of the Enterobacteriaceae and in Pseudomonas as well [65]. There seem to be seven different proteins which can be identified by acrylamide gel electrophoresis. Three of these proteins appear to be important in cell shape, elongation and septation, and some of the differences in the activity of different penicillins are related to the binding of the penicillin to these proteins. Basically, penicillins can be considered from three standpoints: accessibility to target sites, instability of the compound to β-lactamases, and affinity for penicillin-binding proteins. With these concepts in mind it is possible to look at both old and new penicillins.

Penicillin G remains an excellent agent in the treatment of many of the common infections of man produced by streptococci, but major areas of resistance have developed. The first of these is well known; namely *Staphylococcus aureus*. Most *Staph. aureus* which are of hospital origin produce β-lactamases, and fully more than 60% of community staphylococci also are of this same type. *Staph. epidermidis* has characteristically been considered a skin contaminant, and yet this organism has assumed increased importance because of its role as an infecting agent in cardiac surgery or after orthopedic procedures when prosthetic implants are used. Most *Staph. epidermidis* are penicillinase producers and hence resistant to penicillin G. Although streptococci as a group have remained sensitive to penicillin G, *Strep. pneumoniae* have been isolated in South Africa [3] and in the United States which are truly penicillin G-resistant, requiring inhibitory levels of 8–12 μg/ml. This resistance does not seem to be plasmid-mediated. *Neisseria gonorrhoeae* relatively resistant to penicillin G have been known for a number of years [75], but now *N. gonorrhoeae* containing *E. coli* plasmids which mediate resistance via β-lactamase production are found in many countries [4]. All of these caveats about the use of penicillin G apply to penicillin V, and no new natural penicillins which would overcome these problems have been discovered. Surprisingly, one use of penicillin G which has been rediscovered is that against anaerobic bacteria, particularly those of the oral flora [86]. A question which might be logically asked is whether any of the newer penicillins is more effective than penicillin G against susceptible microorganisms. To date there is no evidence to suggest that this is true; so penicillin use in pneumococcal, streptococcal and selected anaerobic infections should continue.

A great deal of research has been devoted to amino penicillins but, except for a couple of compounds, none of the many agents has been a striking improvement over ampicillin [52]. Ampicillin added to the antibacterial activity of penicillin G a number of organisms which are frequent causes of infection in children. These are *Haemophilus influenzae, E. coli,* Salmonella and Shigella. Unfortunately, with the passage of time, isolates of all of these species have become resistant by virtue of the presence of plasmids mediating β-lactamase production [53,97]. Amoxicillin is an amino penicillin which is similar in antibacterial activity to ampicillin, but which has some pharmacologic advantages over ampicillin in view of its more complete absorption after oral ingestion and the higher blood levels produced [48]. However, except in situations in which ampicillin or amoxicillin would have some clear advantage over penicillin G or V, amino penicillins are overused agents. Situations in which use of amino penicillins is indicated would be the treatment of otitis media in individuals under 8–10 years of age, exacerbations of bronchitis in individuals with chronic bronchitis, in selected infections due to Salmonella species, such as arthritis or osteomyelitis, and in Shigellosis in children if the isolates in the community are susceptible.

One oral ampicillin derivative under investigation is bacampicillin. This ester of ampicillin is well absorbed and undergoes immediate conversion to ampicillin as it goes through the intestinal wall and as it enters the serum. Serum levels after a 400 mg oral dose are equivalent to those after a 1 g dose of ampicillin and the absorption occurs more rapidly [80]. Clinical studies have demonstrated the effectiveness of this ester of ampicillin, but there are as yet inadequate comparative data to show that at lower doses bacampicillin is as effective or more effective than the parent compound ampicillin.

A new and unique agent which is analogous in structure to the amino-penicillins is mecillinam. This compound is a β-amidino penicillin and it has some unusual antimicrobial properties [54]. Firstly, it has poor anti-gram-positive activity. Where 0.01 μg/ml of penicillin G would inhibit *Strep. pyogenes,* 4–6 μg/ml of mecillinam are needed to inhibit this organism. It also has much less activity against Haemophilus and Neisseria than does ampicillin. It is against the members of the Entero-bacteriaceae that it is most active. For example, mecillinam can inhibit an *E. coli* at a concentration of 0.4 μg/ml even though the strain is resistant to 100 μg/ml of ampicillin. Although mecillinam is less readily hydrolyzed by the most common plasmid-mediated β-lactamase, the

TEM or Richmond type III variety [54], it is not this slight increase in β-lactamase resistance that is most significant. Rather, mecillinam more readily enters bacterial cells and binds specifically to protein 2 of the penicillin-binding proteins [84]. This binding of mecillinam to protein 2 results in changes in shape of the bacteria, and lysis occurs in a low osmolar, low conductivity environment [54]. Mecillinam has added to the spectrum of ampicillin by inhibiting a significant number of the isolates of Klebsiella and Enterobacter. The activity of mecillinam against *Proteus mirabilis* is variable, and against indole-positive Proteus species the compound is less active than compounds such as carbenicillin. Mecillinam has no antipseudomonas activity. Several groups of investigators have shown that mecillinam acts synergistically with other penicillins such as ampicillin or carbenicillin and with cephalosporins [28,57]. This effect would seem to be due to the fact that the other penicillins cause lysis of cells by binding to penicillin-binding proteins 1b, 2 and 3, while mecillinam binds only to protein 2.

Mecillinam has been made into an ester, pivmecillinam, for oral use and as a salt for parenteral use. To date the clinical studies with the compound are not extensive, but it has been used to treat *E. coli,* Salmonella and other gram-negative infections [11,72]. To determine if mecillinam would show synergy when combined with amoxicillin in urinary tract infections, an experimental model of urine with high inocula of bacteria was studied and synergy could be demonstrated [10]. Clinical studies should resolve whether mecillinam will be effective therapy in man. The animal experiments have shown that mecillinam produces protection in mouse infections either alone or when combined with aminopenicillins [28]. In infections involving abscess formation, where there might be a high oncotic pressure and high conductivity, both conditions which interfere with mecillinam's action, it is possible that the drug would be ineffective. Thus far the brief clinical reports have not shown this to occur. If the activity of mecillinam holds up clinically, it will be an important addition to the penicillin armamentarium.

As already mentioned, the changes in bacterial flora created a need for agents with an increased spectrum over those available. Carbenicillin was introduced in the latter part of the 1960's, and now is considered an integral part of therapy against the *Pseudomonas aeruginosa* infections which are so common in patients with hematologic malignancies, burns and cystic fibrosis. The high serum concentrations of carbenicillin needed to inhibit many Pseudomonas isolates has prompted a continued search for new and better antipseudomonas penicillins and for agents that possess not only the antipseudomonas activity but have activity against organisms such as Klebsiella which are a major group not inhibited by carbenicillin. Ticarcillin, a thienyl malonoyl 6 APA derivative, is similar in activity to carbenicillin except for greater activity, approximately two-fold against Pseudomonas [47]. Unfortunately, ticarcillin has no greater activity than carbenicillin against most of the members of the Enterobacteriaceae, and it is not more stable to the β-lactamases of either gram-positive or gram-negative bacteria. Since ticarcillin can be used at lower doses than carbenicillin, it is possible that it may produce fewer of the serious side effects seen with carbenicillin use. However, in the reported studies, ticarcillin also produces hypokalemia as a result of the large non-reabsorbable anion load, platelet dysfunction, as a result of the binding to platelet ADP, and bacterial overgrowth due to suppression of normal bacteria [69]. Studies of ticarcillin have shown it to be effective in various gram-negative infections due to susceptible Pseudomonas and other gram-negative bacilli [16,69]. In comparative studies, ticarcillin at lower doses is as effective as carbenicillin given in larger amounts, but a clinical superiority of ticarcillin has not been demonstrated and probably never will be, due to the nature of the patients who develop infections for which an agent of this type is used. A comparative study of ticarcillin and tobramycin versus carbenicillin and gentamicin in treatment of respiratory infections did show that ticarcillin-tobramycin was superior [71].

A number of other new penicillins have come and gone. BLP 1654 was a ureido penicillin which was eight-fold more active than carbenicillin if MIC values were considered, but its activity was subject to marked effect from the size of inoculum used in tests and the type of medium used. This agent furthermore showed a marked difference between the MIC and MBC values, so that BLP 1654 was almost bacteriostatic when tested at high colony inoculum with organisms such as Pseudomonas [76]. This agent unfortunately had toxic side effects, and study of it was abandoned. Pirbenicillin, another ureido penicillin which is a monosodium salt, was found to be more active than carbenicillin against *Ps. aeruginosa* and Klebsiella species but less active against Proteus species [8]. Pirbenicillin was not stable in media which were unbuffered, and results of studies from different groups varied widely. Studies of the cidal activity of carbenicillin and pibenicillin revealed that carbenicillin exerted a greater cidal effect [39]. There have been no further studies of this compound.

Two penicillin compounds of interest which may have an eventual role in chemotherapy are azlocillin and mezlocillin. Both of these compounds are semisynthetic acylureido penicillins with *in vitro* activity similar to carbenicillin [23]. Azlocillin is four to eight-fold more active than carbenicillin against *Ps. aeruginosa*. Indeed, as is shown in Table 1, it inhibits some isolates of Pseudomonas resistant to achievable serum

TABLE 1.   Activity of New Penicillins Against Carbenicillin Resistant Bacteria

Organism	Carbenicillin	Azlocillin	Mezlocillin	Piperacillin
		MIC (μg/ml)		
Escherichia coli	>800	12.5	12.5	12.5
Escherichia coli	>800	100	50	50
Klebsiella pneumoniae	>800	100	100	100
Enterobacter cloacae	>800	200	50	50
Serratia marcescens	>800	200	100	100
Proteus morganii	>400		50	25
Pseudomonas aeruginosa	400	50	200	25
Pseudomonas aeruginosa	>800	100	25	12.5
Pseudomonas aeruginosa	>800	50	25	12.5

concentration of carbenicillin, but this is not a predictable phenomenon. Azlocillin and carbenicillin are similar in activity against *E. coli*, Enterobacter, Proteus, including both indole-positive strains as well as *P. mirabilis*, Citrobacter, Acinetobacter and Serratia [23,85]. Azlocillin is much more active than carbenicillin or ampicillin against Klebsiella species, inhibiting 65% of isolates at a concentration of 50 μg/ml. Azlocillin has been combined with aminoglycosides and it acts in a synergistic fashion. For example, when gentamicin or amikacin are combined at a concentration of one-fourth of their MIC value with 25 μg/ml of azlocillin, the isolates inhibited increase from 65% to over 90% [59].

The human pharmacology of azlocillin has not been extensively studied, but the half-life is approximately 75 minutes and the apparent volume of distribution is 20% of the body weight [36]. This is similar to the pharmacokinetic properties of carbenicillin and ticarcillin.

Published clinical experience with azlocillin is minimal [36]. The agent has not undergone extensive investigation in patients with hematologic malignancy and it is unknown whether the synergistic activity it shows when combined with aminoglycosides is of major clinical importance. Nonetheless, azlocillin is an interesting compound in terms of its antibacterial activity, since it seems that its increased activity is secondary to more rapid entry to receptor sites than to resistance to hydrolysis by β-lactamases, since it is not more β-lactamase stable than is carbenicillin [23].

Mezlocillin is similar in structure to azlocillin, differing only by the single mezyl group. Yet it is quite different in antibacterial activity *in vitro* against many of the gram-negative bacilli [9,23]. Mezlocillin has excellent activity against β-hemolytic streptococci, both *Strep. pyogenes* (group A) and *Strep. agalactiae* (group B), inhibiting them by less than 0.5 µg/ml. It also is as active as ampicillin against true enterococci— that is, *Strep. fecalis, Strep. fecium,* etc., inhibiting such organisms at concentrations below 2 µg/ml. Mezlocillin is active against *H. influenzae* and *N. gonorrhoeae,* which contain a TEM type β-lactamase. This is probably due to relative stability of the compound to this enzyme. However, when *E. coli* contain this enzyme, they are usually resistant to mezlocillin. Indeed, the activity of mezlocillin against *E. coli* is trimodal with non-hospital isolates which usually lack β-lactamases inhibited by 0.8 to 6.3 µg/ml, isolates with ampicillin-carbenicillin MIC values 200 µg/ml, inhibited by 25–50 µg/ml, and a third group of *E. coli* isolates as resistant to mezlocillin as they are to ampicillin. Activity of mezlocillin against Salmonella and Shigella is similar to its activity against *E. coli.* Mezlocillin is considerably more active than ampicillin or carbenicillin against Klebsiella. For example, at 25 µg/ml, 75% of isolates are inhibited by mezlocillin, 28% by ampicillin, and 5% by carbenicillin. Mezlocillin is also two-fold more active than carbenicillin against Enterobacter, Citrobacter, indole-positive Proteus, Serratia and Pseudomonas. It also inhibits significantly more *Bacteroides fragilis* isolates [95]. For example, at 25 µg/ml, mezlocillin inhibits 88% as compared with 28% inhibited by carbenicillin. The activity of mezlocillin similar to that of many of the newer penicillins is affected by the size of inoculum used in assay procedures and by the pH and type of medium used in the assay. Furthermore, mezlocillin and azlocillin, mentioned before, when tested against Pseudomonas do have considerable differences between inhibitory and cidal levels. Whether these *in vitro* observations have any relation to clinical states is unclear.

Pharmacokinetic studies of mezlocillin show that it has kinetics similar to other penicillins of this type but with a half-life shorter than that of carbenicillin; namely, 50–60 minutes [38; Pancoast, Jahre, Neu, in preparation]. Clinical studies of the agent are few, but it has proved effective in selected cases of pneumonia and pyelonephritis [38]. But much further work needs to be done before one can make definite statements about its role. The excellent activity against many of the aerobic and anaerobic organisms which comprise the pelvic flora suggests that it might prove to be useful in infections in this sphere.

Piperacillin is a novel piperazine penicillin derivative which is similar in activity to ampicillin against gram-positive organisms and to carbenicillin against gram-negative species [91]. In many aspects, the *in vitro* activity of piperacillin and mezlocillin are similar. It inhibits streptococci at concentrations below 1 µg/ml and inhibits most of the Enterobacteriaceae at concentrations lower than those of carbenicillin. It is the most active penicillin tested against Pseudomonas, inhibiting 60% of isolates at 3 μg/ml and 90% at 12 μg/ml [24]. Indeed, the *in vitro* activity of the compound is similar to that of a number of the aminoglycosides against Pseudomonas. Piperacillin has excellent activity against anaerobic species and inhibits 80% of isolates of *Bacteroides fragilis* at concentrations of 25 μg/ml. Piperacillin is hydrolyzed by various types of β-lactamases, including the most prevalent one, the TEM or Richmond type III enzyme. Nonetheless, hydrolysis is less than that with ampicillin and so piperacillin is active against the so-called fastidious gram-negative species *H. influenzae* and *N. gonorrhoeae,* even when they possess β-lactamases. Piperacillin similar to the other penicillins acts in a synergistic manner with aminoglycosides, such as gentamicin or amikacin [82].

The human pharmacology of piperacillin is similar to that of carbenicillin and the other antipseudomonas penicillins [92]. Extensive studies of the clinical efficacy of piperacillin have been performed in Japan [91]. These have shown that piperacillin is effective in the treatment of infections due to susceptible organisms and that it has no unusual toxicity. Comparative studies are yet to be done.

More recently a semisynthetic penicillin, aplacillin (PC 904), derived from ampicillin, has been undergoing study in Japan. The data about this compound are limited, but of interest since even although the agent is degraded by β-lactamases at a rate similar to carbenicillin, it inhibits many carbenicillin-resistant isolates of Pseudomonas and of the Enterobacteriaceae at low levels [65]. This appears to be due to the fact that the compound is taken up by bacteria much more readily than other penicillins, and that it has a higher affinity for penicillin-binding proteins 3 and 1b than do other penicillins. Aplacillin has proved to be more effective in mouse protection studies than carbenicillin. Although little has been presented or published about the pharmacokinetic parameters of this agent, it is highly protein-bound, approximately 98%, and a large portion of the drug is excreted via the bile [46]. Studies of its affinity for protein indicate that the binding to protein is weak, unlike that seen with some of the semisynthetic antistaphylococcal penicillins. Nonetheless, these pharmacologic aspects of the compound may affect its suitability for use in man. Of some concern would be the effect upon bowel flora in view of the high levels in the intestine.

I have reviewed what is new in the penicillins, attempting to put forward the *in vitro* bacteriologic data and pharmacokinetic parameters which would be of importance with these drugs. There are no indications as to whether any of the drugs under clinical investigation—azlocillin, mezlocillin, piperacillin, or aplacillin—are a major advance over the available carbenicillin and ticarcillin. In truth, many, or even most, community hospitals have little need of such compounds since they are necessary for infections encountered in the large centers where debilitated patients exposed to nosocomial hazards are more apt to be infected by organisms which require slightly greater *in vitro* activity. It is possible that one of these agents could prove superior to the available therapy for abdominal wounds or serious deep pelvic infections. But as we shall see, there are cephamycins which also can play a role in the treatment of such infections and which by virtue of β-lactamase resistance may be preferable.

No new antistaphylococcal penicillins have been developed in the past few years, but there are many unanswered questions about the present antistaphylococcal penicillins. The agents currently available are methicillin, nafcillin and four isoxazolyl penicillins: cloxacillin, dicloxacillin, flucloxacillin and oxacillin. These agents differ minimally in their antibacterial activity, but are markedly different in terms of oral absorption and protein binding [74]. Two questions which I cannot find satisfactory answers to are whether one agent is more efficacious than the others, and whether toxicity is truly greater with one agent. Methicillin has been the agent most associated with toxic side reactions, particularly interstitial nephritis [2]. Nafcillin has been extensively studied in the treatment of experimental staphylococcal endocarditis both alone and combined with aminoglycosides. However, direct comparative studies of oxacillin, methicillin and nafcillin have yet to be performed. Selection of an oral antistaphylococcal penicillin agent is also difficult since even though one agent may have higher oral absorption, its higher protein binding results in serum values which are equivalent. Thus at the present time, selection of an antistaphylococcal β-lactamase-resistant penicillin, whether for oral or parenteral use, can be based on financial considerations.

There are several different oral esters of carbenicillin which are used in the treatment of urinary tract infections due to Pseudomonas or to indole-positive Proteus. The most widely known of these is indanylcarbenicillin, which has been used clinically for several years. Carfecillin is another ester. A study by the group of the Institute Jules Bordet, comparing indanylcarbenicillin and carfecillin, showed a lower recurrence rate in the carfecillin treated group as well as fewer side effects [32]. Further studies are indicated to determine if this is in fact the case. However, both agents are of limited use in the hospitalized patient.

Unquestionably, new insights into the action of penicillins will result in continued development of penicillins which show increased activity against the common resistant organisms. Whether major improvements in the pharmacology of penicillins are possible is unknown. None of the newer agents has been shown to be a less likely cause of the most serious side effect of penicillin therapy; namely, allergic reactions. Even though the spectrum of the newer penicillins has been widely broadened, there are serious gaps which require the use of cephalosporins or aminoglycosides. Nonetheless, it is apparent that, as our knowledge of the sites of action of penicillins has increased and as our knowledge of the type of β-lactamases has improved, we have been able to more carefully direct the goals that new penicillins must fulfill.

CEPHALOSPORINS AND CEPHAMYCINS

Cephalosporin antibiotics have increased in number in the past few years, and in addition to the several agents which are soon to become available commercially, cephalosporins with markedly different spectra of activity are under study. The cephalosporin nucleus can be modified at several sites, but modifications at position 7 of the β-lactam ring seem to be associated with alteration in antibacterial activity and substitutions at position 3 of the dihydrohythiazine ring associated with changes in pharmacokinetic properties and metabolism. Clearly, substitutions at both positions can alter these general concepts of structure and function. In general, the antibacterial activity of cephalosporins commercially available has been similar with all of the agents having activity against many of the major gram-positive and gram-negative species, such that the agents were active against staphylococci, streptococci (except enterococci), *E. coli,* Klebsiella and *Proteus mirabilis* [93]. None of the original agents was active against Enterobacter, indole-positive Proteus, Pseudomonas, Serratia or *Bacteroides fragilis.* Furthermore, there have been reports of increasing numbers of *E. coli* and Klebsiella which contained β-lactamases which made the strains resistant to compounds such as cephalothin, cefazolin and cephalexin. For this reason, new agents have been sought to overcome these deficiencies. Before considering these newer agents it may be of value to consider the position of the older compounds.

There are three major acetoxymethyl cephalosporins: cephalothin, cephapirin and cefacetrile. The only antibacterial difference between the three is the greater activity of cefacetrile against enterococci and slightly greater stability of cephalothin to the *Staph. aureus* β-lactamase [19]. All three compounds are metabolized in man to desacetyl derivatives which are of lower antibacterial activity. All are approximately 70% bound to protein. These agents, for practical purposes, can be given only by intravenous injection, since intramuscular injection is quite painful and serum levels after 1 g are only 20 μg/ml. The half-life of all three is approximately 30–40 minutes. Therapeutically the compounds appear to be quite similar, and cephalothin particularly has been used to treat serious infections ranging from endocarditis to osteomyelitis [45].

In 1966 cephaloridine was introduced. This agent, which lacks a acetoxy group at position 3, is metabolically stable, well tolerated by IM injection, produces serum levels twice those of the previous compounds, and has a half-life of 90 minutes. There are, however, two unfortunate aspects to this agent, which is used minimally in the United States but widely in Europe. Cephaloridine is less stable to the β-lactamases of gram-positive and gram-negative organisms and at doses above 4 g per day it produces renal toxicity [2]. Thus there seems little rationale for its continued use. On the other hand, cefazolin, which has a mercapo-thiadiazole group at position 3, seems to have overcome many of the problems of the earlier agents. This compound has the same antibacterial activity of the earlier cephalosporins but is well tolerated by either IM or IV injection. It also has a half-life of nearly two hours and produces serum levels four-fold greater than those of the acetoxy cephalosporins [62]. Cefazolin appears to achieve high biliary levels as well. Cefazolin is 85% protein bound and hence there is less free drug to be antibacterially active. This agent has proved to be useful in many settings; hence, it would seem to be an appropriate cephalosporin for the hospital in which drug resistance is not a problem.

There are three new parenterally administered cephalosporin-cephamycin compounds which have undergone extensive *in vitro*, pharmacokinetic and clinical trial analysis. These agents all are β-lactamase-resistant and offer a greater potential of use for cephalosporin-cephamycin compounds. Interestingly, each of the agents has a slightly different spectrum of antibacterial activity, making it difficult to say that one of them is the second generation cephalosporin of choice. Cefamandole has an antibacterial activity against gram-positive staphylococci and streptococci very similar to cephalothin [25]. It has, however, much greater activity against Haemophilus and Neisseria, including β-lactamase-producing strains. It is active against many of the β-lactamase-producing cephalothin-resistant *E. coli* and against Enterobacters [49]. It lacks activity against some β-lactamase-producing Klebsiella and is inactive against many of the highly resistant Serratia and Providencia. It has no appreciable activity against Pseudomonas and has relatively weak activity against *Bacteroides fragilis*.

Cefuroxime has activity comparable to cephalothin and cefamandole against staphylococcal and streptococcal species [31,60,66]. It also inhibits β-lactamase-producing Neisseria and Haemophilus. It has greater *in vitro* activity than cefamandole against β-lactamase-producing *E. coli*, Klebsiella and some Proteus and is as active against Enterobacter. Cefuroxime inhibits a number of the isolates of *E. coli* and Klebsiella resistant to cefamandole and inhibits Enterobacter and Citrobacter resistant to cefoxitin. It lacks activity against many Serratia, some indole-positive Proteus and *B. fragilis* [60].

Cefoxitin is a truly β-lactamase-resistant compound. Strictly speaking, it is a cephamycin, a fermentation product of streptomyces. It is resistant to hydrolysis by β-lactamases by virtue of the methoxy substituent attached to the β-lactam ring at position 7 which provided steric hinderance [68]. Although cefoxitin has a carbamate substituent at position 3 of the structure, this is not as susceptible to mammalian esterases as is the acetoxy group. Cefoxitin is much less active than are the other parenteral cephalosporins against staphylococci and streptococci. The concentrations of cefoxitin needed to inhibit such organisms are at least ten-fold higher than that of cephalothin, cefuroxime or cefamandole. Against gram-negative bacteria, however, cefoxitin has activity equal to the older compounds against usual isolates of *E. coli* or Proteus. Furthermore, it is active against Klebsiella, Providencia and indole-positive Proteus resistant to all other cephalosporins. It is also active against the majority of *B. fragilis* at concentrations which could be achieved in man. Cefoxitin is not active against Enterobacter or Pseudomonas [50,89].

Pharmacologically, cefamandole and cefoxitin are quite similar in terms of protein binding, peak serum levels and distributions in the body [12,27,61]. Cefamandole can be administered by IM injection, whereas cefoxitin cannot unless diluted in lidocaine. The half-life of both agents is short, 40–50 minutes, so that both agents in serious infections would need to be given every four hours. In contrast, cefuroxime, although somewhat less protein bound, has a longer half-life, reaches higher serum levels and is well tolerated by either IM or IV injection [20].

All of the agents have been studied in large clinical trials. Cefamandole has proved effective in pneumonitis, urinary tract infections, osteomyelitis and endocarditis [44,70]. Cefuroxime has had a similar record of study in Europe, and cefoxitin has been studied in all the aforementioned conditions as well as in infections due to cephalothin-resistant Enterobacteriaceae and those due to anaerobic species [41,88]. Either cefamandole or cefuroxime would seem to be appropriate to use in respiratory infections due to Haemophilus, *Streptococcus pneumoniae* or *Staph. aureus*, with the realization that a number of older penicillins or cephalosporins work as effectively. In treatment of gram-negative infections due to the β-lactamase-producing Enterobacteriaceae, any of the three agents could be used, and in this regard these agents, particularly the highly β-lactamase-resistant cefoxitin, offer an alternative to the aminoglycosides. In abdominal and gynecologic infections due to a mixture of aerobic and anaerobic organisms, cefoxitin seems to offer the possibility of use as a single agent. It is wise, however, to realize that the use of these agents has been limited and it is possible that some heretofor unsuspected toxicity could surface in the next few years while these agents are first being used.

Several other cephalosporin compounds have recently undergone investigation. Ceftezole is a demethyl cefazolin which has antibacterial activity similar to cephalothin and cefazolin [63]. It is less protein bound than cefazolin, but it has lower peak serum levels and a shorter half-life than cefazolin. It seems doubtful that this agent would be a significant addition to the therapeutic armamentarium, although it has proven useful in extensive clinical trails in Japan. Cefazaflur has similar *in vitro* activity to cephalothin and cefazolin and is active against some strains resistant to these agents [1,15]. Its pharmacokinetic properties are not a major advance, so that this agent does not seem to compare to the three compounds mentioned earlier. A cephalosporin with two previously unused side chains of O-aminomethylphenylacetyl and carboxy methyl tetrazolethio is BLS-786 [37]. This agent has *in vitro* activity against gram-negative species similar to cefamandole and cefuroxime but is less active against gram-positive organisms. It is not as stable to β-lactamases as is cefoxitin or other 7-methoxycephem derivatives, but pharmacologically it is unusual because of an extremely long half-life. The agent has worked well in mouse protection tests and human studies are in progress. The *in vitro* activity and the long half-life may make this compound useful, provided it has no toxicities of a hepatic or renal nature.

Two cephalosporins active against Pseudomonas have been produced. The one, SCE-129, is quite unusual in that this compound is active against only Pseudomonas and gram-positive cocci [26]. The agent is resistant to the common β-lactamase found in Pseudomonas but is hydrolyzed by type III, TEM enzyme, or by the type V β-lactamase capable of hydrolyzing cloxacillin if these plasmid-mediated enzymes are present in the Pseudomonas [67]. This compound has a low protein binding and half-life of 1.4 hours [43]. Clinical studies are not available, although animal protection experiments have indicated that the compound is protective *in vivo*.

HR 756 is another cephalothin which is active against Pseudomonas but also is active against most gram-positive and gram-negative Enterobacteriaceae at very low concentrations [29]. Its activity against Pseudomonas is several fold greater than that of carbenicillin. Preliminary studies show minimal effect of pH, inoculum size or serum upon the *in vitro* activity of the compound, and it is protective in mouse infection tests [29; Neu, Fu, Aswapokee, et al. in preparation].

It should be apparent from this overview that the physician will be faced with many new agents in the coming decade. The β-lactamase-resistant cephalosporins, cefamandole, cefuroxime and cefoxitin, are soon to be made available commercially. Choice of which one to use should be based on consideration of resistant patterns in a particular hospital as well as the type of flora suspected. Clearly in many smaller hospitals these new parenteral cephalosporins may not be needed. The third generation of cephalosporins will be those which have added Pseudomonas activity. The utility of such agents can be determined only after extensive clinical trials.

There have been fewer oral cephalosporins studied. The most widely used oral compound is cephalexin. Cephradine is, for practical purposes, identical in antibacterial and pharmacologic properties [45,62]. New oral compounds are cefatrizine, cefadroxil, cefaclor and CGP 9000 [6,7,14,78,98]. The *in vitro* activity of all of the compounds is quite similar except for that of cefaclor which is considerably more active against Haemophilus. None of the compounds has increased resistance against β-lactamases nor do they possess Pseudomonas or Bacteroides activity. The human pharmacology of all of the oral preparations is fairly similar to that of cephalexin. Studies of cefaclor have shown that it achieves reasonable levels in middle ear fluid [42]. If cefaclor proves to be of value in otitis media, it may be a worthwhile new compound. As for the other agents, unless some unusual properties appear in further studies, the agents have added little to the oral cephalosporins.

AMINOGLYCOSIDES

The aminoglycoside antibiotics are actually among the older agents used to treat infection, if one considers that streptomycin was discovered in 1944, neomycin in 1949 and kanamycin in 1957. Progress in the treatment of hematologic diseases as well as the concept of intensive care medicine has made agents in this class extremely important in the management of infectious complications of other therapy. Kanamycin might be looked at as an agent which illustrates the problems of this class of compounds. This agent, which was actually first used because of its activity against staphylococci in an era in which antistaphylococcal penicillins were not yet available, was soon used to treat serious gram-negative infections. Two problems appeared. The one was bacterial resistance and the other toxicity, specifically ototoxicity [18]. At present, the commercially available aminoglycosides differ in antibacterial activity, depending upon factors peculiar to each institution. All aminoglycosides have a low therapeutic index; that is, the ratio between effective dose and toxicity is narrow.

All aminoglycosides are bactericidal compounds that inhibit protein biosynthesis through binding to specific receptor sites on the 30s ribosomes. There are a number of mechanisms of bacterial resistance to aminoglycosides, but the most commonly encountered one is due to the fact that the microorganism contains a plasmid that mediates production of enzymes which adenylate, phosphorylate or acetylate the amino or hydroxyl groups present on all aminoglycosides. Modification of these sites on the molecule prevents binding to the 30s receptor site proteins [51].

Kanamycin is not active against *Pseudomonas aeruginosa* since most of the Pseudomonas contain plasmids mediating production of phosphorylating enzymes. In many institutions, resistance of a considerable fraction of the *E. coli* and Klebsiella isolates have developed in the last ten years. If the institution is one in which Serratia and Providencia are prevalent, these organisms usually also are resistant to kanamycin. Thus, because of this bacterial resistance, the clinical use of kanamycin has declined.

Gentamicin and tobramycin, which has been in use for only about four years, are quite similar in their antibacterial spectrum. Both agents are active against Pseudomonas, most of the members of the Enterobacteriaceae and most staphylococci. Minor differences are the consistently two-fold greater activity of tobramycin against Pseudomonas and the greater activity of gentamicin against some Serratia and Proteus [55]. Again, however, resistance has been gradually increasing, and in some parts of the world resistance of Klebsiella, Pseudomonas and particularly Serratia has reached a level of significance. In general, gentamicin and tobramycin have been inactive against a strain resistant to either agent; the exception is some strains of *Pseudomonas aeruginosa* which are resistant to gentamicin but sensitive to tobramycin. The agent that overcame this resistance problem to some extent has been amikacin. Amikacin has a replacement of the amino groups at position 1 of the streptamine nucleus with an L-α-amino-α-hydroxybutyric acid side chain [33]. This modification has protected amikacin against attack by most of the common inactivating enzymes which are present in the Enterobacteriaceae and Pseudomonas [73]. Recently, strains of a number of species resistant to amikacin have been encountered. Most of these bacteria are resistant not by virtue of inactivating enzymes, but because of failure to transport the compound within the bacterial cell to its site of action. Such organisms are resistant to all of the aminoglycosides. Some of these organisms have developed this form of resistance as a mutational event, but some appear to contain plasmids which convey this property.

There are several new aminoglycosides which are either under study or currently available in other countries. Sisomicin is a compound which could be viewed as a dehydrogenated C_{1a} gentamicin. It is more active than the gentamicin complex against many bacteria, particularly Pseudomonas and *E. coli* [92]. It seems to kill organisms more rapidly than other aminoglycosides, perhaps due to a more rapid uptake by the bacterial cells. Unfortunately, it is not effective against organisms resistant to gentamicin. Netilmicin, on the other hand, which is similar in structure to sisomicin except for an ethyl group at position 1 of the streptamine nucleus, is resistant to inactivation by many of the adenylating and phosphorylating enzymes in *E. coli,* Klebsiella, Enterobacter and Proteus, but it is inactivated by some gentamicin-resistant Pseudomonas, Serratia and Providencia which contain certain acetylating enzymes [21]. Two other agents which look promising as compounds which are resistant to inactivating enzymes are episisomicin (SCH 22591) and a hydroxyaminopropyl derivative of gentamicin B, SCH 21420. These agents are comparable in activity to gentamicin, netilmicin and amikacin against the usual isolates of *E. coli*, Enterobacter and Klebsiella, and both agents inhibit many gentamicin-resistant species, including a number of Serratia and Providencia [22]. The gentamicin B derivative is active by virtue of the steric hinderance conveyed by the propyl side chain, but the episisomicin, even though inactivated by some of the isolated enymes, seems to enter some bacteria so rapidly that it can kill bacteria-containing enzymes which normally would destroy the antibiotic. Thus there appears to be continued progress in the development of agents to overcome aminoglycoside resistance, although the bacteria seem to always have a slight advantage.

From a pharmacologic viewpoint, all of the agents of this class are quite similar. None of the compounds are appreciably absorbed when given by the oral route so they must be administered parenterally. Adequate serum levels are achieved by either intramuscular or intravenous administration. None of the aminoglycosides is bound to plasma proteins, and the apparent volume of distribution of all of the drug is similar to the extracellular space (20–30%) of body weight. Even in the presence of meningeal inflammation, penetration of the aminoglycosides into the cerebrospinal fluid is inadequate to achieve therapeutic levels. Penetration into bile, synovial fluid, pleural and pericardial fluid is similar for the agents. Gentamicin, sisomicin, tobramycin and netilmicin yield serum levels which are nearly identical when given at equivalent mg/kg dosage programs [79]. Thus, 1 mg/kg yields a blood level of 4 μg/ml when these agents are given by IM injection. Kanamycin, amikacin and probably the HAPA-gentamicin B derivative yield equivalent serum levels which are higher than the levels of the previous agents, due to the larger amount of drug which can be given. Thus, when 7.5 mg/kg of these agents is given by IM injection, serum levels of 15–20 μg/ml are achieved [34].

In terms of the elimination of the compounds, there are subtle differences. Most of the data is based upon rat experiments. Recent reports have shown that gentamicin accumulations within the tissues of the kidney and renal concentrations of the drug are many times greater than the plasma levels [94]. Gentamicin has been recovered from the urine of man up to 20 days after a week of therapy. Tobramycin and netilmicin do not accumulate to the same degree in the renal cortex, and as a consequence much higher doses are needed to achieve the same degree of toxicity found with gentamicin [40,90].

Ototoxicity has been a prominent problem side effect of aminoglycoside therapy, even though the incidence of toxicity is low [30,56]. Both vestibular and cochlear damage can be produced in animals through the administration of high doses of the compounds. Clinical reports suggest that one aminoglycoside produces more vestibular toxicity and another greater auditory loss. But either toxicity or both can occur with any of the agents. The basic cellular mechanism of the ototoxicity is still unknown. In animal models, tobramycin and netilmicin produce much less toxicity than does gentamicin, sisomicin or kanamycin or amikacin [13].

Comments on the Usage of Aminoglycoside

To date it has been difficult to translate the aforementioned animal experiments to man. Clinical studies comparing aminoglycosides one with the other have not convincingly shown that one agent is either more efficacious or less toxic than another when used alone [21,81]. In life-threatening infections, particularly in individuals with underlying diseases which compromise host defense, aminoglycosides are rarely used as single agents, making even more complex the analysis of which agent is best [35]. All of the older aminoglycosides as well as the agents still under study have been effective in the treatment of experimental infections in animals and infections in man if the organism producing the infection is susceptible to the particular agent. Failure of aminoglycosides to clear an infection because of inadequate serum levels can occur with any of the agents if there is not close attention to doses used and the interval between doses [5].

At present in institutions in which there is a high level of gentamicin resistance, amikacin would be the agent of choice in high risk patients who have been hospitalized for a period and hence colonized by resistant bacteria. In proven Pseudomonas infections where resistance is not a problem, tobramycin may offer some advantage. The differences in ototoxicity and nephrotoxicity of gentamicin and tobramycin are still under exploration. It would seem reasonable, however, that in patients in whom a long period of therapy (> 10 days) is contemplated, tobramycin may be preferable. Hard and fast rules cannot be given. Where netilmicin and some of the other derivatives will fit in this picture depends on both trends in bacterial resistance and further studies of the comparative toxicity of the agents of this class. In the preliminary clinical studies of netilmicin, the incidence of toxicity has ranged from minimal to a level reported for the older agents.

The restriction of the use of particular aminoglycosides in the hospital is an issue that elicits widely disparate responses by general physicians, members of the pharmaceutical industry and infectious disease specialists. It is not established whether restriction of the use of agents such as amikacin or netilmicin will decrease the appearance of resistant isolates. Earlier indiscriminate use of gentamicin as a topical agent did produce serious resistance problems. If permeability changes can be mediated by plasmids, it would seem advisable to save certain agents. If, however, resistance will appear regardless of the volume of use, such policy has little sense. There are, however, reasons to make physicians learn how to use aminoglycosides in a more rational manner. Much of the early poor response to therapy with these agents is due to the low levels of drug achieved in serum and tissue because of underdosing. Similarly, many of the recent cases of toxicity are due to maintenance of high doses later in an illness when the level of the drug needed is less, since the agents accumulate in the kidney. Perhaps with the general availability of serum levels some of these problems will be solved, and we will be able to deliniate differences in the compounds which now remain blurred except for the differences in their antibacterial activity.

Comment on Other Agents

I have chosen in this review not to consider in any detail agents belonging to the macrolide, lincinoid, or sulfonamide groups. Developments in macrolide chemistry have been small. Jocamycin and rosamicin

are similar in *in vitro* activity and human pharmacology to erythromycin, but they have not so far been shown to have unusual properties
that would cause them to be considered as replacements of erythromycin
[77,87,96].

There have been no new compounds similar to clindamycin. The agent
has had two periods of use. The first was one in which there clearly was
indiscriminate use of clindamycin. The second period was that in which
fear of the toxicity of enterocolitis made many physicians reluctant to
use the compound. At present, enterocolitis appears to be a most
infrequent occurrence [58]. Careful selection of patients, early discon-
tinuation of the drug and not using agents which decrease gut motility all
may have been important. The studies of the overgrowth of a bacterial
flora in the gut may aid in our understanding of all forms of enterocolitis
produced by antimicrobial agents. Major resistance of Bacteroides to
clindamycin has not developed to date, and this agent is a useful compound in the treatment of anaerobic pleuropulmonary, abdominal and
gynecologic infections.

The use of chloramphenicol has increased with the awareness of problems attendent upon anaerobic infections. Resistance of anaerobic
species to chloramphenicol is minimal, but the Enterobacteriaceae have
shown increased resistance because of the plasmid-mediated enzyme,
chloramphenicol transacetylase. This has been particularly notable for
the high resistance of *Salmonella typhii* in some parts of the world where
typhoid is still a problem. Chloramphenicol-resistant *Strep. pneumoniae*
have been found in several countries, making this a concern, since
chloramphenicol, because of its ready entry into the spinal fluid, has
been the agent of choice in meningitis if penicillin resistance is suspected
or there is known allergy to penicillin. Resistance of Haemophilus to
chloramphenicol is rare, but already encountered in the United States. It
is probable that modification of the chloramphenicol nucleus could be
achieved in the light of certain advances in organic chemistry. It would
be extremely difficult, however, to test such agents clinically to be
certain that their toxicity is not greater than chloramphenicol itself, since
there are no adequate models of hematologic toxicity.

Recently, studies of trimethoprim alone, as compared with the trimethoprim-sulfamethoxazole combination, have been undertaken. It will
be of great interest to see if use of trimethoprim alone will result in more
rapid development of resistance or if it will have fewer side effects than
the combination. Resistance has been slow to develop, but already we
have encountered Serratia and Enterobacter isolates which are resistant
to trimethoprim. The use of the combination in patients with urologic
infections probably contributes to the resistance, since these patients

often have urethral catheters and the foreign body causes persistance of organisms which develop resistance. Trimethoprim-sulfamethoxazole has proved to be extremely useful in many life-threatening infections, and the future availability of an easily administered parenteral form will widen the possible uses of the combination.

SUMMARY

Many advances have been made in creating structures which will circumvent the increasing problems of bacterial resistance to antibiotics. Advances of a pharmacologic or toxicologic nature have been less frequent, as this review has illustrated. A number of new penicillins, cephalosporins and aminoglycosides will become available in the next few years. The choice of one compound over another will be difficult, since the advantages of a compound in one area are often mitigated by reduction of antimicrobial activity in another or a new form of toxicity. The selection of the most appropriate agent with which to initiate therapy is still based on the principles of using the well established drug that is still effective, the drug with the fewest side effects and the least expensive agent. This last factor should be carefully noted, since there is a tendency to select agents which offer an advance in the therapy of infection due to multiresistant bacteria when these bacteria may not be truly important in the environment in which one operates. Thus, even though in this review I have discussed at length new agents, I would caution the reader to consider that the old penicillins, the old cephalosporins and the old aminoglycosides may be more than adequate for his specific needs. A better understanding of the antibacterial spectrum, pharmacologic properties and toxicities of antibiotics may obviate the desire to use the newest agent.

REFERENCES

1. Actor P, Uri JV, Guarini JR, et al: A new parenteral cephalosporin SKF 59962: *in vitro* and *in vivo* antibacterial activity and serum levels in experimental animals. J Antibiot (Tokyo) 28:471–476, 1977.
2. Appel GB, Neu HC: The nephrotoxicity of antimicrobial agents. N Engl J Med 296:663–671, 722–728, 784–787, 1977.
3. Appelbaum PC, Hallett AF, Bhamjee A, et al: Penicillin and chloramphenicol resistant *Streptococcus* pneumonia from clinical specimens. 10th Int'l. Cong. Chemother. No. 179, September, 1975.

4. Ashford WA, Golash RG, Hemming VG: Penicillinase producing Neisseria gonorrhoeae. Lancet 2:657, 1976.

5. Barza M, Brown RB, Shen D, et al: Predictability of blood levels of gentamicin in man. J Infect Dis 132:165–174, 1975.

6. Bill NJ, Washington JA III: Comparison of *in vitro* activity of cephalexin, cephradine and cefaclor. Antimicrob Agents Chemother. 11:470–474, 1977.

7. Blackwell CC, Freimer EH, Tuke GC: *In vitro* evaluation of the new oral cephalosporin cefatrizine; comparison with other cephalosporins. Antimicrob Agents Chemother 10:288–292, 1976.

8. Bodey GP, Rodriguez V, Weaver S: Pirbenicillin, a new semisynthetic penicillin with broad spectrum activity. Antimicrob Agents Chemother 9:668–673, 1976.

9. Bodey GP, Tan T: Mezlocillin: *in vitro* studies of a new broad spectrum penicillin. Antimicrob Agents Chemother 11:74–79, 1977.

10. Bohni E: Kinetics of bactericidal effect in human urine during treatment with pivmecillinam and amoxycillin alone and combined. 10th Int'l Cong. Chemother No. 191, 1977.

11. Bresky B: Controlled randomized study comparing amoxycillin and pivmecillinam in adult out-patients presenting with symptoms of acute urinary tract infection. J Antimicrob Chemother 3 (Supp):121–127, 1977.

12. Brumfitt WJ, Kosmidis J, Hamilton-Miller JMT, Gilchrist JNG: Cefoxitin and cephalothin—antimicrobial activity, human pharmacokinetics and toxicology. Antimicrob Agents Chemother 6:290–299, 1974.

13. Brummett RE, Fox KE, Bendrick T, Hines D: Comparative ototoxicity of tobramycin, gentamicin, sisomicin and amikacin. 10th Int'l. Cong. Chemother. No. 207, 1977.

14. Buck RE, Price KE: Cefadroxil, a new broad spectrum cephalosporin. Antimicrob Agents Chemother 11:324–330, 1977.

15. Counts GW, Gregory D, Zeleznik D, Turck M: Cefazaflur a new parenteral cephalosporin *in vitro* studies. Antimicrob Agents Chemother 11:708–711, 1977.

16. Erwin FR, Bullock WE: Clinical and pharmacological studies of ticarcillin in gram-negative infections. Antimicrob Agents Chemother 9:94–101, 1976.

17. Feld R, Valdivieso M, Bodey GP, et al. Comparison of amikacin and tobramycin in the treatment of infection in patients with cancer. J Infect Dis 135:61–66, 1977.

18. Finland M: Summary of the conference on kanamycin: appraisal after eight years of clinical application. Ann NY Acad Sci 132:1045–1090, 1966.

19. Fong IW, Engelking ER, Kirby WMM: Relative inactivation by *Staphylococcal* aureus of eight cephalosporin antibiotics. Antimicrob Agents Chemother 9:939–944, 1976.

20. Foord RD: Cefuroxime, human pharmacokinetics. Antimicrob Agents Chemother 9:741–747, 1976.

21. Fu KP, Neu HC: *In vitro* study of netilmicin compared with other aminoglycosides. Antimicrob Agents Chemother 10:526–534, 1976.

22. Fu KP, Neu HC: The *in vitro* activity of 1-N HAPA gentamicin B and 5—sisomicin compared to other aminoglycosides. 17th Interscience Conf. Antimicrob. Ag. Chemother. No. 250, 1977.

23. Fu KP, Neu HC: Azlocillin and mezlocillin-new ureido penicillins. Antimicrob Agents Chemother (in press, 1978).

24. Fu KP, Neu HC: Piperacillin—a new penicillin active against many bacteria resistant to other penicillins. Antimicrob Agents Chemother (in press, 1978).

25. Fu KP, Neu HC: A comparative study of the activity of cefamandole and other

cephalosporin antibiotics with analysis of beta-lactamase stability and synergy of cefamandole with aminoglycosides J Infect Dis (in press, 1978).

26. Goto S, Ogawa M, Kaneko Y, et al: SCE-129, a new antipseudomonas cephalosporin I *in vitro* and *in vivo* properties. 10th Int'l. Cong. Chemother. No. 373, 1977.

27. Griffith RS, Black HR, Brier GL, Wolny JD: Cefamandole *in vitro* and clinical pharmacokinetics. Antimicrob Agents Chemother 10:814–823, 1976.

28. Grumberg E, Cleeland R, Beskid G, DeLorenzo WF: *In vitro* synergy between 6 B-amidinopenicillanic acid derivatives and other antibiotics. Antimicrob Agents Chemother 9:589–594, 1976.

29. Heymes R, Lutz A, Schrinner E: Experimental evaluation of HR 756 a new cephalosporin derivative. 10th Int'l. Cong. Chemother. No. 321, 1977.

30. Jackson GG, Arcieri G: Ototoxicity of gentamicin in man. A survey and controlled analysis of clinical experience in the United States. J Infect Dis 124:130–137, 1971.

31. Jones RN, Fuchs PC, Gavan TL, et al: Cefuroxine, a new parenteral cephalosporin: collaborative *in vitro* susceptibility comparison with cephalothin against 5,887 clinical bacterial isolates. Antimicrob Agents Chemother 12:47–50, 1977.

32. Kahan-Coppens L, Klastersky J: Comparative study of carfecillin and indanyl-carbenicillin in patients with complicated urinary tract infections. 10th Int'l Cong. Chemother. No. 24, 1977.

33. Kawaguchi H: BB-K8 (Amikacin) a semisynthetic kanamycin derivative. *In:* Mitsuhashi S (Ed): Drug Action and Drug Resistance in Bacteria. Tokyo, Univ. Tokyo Press, 1975, pp 45–76.

34. Kirby WMM, Clarke JT, Libke RD, et al: Clinical pharmacology of amikacin and kanamycin. J Infect Dis 134:312–315 (Suppl), 1976.

35. Klastersky J, Hensgens C, Debusscher L: Emperic therapy for cancer patients: comparative study of ticarcillin-tobramycin, ticarcillin-cephalothin and cephalothin-tobramycin. Antimicrob Agents Chemother 7:640–645, 1975.

36. Konig HB, Metzger KG, Murmann RP, et al: Azlocillin—ein neues penicillin gegen Pseudomonas aeruginosa und andere gramnegative bakterien. Infection 5:170–182, 1977.

37. Leitner F, Misiek M, Purisiano TA, et al: Laboratory evaluation of BL-S786, a cephalosporin with broad spectrum antibacterial activity. Antimicrob Agents Chemother 10:426–435, 1976.

38. Lode H, Niestrah U, Koeppe P, Langmaack H: Azlocillin und Mezlocillin zwei neue semisynthetische acylureidopeniciline. Infection 5:163–169, 1977.

39. Lopez DE, Standiford HC, Tatem BA, et al: Pirbenicillin: comparison with carbenicillin and BL-P1654 alone and with gentamicin against Pseudomonas aeruginosa. Antimicrob Agents Chemother 11:441–448, 1977.

40. Luft FC, Yum MN, Kleit SA: Comparative nephrotoxicities of netilmicin and gentamicin in rats. Antimicrob Agents Chemother 10:845–949, 1977.

41. McCloskey R: Results of a clinical trial of cefoxitin—a new cephamycin antibiotic. Antimicrob Agents Chemother 12:636–641, 1977.

42. McLinn SE: A comparative study of cefaclor a new cephalosporin and amoxicillin in the treatment of acute otitis media in children. Relationship of antibiotic concentrations of cefaclor and amoxicillin found in the middle ear effusions and their *in vitro* activity. 10th Int'l. Cong. Chemother. No. 4, 1977.

43. Mashimo K, Taguchi T, Nakang Y, Yamaguchi N: Pharmacology of SCE-129, a new cephalosporin antibiotic in human volunteers. 10th Int'l. Cong. Chemother. No. 375, 1977.

44. Meyers BR, Wormser G, Gartenberg G, et al: Cefamandole therapy in the seriously ill hospitalized patient. 10th Int'l. Cong. Chemother. No. 387, 1977.

45. Moellering RC Jr, Swartz MN: The newer cephalosporins. N Engl J Med 294:24–28, 1976.

46. Nagata A, Iba K, Ohbe Y., et al: Metabolism of a new semisynthetic penicillin PC-904. 10th Int'l. Cong. Chemother. No. 195, 1977.

47. Neu HC, Garvey GJ: Comparative *in vitro* activity and clinical pharmacology of ticarcillin and carbenicillin. Antimicrob Agents Chemother 8:457–462, 1972.

48. Neu HC: Antimicrobial activity and human pharmacology of amoxicillin. J Infect Dis (Suppl) 129:123–131, 1974.

49. Neu HC: Cefamandole, a cephalosporin antibiotic with an unusually wide spectrum of activity. Antimicrob Agents Chemother 6:177–182, 1974.

50. Neu HC: Cefoxitin, a semisynthetic cephamycin antibiotic—antibacterial spectrum and resistance to hydrolysis by gram-negative B-lactamases. Antimicrob Agents Chemother 6:170–176, 1974.

51. Neu HC: Molecular modifications of antimicrobial agents to overcome drug resistance. Antibiot Chemother 20:87–111, 1975.

52. Neu HC: Aminopenicillins—clinical pharmacology and use in disease states. Int J Clin Pharmacol Biopharm 11:132–143, 1975.

53. Neu HC, Cherubin CE, Longo ED, Winter J: Antimicrobial resistance of shigella isolated in New York City. Antimicrob Agents Chemother 7:833–836, 1975.

54. Neu HC: Mecillinam, a novel penicillanic acid derivative with unusual activity against gram-negative bacteria. Antimicrob Agents Chemother 9:793–799, 1976.

55. Neu HC: Tobramycin: An overview. J Infect Dis (Suppl) 134:3–19, 1976.

56. Neu HC, Bendush CL: Ototoxicity of tobramycin: A clinical overview. J Infect Dis (Suppl) 134:206–218, 1976.

57. Neu HC: Mecillinam—an amidino penicillin which acts synergistically with other B-lactam compounds. J Antimicrob Chemother (Suppl) 3:43–58, 1977.

58. Neu HC, Prince A, Ortiz-Neu C, Garvey GJ: Incidence of diarrhea and colitis associated with clindamycin therapy. J Infect Dis 135:120–125, 1977.

59. Neu HC, Fu KP: The synergy of azlocillin and mezlocillin combined with aminoglycoside antibiotics and cephalosporins. Antimicrob Agents Chemother (in press, 1978).

60. Neu HC, Fu KP: Cefuroxime—a B-lactamase resistant cephalosporin with a broad spectrum of gram-positive and gram-negative activity. Antimicrob Agents Chemother (in press, 1978).

61. Neu HC: Pharmacokinetics of cefamandole alone and compared with other cephalosporin compounds. J Infect Dis (in press, 1978).

62. Nightingale CH, Greene DS, Quintilanni R: Pharmacokinetics and clinical use of cephalosporin antibiotics. J Pharm Sci 64:1899–1927, 1975.

63. Nishida M, Murakawa T, Kamimura T, et al: *In vitro* and *in vivo* evaluation of ceftezole a new cephalosporin derivative. Antimicrob Agents Chemother 10:1–13, 1976.

64. Noguchi H, Mitsuhashi S: Bacteriological and biochemical approaches to antipseudomonal activity of PC-904. 10th Int'l. Cong. Chemother. No. 193, 1977.

65. Noguchi H, Kubo M, Komatsu T: Bacteriological and biochemical approaches to apalcillin (PC-904), a new broad spectrum semisynthetic penicillin. Second Tokyo Symposium—Microl. Drug-resistance. III D-6, October, 1977.

66. O'Callaghan CH, Sykes RB, Griffiths A, Thorton JC: Cefuroxime, a new cephalosporin antibiotic; activity *in vitro*. Antimicrob Agents Chemother 9:511–519, 1976.

67. Okonogi K, Kida M, Yoneda M, Mitsuhashi S: SCE-129, a new antipseudomonal

cephalosporin resistance to hydrolysis by beta-lactamase. 10th Inter'l. Cong. Chemother. No. 374, 1977.

68. Onishi HR, Daoust DR, Zimmerman SB, et al: Cefoxitin, a semisynthetic cephamycin antibiotic: resistance to beta-lactamase inactivation. Antimicrob Agents Chemother 5:38–48, 1974.

69. Parry MF, Neu HC: Ticarcillin for treatment of serious gram-negative infections with gram-negative bacteria. J Infect Dis 134:476–485, 1976.

70. Parry MF, Garvey GJ, Goldberger M, Neu HC: Therapy of serious infection with cefamandole. 10th Int'l. Cong. Chemother. No. 388, 1977.

71. Parry MF, Neu HC: A comparative study of ticarcillin plus tobramycin versus carbenicillin plus gentamicin for the treatment of serious infections due to gram negative bacilli. Am J Med (in press, 1978).

72. Pines A, Nandi AR, Raafat H, Rahman M: Pivmecillinam and amoxycillin as combined treatment in purulent exacerbations of chronic bronchitis. J Antimicrob Chemother (Suppl) 3:141–148, 1977.

73. Price KE, DeFuria MD, Purisano TA: Amikacin an aminoglycoside with marked activity against antibiotic resistant clinical isolates. J Infect Dis (Suppl) 134:249–261, 1976.

74. Rolinson GN, Sutherland R: Semisynthetic penicillins. Adv Pharmacol Chemother 11:151–172, 1973.

75. Powell JT, Bond JH: Multiple antibiotic resistance of clinical strains of Neisseria gonorrhoeae isolated in South Carolina. Antimicrob Agents Chemother 10:639–643, 1976.

76. Sanders CC, Sanders WE Jr: BL-P1654: Abacteriostatic penicilin? Antimicrob Agents Chemother 7:435–440, 1975.

77. Shadomy S, Tipple M, Pazton L: Josamycin and rosamicin; in vitro comparisons with erythromycin and clindamycin. Antimicrob Agents Chemother 90:773–775, 1976.

78. Shadomy S, Wagner G, Carver M: In vitro activities of five oral cephalosporins against aerobic pathogenic bacteria. Antimicrob Agents Chemother 12:609–613, 1977.

79. Simon VK, Mosinger EV, Malerczy V: Pharmacokinetic studies of tobramycin and gentamicin. Antimicrob Agents Chemother 3:445–450, 1973.

80. Sjovall J, Magni L: Comparative clinical pharmacology of bacampicillin and high oral doses of ampicillin. 10th Int'l. Cong. Chemother. No. 130, 1977.

81. Smith CR, Baughman KL, Edwards CQ, et al: Controlled comparison of amikacin and gentamicin. N Engl J Med 296:349–353, 1977.

82. Soejima R, Naoe H, Matsushima T, et al: Laboratory and clinical studies on T 1220. Chemotherapy (Japan) 25:1087–1093, 1977.

83. Spratt BG: Distinct penicillin binding proteins involved in the division, elongation and shape of Escherichia coli K12. Proc Natl Acad Sci USA 72:2999–3005, 1975.

84. Spratt BG: The mechanism of action of mecillinam. J Antimicrob Chemother (Suppl) 3:13–19, 1977.

85. Stewart D, Bodey GP: Azlocillin: in vitro studies of a new semisynthetic penicillin. Antimicrob Agents Chemother 11:865–870, 1976.

86. Sutter VL, Finegold SM: Susceptibility of anaerobic bacteria to 23 antimicrobial agents. Antimicrob Agents Chemother 10:736–741, 1976.

87. Sutter VL, Finegold SM: Rosamicin: in vitro activity against anaerobes and comparisons with erythromycin. Antimicrob Agents Chemother 9:350–354, 1976.

88. Sweet RL, Hadley KW, Mills J, Robbie M: Cefoxitin in the treatment of pelvic infections. 10th Int'l. Cong. Chemother. No. 85, 1977.

89. Tally FP, Jacobu NV, Bartlett JG, et al: Susceptibility of anaerobes to cefoxitin and other cephalosporins. Antimicrob Agents Chemother 7:128–132, 1975.
90. Trottier S, Bergeron MG, Gauvreau L: Intrarenal concentrations of netilmicin and gentamicin. 10th Int'l Cong. Chemother. No. 264, 1977.
91. Ueda Y: Summary of fundamental and clinical studies on T-1220, a broad spectrum penicillin derivative. Chemotherapy (Japan) 25:683–699, 1977.
92. Waitz JA, Moss EL Jr, Drube CG, Weinstein MJ: Comparative activity of sisomicin, gentamicin, kanamycin and tobramycin. Antimicrob Agents Chemother 2:431–437, 1972.
93. Washington JA II: The *in vitro* spectrum of the cephalosporins Mayo Clin Proc 51:237–250, 1976.
94. Welton A, Carter GG, Bryant HH, et al: Tobramycin and gentamicin intrarenal kinetic comparisons therapeutic and toxicological answers. 10th Int'l. Cong. Chemother. No. 263, 1977.
95. Werner H, Krasemann C: Susceptibility of Bacteroidaceae to mezlocillin, azlocillin, carbenicillin 16th Intersci. Conf. Antimicrob Agents Chemother No. 347, 1976.
96. Westerman EL, Williams TW Jr, Moreland N: *In vitro* activity of josamycin against aerobic gram-positive cocci and anaerobes. Antimicrob Agents Chemother 9:988–993, 1976.
97. Williams JD, Andrews J: Sensitivity of *Haemophilus influenzae* to antibiotics. Br Med J 1:134–137, 1974.
98. Zak O, Tosch W, Vischer WA, Kradolfer F: Comparative experimental studies of 3-methoxy and 3-methyl cephems. Drugs Exp Clin Res 3:11–20, 1977.

CHAPTER 5

CURRENT ANTIFUNGAL THERAPY

Allan J. Weinstein, M.D.

In recent years there has been a dramatic increase in the incidence of fungal infection observed in clinical practice [1]. This has been due, in part, to advances in the modern practice of medicine. Improvements in the diagnosis and therapy of malignant [23,24,79,91] and immunosuppressive [12,26,116] diseases have permitted patients to survive for longer periods of time and to develop infections which previously occurred only infrequently. Similar changes have resulted from the increasing use of pharmacologic agents which are immunosuppressive and cytotoxic. There can be little doubt that the greater incidence of serious fungal infections observed in recent years has been the result of such changes in medical practice. This has led to a better understanding of the pathogenesis and therapy of local and systemic fungal infections, and has also resulted in the description of diseases which previously were unknown. The use of immunosuppressive and cytotoxic chemotherapy and advances in the intravenous administration of fluids for nutritional supplementation have been responsible, in large part, for the frequent observation of Candida endophthalmitis [34,38,68], an infection which had only occasionally been described prior to the advent of such therapy. It is important, therefore, that the practitioner be aware of those therapeutic agents available for the treatment of serious fungal infection. Although the number of such compounds is small, the varied indications for their use and the multiplicity of the untoward effects with which they are associated require that the physician understand the precise role of each in the modern therapy of fungal infection.

It is the purpose of this chapter to discuss in detail clinical aspects of the use of the currently available antifungal agents. Major emphasis will be placed on those preparations which are administered parenterally in the therapy of serious mycotic infections. There will, however, also be a brief discussion of the topical antifungal preparations.

From the Department of Infectious Disease, Cleveland Clinic Foundation, Cleveland, Ohio.

5-Fluorocytosine

5-fluorocytosine is a fluorinated pyrimidine that is well absorbed from the human gastrointestinal tract [95]. It is not toxic to mammalian cells. Within twenty-four hours of being taken orally, 85 to 95 per cent of the drug is excreted unchanged in the urine [9].

The precise mechanism of action of 5-fluorocytosine is unknown. However, fungi that are susceptible to 5-fluorocytosine contain cytosine deaminase, an enzyme which is not present in mammalian cells. This enzyme converts 5-fluorocytosine to 5-fluorouracil. 5-fluorouracil is subsequently incorporated into fungal RNA. It has been suggested that this may be responsible for changes in protein synthesis in the fungal cell [73,75,76]. However, it is possible that the antifungal effect of 5-fluorocytosine is achieved in some other fashion.

5-fluorocytosine has activity against most strains of *Cryptococcus neoformans*, candida, *Torulopsis glabrata*, and aspergillus. Most other fungi are highly resistant to 5-fluorocytosine [45,89,90,95].

A wide range of untoward effects has been associated with the administration of 5-fluorocytosine. Abnormalities in hepatic function, manifest by elevated transaminases or alkaline phosphatase, have been observed in approximately 5 per cent of patients [6,95,110]. In most cases the patients have been asymptomatic. It has been recommended that liver function tests be monitored once-weekly in patients receiving 5-fluorocytosine.

Abnormalities of the blood-forming elements, primarily leukopenia and thrombocytopenia, have followed the use of 5-fluorocytosine [6,56,67,78]. When the compound has been administered alone, the abnormalities have almost always been confined to patients with azotemia. However, such changes also appear to be more common in patients who are given 5-fluorocytosine in combination with amphotericin B. This may be due, in part, to the production of azotemia by amphotericin B. It has been recommended that the complete blood count be monitored twice-weekly in patients receiving 5-fluorocytosine, and that there be a reduction in dosage when there is evidence of a decrease in white blood cell count or platelet count [6].

Approximately 6 per cent of patients given 5-fluorocytosine develop some form of gastrointestinal intolerance [6]. This includes nausea, vomiting, anorexia, abdominal pain, and diarrhea. Intestinal perforation has been rarely observed [46,104].

The clinical indications for the use of 5-fluorocytosine are limited. While the compound is effective in the treatment of serious cryptococcal infection, including cryptococcal meningitis [108], the rate of response is probably less than that observed when amphotericin B is administered.

In addition, the use of 5-fluorocytosine has been associated with the development of drug resistance in cryptococci [11]. Because of these factors, the most obvious use of 5-fluorocytosine in the therapy of cryptococcal infections is in combination with amphotericin B [107]. Such combination therapy has produced cure rates equal to or higher than those produced by previously utilized regimens for cryptococcal meningitis, and has only rarely been associated with the development of 5-fluorocytosine resistance. It is anticipated that, as a result of the lower doses that are used, such a program of combined therapy will be associated with a lower incidence of 5-fluorocytosine-induced untoward effects [6]. There also appears to be less amphotericin B toxicity in patients receiving such therapy, probably because of the reduced doses of amphotericin B that are administered [6].

Because of the possibility of the development of drug resistance, there is no situation in which candida infection should be treated with 5-fluorocytosine alone. In addition, the response rate of patients with candida infections treated with 5-fluorocytosine alone is lower than that of patients treated with amphotericin B [6]. It has been recommended that in serious candida infections (i.e., those in which intravenous use of amphotericin B would ordinarily be administered) it is reasonable to consider the addition of 5-fluorocytosine to amphotericin B, except when the infection is due to a strain which is highly resistant to 5-fluorocytosine [6]. There are, at present, no data available which will permit the use of 5-fluorocytosine alone in clinical fungal infections.

Although most strains of *Torulopsis glabrata* are susceptible to 5-fluorocytosine, there is, at present, only meager evidence to suggest that this agent is beneficial in infections produced by this organism [6,95]. Amphotericin B is the drug of first choice in infections due to *Torulopsis glabrata*. Similarly, while many strains of aspergillus are susceptible to 5-fluorocytosine, the clinical experience with this compound in aspergillosis is extremely limited [5,95,110].

The currently recommended dose of 5-fluorocytosine, specifically when used in combination with amphotericin B, is 37.5 mg/kg of body weight every six hours by mouth [6]. Because the compound is almost entirely excreted unchanged in the urine, reduced doses must be employed when renal function is impaired. It has been recommended that one dose every six hours be administered to patients with creatinine clearances of at least 40 ml/min; one dose every 12 hours for clearances of 20–40 ml/min, and one dose every 24 hours for clearances of 10–20 ml/min [87]. There are, at present, no specific recommendations for the administration of this agent to individuals with more severe degrees of renal failure or with changing renal function. 5-fluorocytosine can be removed both by peritoneal dialysis and hemodialysis [5,10].

While 5-fluorocytosine possesses *in vitro* activity against four fungi of major clinical significance (*Cryptococcus,* candida, *Torulopsis glabrata,* and aspergillus), this compound has enjoyed only limited use since its introduction in 1972. Such restrictions in use are due to the development of 5-fluorocytosine resistance among fungi, and to the occurrence of drug-induced untoward effects. At the present time, the clinical use of 5-fluorocytosine is limited to combination therapy with amphotericin B in certain patients with cryptococcal and candidal infections.

Clotrimazole

Clotrimazole is a compound which has recently become available for the therapy of fungal infections. Little is known about the mechanism of action of this drug, but is has been suggested that relatively high concentrations of clotrimazole may preferentially damage fungal cell membranes, making them permeable to intracellular phosphates and potassium, thus inhibiting intracellular macromolecular synthesis. Such a mechanism of action is similar to that which has been described for amphotericin B [106].

A large number of fungi are susceptible to clotrimazole. These include aspergillus species, candida species, *Histoplasma capsulatum, Blastomyces dermatitidis, Cryptococcus neoformans, Sporotrichum schenkii,* and *Coccidioides immitis. In vitro* resistance to clotrimazole has not been observed [53,105].

Clotrimazole is absorbed poorly from the human gastrointestinal tract. Urinary levels are approximately four times those of serum [106]. Untoward effects have been noted in a high percentage of patients given this compound. Gastrointestinal abnormalities, including nausea, vomiting, abdominal pain, and diarrhea, are common [19]. Hallucinations and disorientation have been observed [106]. The frequency of such toxicity and a rather limited rate of clinical efficacy have led some to suggest that there are no indications for the systemic use of clotrimazole [106]. There are, however, a number of conditions in which this agent can be used topically [57,60,63,70,92,94].

When clotrimazole is prepared as either a 1 per cent solution or as a 1 per cent cream, no substantial dermal irritation or phototoxicity has been observed [94]. In view of its wide range of activity against dermatophytes (trichophyton, epidermophyton, and microsporum) and its activity against *Candida albicans*, this agent has an important role in the therapy of superficial fungal infections. Usefulness in the topical therapy of dermatophytoses has been established [57,92,94]. It has also been demonstrated that clotrimazole is highly effective in the topical therapy of candidal vulvovaginitis [63], and can eradicate infection when administered over a short treatment period (three days). Similarly, clotrimazole troches have been successfully employed in oral candidiasis [70].

Although clotrimazole was effective in the treatment of chronic mucocutaneous candidiasis in one patient [60], it appears, at present, that the major use of this compound will be in the therapy of superficial mycotic infections.

Miconazole

Miconazole is a new broad-spectrum antifungal agent [16,109]. Most strains of *Cryptococcus neoformans, Candida albicans,* and *Coccidioides immitis* can be inhibited by clinically achievable concentrations of miconazole. At present in the United States, miconazole is being used experimentally in the therapy of candidiasis, coccidioidomycosis, cryptococcosis, histoplasmosis, and other deep fungal infections [54,86,96,97].

Miconazole resembles clotrimazole in certain characteristics: Both have broad antifungal activity; both have similar effects on fungi, possibly on purine or pyrimidine metabolism or both; both have efficacy when administered locally or topically [25]. The drugs are dissimilar, however, in that miconazole may be administered intravenously, while clotrimazole can be used only in oral or topical form. It has been suggested that miconazole is eliminated from the body by nonrenal pathways [96]. Information concerning penetration of miconazole into body fluids is sparse. However, it does cross the blood-brain barrier to some extent [98].

Because the use of miconazole in serious fungal infections has been limited, the true incidence and precise nature of untoward effects related to its administration are not known. However, phlebitis has been commonly associated with intravenous administration of miconazole [96], and anemia has occasionally been noted following its use [62,96], Transient nausea, rash, and arthralgias have occurred. Some investigators have noted aggregation of patients' erythrocytes, visible macroscopically on peripheral blood smears. This is apprently related to abnormalities which occur in the serum of patients receiving miconazole [96]. An unusual serum lipoprotein abnormality has been observed to be produced by the vehicle of miconazole [4]. Extremely high concentrations of serum cholesterol and triglycerides were noted, with an unusual lipoprotein pattern showing a lipid-stained band with the electrophoretic mobility of gamma-2 globulin and none of the usual characteristics of normal serum lipoproteins.

The broad spectrum of antifungal activity, and an apparently low incidence of significant untoward effects, have stimulated extensive study of miconazole during the past few years. Miconazole has been demonstrated to be effective in chronic coccidioidomycosis, South American blastomycosis, disseminated candidiasis, pulmonary aspergillosis, and cryptococcal meningitis [54,72,86,96,97,98]. In addition, topical administration of miconazole has been successful in oral candidiasis, cutaneous candidiasis, and both gastrointestinal and vulvovaginal candidiasis [15,28,84,99].

At present, the precise role of miconazole in the therapy of deep fungal infections remains to be determined. However, because of its activity against candida and a wide variety of dermatophytes (trichophyton, epidermophyton, and microsporum) [17], miconazole has already become an important agent in the therapy of superficial fungal infections.

Griseofulvin

Griseofulvin is an oral antifungal agent which is very effective in certain types of dermatophytoses [35,44]. While details of the mechanism of action of this agent are unclear, fungal cultures actively take up large quantities of griseofulvin and the drug is bound to cellular lipids [55]. Griseofulvin is active against microsporum, epidermophyton, and trichophyton species. It has no effect on other fungi, including candida species. The development of resistance to griseofulvin among fungal isolates from humans is very rare.

Griseofulvin rarely produces untoward effects and such reactions are usually transient and reversible [8,41,43]. Among the side effects of griseofulvin is headache, which may be severe but usually disappears even with the continuance of therapy. Other nervous system manifestations, such as lethargy, mental confusion and vertigo, may occur. Leukopenia, neutropenia, and monocytosis have developed rarely in patients receiving griseofulvin. Although the compound has not been associated with the production of renal insufficiency, albuminuria and cylindruria have been noted. Griseofulvin has been associated with the production of urticaria, erythema, and vesicular and morbilliform eruptions. Serum sickness and angioedema occasionally develop. Nausea, vomiting, diarrhea, and hepatotoxicity have occurred following the administration of griseofulvin.

Although griseofulvin should not be given to patients with porphyria, since it causes increased synthesis of delta aminolevulinic acid, in normal patients it only rarely produces an inrease in stool porphyrin, without evidence of clinical disease [111]. Patients receiving anticoagulants should not receive griseofulvin, since the hepatic enzymes activated by griseofulvin also cause degradation of warfarin, and the increased dose of warfarin required during concomitant griseofulvin administration may prove excessive once griseofulvin has been discontinued [29].

Griseofulvin is available in oral form only. The recommended daily dose for children is 10 mg/kg. For adults, 500 mg to 1 gram per day is usually administered, with the dose divided into four equal parts and given at six-hour intervals.

Fungal infection of the skin, hair, and nails, due to microsporum, trichophyton, or epidermophyton species may be successfully treated with griseofulvin [8,41,43]. Although symptomatic relief of skin infections may occur within 48 hours following the institution of griseofulvin therapy, effective therapy usually requires extended periods of time. Infections in intertriginous areas may require two to four weeks, those involving palms and soles four to eight weeks, and infections involving fingernails or toenails from four months to twelve months.

Griseofulvin is a highly effective and relatively nontoxic agent for the therapy of superficial fungal infections.

Hamycin

Hamycin is an orally administered polyene antifungal antibiotic which is highly active against *Candida albicans* [74]. This compound also has activity against several species of aspergillus, *Histoplasma capsulatum,* and *Blastomyces dermatitidis* [101]. It has been suggested that, unlike amphotericin B, hamycin may not be associated with a significant incidence of nephrotoxicity [102]. It has been observed that hamycin may be more effective than amphotericin B in the treatment of blastomycosis [51]. This agent has been used successfully in the local therapy of vaginal candidiasis. Hamycin is not available for use in the United States.

Tolnaftate

Tolnaftate is a topical fungicidal agent. This compound is useful in dermatophytoses due to trichophyton, microsporum, and epidermophyton species. It is without effect on candida species [2,80,81]. There has been no evidence of the development of drug resistance to tolnaftate.

The clinical results of therapy with tolnaftate are most dramatic in skin disease. The agent is less effective in infections involving the scalp and nails. Tolnaftate is relatively free of untoward effects [42]. However, contact allergy to tolnaftate has been observed [40]. Tolnaftate is available in cream, powder, and solution containing 1 per cent of the drug. It is usually applied to the affected area twice-daily, and successful therapy is usually achieved within seven to twenty-one days.

Candicidin
Candicidin is a polyene antibiotic which is effective only in the therapy of vaginal candidiasis. This agent is administered topically, and has rarely been associated with adverse effects.

Hydroxystilbamidine Isethionate
Hydroxystilbamidine isethionate is effective *in vitro* against *Blastomyces dermititidis*, and there have been favorable results when it has been employed in the treatment of human systemic and pulmonary North American blastomycosis [20,61]. However, two effects of the administration of this agent have led to the recommendation that it be used only in unusual circumstances. First, when hydroxystilbamidine isethionate has been used in North American blastomycosis, the incidence of relapse has been high [20]. Second, administration of this compound has been associated with a wide variety of untoward effects, similar to those produced by its congener, pentamidine. Intravenous administration of hydroxystilbamidine isethionate has led to the rapid development of breathlessness, tachycardia, dizziness, headache, and fainting. Such effects are most probably related to the sharp decreases in blood pressure which are associated with the rapid administration of this drug [82]. In addition, neuropathy has occurred frequently following the adminstration of this compound. Hypoglycemia and, paradoxically, hyperglycemia have resulted from the administration of hydroxystilbamidine isethionate. Reversible renal dysfunction has also been observed.

In view of the high relapse rate, and the considerable incidence of untoward effects associated with hydroxystilbamidine isethionate therapy, the use of this agent must be limited to those situations in which no other therapeutic alternatives are available.

Haloprigin
Haloprigin is halogenated phenolic ether which is fungicidal to various species of epidermophyton, microsporum, trichophyton, and *Candida albicans* [47,88]. Haloprigin acts by inhibiting oxygen uptake by the fungal cell and by disrupting the fungal cell membrane. In addition, it interferes with protein and nucleic acid synthesis [48]. The use of haloprigin has not been associated with the development of resistant strains of fungi (47).

Haloprigin is administered topically. It is available in a 1 per cent solution or cream. Haloprigin occasionally produces irritation and maceration, especially in acute and secondarily infected tinea infections. Occasionally, exacerbation of the lesion being treated has been observed when haloprigin has been applied to skin lesions; this occurs most prominently when the lesion is located on the foot and occlusive footwear is worn [50]. Photosensitivity does not occur. Systemic toxicity has not been observed.

Haloprigin is effective in the treatment of fungal infections of the skin, including those due to *Candida albicans*. However, controlled studies have shown no significant difference between the efficacy of haloprigin and that of tolnaftate in the treatment of tinea pedis [22], and similar results occur when haloprigin and nystatin are employed in the therapy of cutaneous candidiasis [23].

Nystatin

Nystatin is a polyene antibiotic with a broad antifungal spectrum that includes candida species, the fungi causing dermatophytic infection, and those causing systemic fungal infections [52]. Nystatin is bound by drug-sensitive yeasts and fungi, but not by resistant microorganisms. The antifungal activity of nystatin is due to its ability to interfere with cholesterol-containing cell membrane function and to alter potassium and sodium cellular exchange, producing fungal cell disruption. Because of this mode of action, resistant strains are difficult to induce *in vivo* [58,103,115].

Nystatin is effective against candida, *Cryptococcus neoformans, Histoplasma capsulatum, Blastomyces dermatitidis,* trichophyton, epidermophyton, and microsporum. There are, however, a number of strains of candida, other than albicans, which are quite resistant to nystatin [112].

Nystatin is not absorbed from the gastrointestinal tract, the skin, or mucous membranes. Significant plasma concentrations of nystatin are occasionally produced in patients with renal insufficiency who are taking conventional doses by mouth [112].

Nystatin is uncommonly associated with untoward effects. Nausea, vomiting, and diarrhea may occur following oral adminstration. No other local or systemic untoward effects have been reported.

Nystatin is available in ointments, oral suspensions, oral tablets, creams, and powders. The oral dose is 500,000 to 1,000,000 units three times per day for adults, and 100,000 units three to four times per day for children. Topical application is performed two to three times daily, and vaginal tablets are inserted once or twice daily.

Nystatin is effective in the treatment of localized candida infections of the vagina, skin, and mouth. Superficial monilial infections in inter-triginous areas, vagina, mouth, the angles of the mouth, between the fingers, and in the nail folds respond to topical nystatin therapy. Nail involvement due to *Candida albicans* is not affected. Monilial infections of the lungs, liver, and other organs respond poorly to systemic nystatin because of inadequate absorption from the gastrointestinal tract [52]. Response to topical nystatin is rapid. However, some patients with oral, esophageal, or vaginal candidiasis fail to improve when treated with nystatin. This occurs most commonly in individuals who have developed monilial infection as the result of suprainfection following broad-spectrum antimicrobial therapy. Because of its high rate of efficacy and low incidence of untoward effects, nystatin must be considered to be one of the agents of first choice in the treatment of most superficial candida infections.

Amphotericin B

Amphotericin B is a polyene antifungal agent which is the most widely used and most effective compound currently available for the therapy of serious fungal infections. Amphotericin B interferes with cell membrane function. It reduces the capacity of plasma membranes to maintain intracellular ionic gradients. Amphotericin B interferes with membrane-bound sterols and produces multimolecular complexes which enhance the permeability of the membranes to anions and, to a lesser degree, cations [106]. This action allows sodium and water to enter the cell, with con-sequent swelling of the cytoplasmic ground substance and endoplasmic reticulum, and ultimate destruction of the cell [85]. Amphotericin B also disrupts lysosomes; some of the toxic reactions produced by it may be related to such disruption [114].

The minimal inhibitory concentrtions of those fungi susceptible to amphotericin B range from 0.02 to 1.00 μg/ml, levels that can readily be obtained in serum after intravenous administration [7]. The minimum fungicidal concentration does not usually vary by more than two-fold from the minimal inhibitory concentration [106]. The results of *in vivo* studies in animals generally parallel the *in vitro* values.

In declining order of sensitivity to amphotericin B, the susceptible fungi are *Blastomyces dermatitidis, Histoplasma capsulatum, Cryptococ-cus neoformans,* candida species, *Sporotrichum schenkii,* and *Coccidi-oides immitis.* Aspergillus species are frequently resistant, while phycomyces species are highly variable, ranging from exquisitely sensi-tive to highly resistant [32,37].

When strains of *Candida albicans* and *Coccidioides immitis* are serially subcultured in increasing concentrations of amphotericin B, resistance to the drug may develop. However, apart from those exceptions noted above, amphotericin B-resistant strains are infrequently encountered. Even when a patient has suffered a relapse following a course of chemotherapy, the most recent isolate usually is as susceptible to amphotericin B as was the first [106]. There is no evidence that resistance to amphotericin B develops *in vivo*.

Amphotericin B is poorly absorbed from the human gastrointestinal tract. Maximum serum levels following oral administration have ranged from no detectable amphotericin B to 0.5 μg/ml [7]. Details of the tissue distribution of amphotericin B are unknown. Amphotericin B is administered primarily by the intravenous route. However, after intravenous administration, the plasma level is only 10 per cent of the predicted value [7]. Even if equal diffusion into the extracellular space is assumed, it is possible to account for only 40 percent of the administered amphotericin B. Levels in the cerebrospinal fluid are approximately 1/40 those in serum [30]. Smaller amounts are present in bronchial secretions, saliva, and aqueous humor.

Amphotericin B is excreted very slowly in the urine, with only a small fraction present in active form. With repeated daily infusions, only about 5 per cent of the administered dose is excreted daily in the urine. The drug continues to be excreted up to three weeks following the cessation of therapy. Because of the low rate of urinary excretion, there is no accumulation of amphotericin B in the serum of patients with renal failure [5,36].

Amphotericin B may be administered topically, locally, and intravenously. Topical amphotericin B has been utilized in cutaneous and mucocutaneous moniliasis [69], including intertriginous, interdigital, and oral infections. It is particularly effective in treating monilial infections of the diaper area.

Local instillation of amphotericin B is infrequently required. However, intrathecal administration has been employed in the treatment of coccidioidal meningitis and in some refractory cases of cryptococcal meningitis. Injection may be made into the lumbar area, cisterna magna, or, by the use of a prosthesis, into the cerebral ventricles [30,71,93]. Bladder irrigation with amphotericin B has been used in candidal cystitis. Intraarticular injections of amphotericin B are sometimes useful in coccidioidal arthritis and in some patients with osteoarticular sporotrichosis [5]. Cutaneous lesions of chromoblastomycosis may occasionally respond to the repeated injections of amphotericin B [5]. Local irritation may follow the direct installation of amphotericin B; however, this is unusual.

The usual method of administration of amphotericin B is by the intravenous route. At least four different schedules have been recommended for the administration of this compound. They are as follows [3,5,7,33]:

1. Administration of 0.25 mg/kg the first day, followed by an increase of 0.25 mg/kg each day until the daily maintenance dose of 1 mg/kg is reached.

2. Administration of 1 mg of amphotericin B on day one, 5 mg on the second day, 10 mg on the third day, with subsequent daily increases of 5 to 10 mg until 1 mg/kg is being administered daily.

3. One mg of amphotericin B is administered intravenously on the first day. This is followed by gradual daily increases until the peak plasma amphotericin B concentration is at least twice that required for the *in vitro* inhibition of the organism isolated from the patient.

4. Amphotericin B administration is instituted at the maintenance dose of 0.3 to 0.6 mg/kg on the first day.

In all of the recommended programs for the administration of amphotericin B, a "test dose" is given prior to the initiation of therapy [5]. The "test dose" consists of 1 mg of amphotericin B infused intravenously over four to six hours. The purpose of the "test dose" is to determine whether chills, vomiting, fever, and/or headache will occur in the patient being treated. When such reactions develop following the "test dose," subsequent doses of amphotericin B must be preceded by the administration of salicylates, antihistamines, and/or corticosteroids.

A number of untoward effects have been associated with the use of amphotericin B [112]. Hypersensitivity reactions, manifest by anaphylaxis, thrombocytopenia, and convulsions, occasionally occur. Local irritative effects, such as headache, fever, chills, and vomiting, develop in a significant percentage of patients receiving amphotericin B, but in most cases pretreatment with or simultaneous administration of salicylates, antihistamines, and/or corticosterioids will prevent such reactions.

Because rapid administration of amphotericin B may produce ventricular arrhythmias in animals, the agent is conventionally given over a four to six hour period in man [21]. Hepatotoxicity with jaundice is so infrequently encountered with amphotericin B therapy that it has been suggested that this may be an idiosyncratic reaction [5]. Anemia frequently follows the administration of amphotericin B. The hematocrit slowly falls to a stable value, usually between 22 and 35 per cent. The bone marrow appears normal. Transfusion is usually unnecessary. Leukopenia and thrombocytopenia are rare [65].

The most common untoward effect of amphotericin B is the development of renal dysfunction. The histologic changes in the kidney which are produced by amphotericin B are variable and are, most probably, dose-related. Amphotericin B causes thickening and fragmentation of the glomerular basement membranes and hypercellularity, fibrosis, and hyalinization of glomeruli. Focal and generalized degeneration and atrophy of tubules, especially the ascending loop of Henle and distal convoluted tubule, have been observed. Nephrocalcinosis occurs in both the proximal and distal convoluted tubules: divalent calcium is present intraluminally, intercellularly, and interstitially, and the highest concentration is at the corticomedullary junctions [113].

Functional renal changes occur earlier than anatomic ones and include decreased glomerular filtration rate, renal plasma flow, and filtration fraction. With the exception of renal blood flow, the values return to normal when therapy is discontinued. A decrease in concentrating ability and increased serum levels of creatinine and blood urea nitrogen also occur during treatment.

The mechanisms thought to be responsible for decreased renal function are arteriolar spasm, deposition of calcium during periods of ischemia, which leads to altered permeability of membranes and electrolyte abnormalities, imbalance of fluid and electrolytes, and lysis of the membranes of cellular lysosomes, leading to injury of renal cells. The most consistent change in renal tubular function produced by amphotericin B is an increase in the clearance of uric acid; this is directly related to dose and inversely related to the glomerular filtration rate [18].

Renal tubular acidosis is a common dose-related effect of amphotericin B therapy. The most frequent biochemical abnormality associated with the use of amphotericin B is hypokalemia. It has been suggested that this may be due either to wasting of sodium and potassium, which occurs only in the presence of renal tubular acidosis, or to a direct toxic effect on the permeability of renal tubular epithelium [113].

Mild renal functional abnormalities usually disappear when amphotericin B therapy is discontinued and do not contraindicate retreatment. Irreversible renal failure is unusual. It has been suggested that administration of alkali may be helpful in preventing renal dysfunction during prolonged treatment [31,64]. More recently, it has been noted that concurrent use of mannitol may result in a significant decrease in the incidence of amphotericin B-induced nephrotoxicity [83]. When administered intravenously, mannitol increases renal blood flow and glomerular filtration [77], and in animals prevents the tubular vacuolization and azotemia produced by amphotericin B [49]. Limited data suggest that similar effects may occur in man. In some patients who develop renal failure while receiving amphotericin B, stabilization and, occasionally, improvement of renal function has been noted when the agent is administered every other day, rather than once-daily.

While the incidence and severity of amphotericin B-induced toxicity can be considerable, concern regarding untoward effects must not prevent the physician from administering the agent when its use is required. Because of its broad antifungal activity, there are many patients whose infections can be cured only by amphotericin B. While a few of these patients may be endangered by the toxicity of the drug, the risks are usually far outweighed by the potential benefits of such therapy, and one must not allow "amphotericin B pharmacophobia" [100] to delay the institution of proper treatment. In addition, the use of the newer schedules of amphotericin B administration (i.e., those listed as numbers 3 and 4, above) has been associated with a lower incidence of untoward effects.

Intravenous administration of amphotericin B may involve either "short" or "long" courses of therapy. "Short" courses of "low dose" intravenous amphotericin B have been extremely effective in the therapy of resistant mucosal candidal infections. Patients with candida laryngitis, esophagitis, pharyngitis, and cystitis who have failed to respond to local administration of antifungal agents, such as nystatin, have had striking clinical responses to small total doses (10 to 355 mg) of amphotericin B administered over brief periods of time (4 to 18 days) [66].

The duration of amphotericin B administration for deep mycotic infections varies with the nature, severity, and location of the infection. It is also influenced by the development of untoward effects. Patients usually are treated for between six weeks and four months. The total quantity of amphotericin B required for the eradication of most deep mycotic infections is 2 to 3 grams [112].

Because of its wide range of activity, amphotericin B is the keystone of modern antifungal chemotherapy. It is the agent of first choice in all forms of blastomycosis. Patients with acute, disseminated, or active chronic cavitary histoplasmosis should receive amphotericin B. Individuals with meningitis, pyelonephritis, or osteomyelitis due to *Cryptococcus neoformans* should be treated with this agent. Although the rate of success with amphotericin B in the therapy of coccidioidomycosis is variable, the absence of more effective compounds requires that it be the primary mode of therapy in this illness.

Although, as noted previously, amphotericin B is sometimes required in mucosal candidal infections, it is in the therapy of deep candida infections (e.g., septicemia, endocarditis, and the recently described endophthalmitis) that it is most clearly indicated. It is also effective in the therapy of pulmonary and synovial sporotrichosis. Amphotericin B is used in infections due to phycomycetes, because it is the only potentially effective agent.

Despite its efficacy, major concern about amphotericin B persists because of its potential untoward effects. Recently, there have been two developments which may modulate such concern. The methyl ester of amphotericin B is currently under investigation [14,39]. This water-soluble derivative of amphotericin B possesses significant antifungal activity, and, based on preliminary studies, may be associated with a lower incidence of toxicity when compared with that produced by amphotericin B itself. In addition, newer programs are being developed for the therapy of systemic mycotic infections, which involve the concurrent administration of amphotericin B with another antifungal agent. For example, in cryptococcal meningitis, the use of amphotericin B with 5-fluorocytosine may permit lower doses of amphotericin B to be employed, and, thus, diminish the incidence of amphotericin B-induced untoward effects [107]. Similarly, combinations of amphotericin B with other agents such as rifampin [59] and polymyxin B [27] have been observed to be possibly more effective, and potentially less toxic, modes of therapy for histoplasmosis, blastomycosis, and coccidioidomycosis.

Local and systemic mycoses have become increasingly important clinical problems in the recent past. Advances in the diagnosis and therapy of diseases which formerly would have been rapidly fatal have been attended by an increase in the incidence of such potentially lethal infections. While the therapeutic options in the management of these infections are limited, the currently available antifungal preparations are highly effective in many of the conditions with which the practitioner is commonly confronted. It is only with a clear understanding of the indications for their use, their untoward effects, and the intricacies of their administration that this group of compounds can be successfully employed.

REFERENCES

1. Abernathy RS: Treatment of systemic mycoses. Medicine 52:385–394, 1973.
2. Adam JE, Cory GE: Tolnaftate (Tinactin) a new topical antifungal agent. Can Med Assoc J 93:1004–1005, 1965.
3. Andriole VT, Kravetz HM: The use of amphotericin B in man. JAMA 180:269–272, 1962.
4. Bagnarello AG, Lewis LA, McHenry MC et al: Unusual serum lipoprotein abnormality induced by the vehicle of miconazole. N Engl J Med 296:497–499, 1977.
5. Bennett JE: Chemotherapy of systemic mycoses. N Engl J Med 290:30–32; 320–323, 1974.
6. Bennett JE: Flucytosine. Ann Intern Med 86:319–322, 1977.
7. Bindschadler DD, Bennett JE: A pharmacologic guide to the clinical use of amphotericin B. J Infect Dis 120:427–436, 1969.

8. Blank H, Smith JG, Jr, Roth FJ, Jr et al: Griseofulvin for the systemic treatment of dermatomycoses. JAMA 171:2168–2173, 1959.

9. Block ER, Bennett JE: Pharmacological studies with 5-fluorocytosine. Antimicrob Agents Chemother 1:476–482, 1972.

10. Block ER, Bennett JE, Livoti LG et al: Flucytosine and amphotericin B: Hemodialysis effects on the plasma concentration and clearance. Studies in man. Ann Intern Med 80:613–617, 1974.

11. Block ER, Jennings AE, Bennett JE: 5-fluorocytosine resistance in Cryptococcus neoformans. Antimicrob Agents Chemother 3:649–656, 1973.

12. Bode FR, Pare JAP, Fraser RG: Pulmonary diseases in the compromised host. Medicine 53:255–293, 1974.

13. Bodey GP: Infections in cancer patients. Cancer Treat Rev 2:89–128, 1975.

14. Bonner DD, Tewar RP, Solotorovsky M et al: Comparative chemotherapeutic activity of amphotericin B and amphotericin B methyl ester. Antimicrob Agents Chemother 7:724–729, 1975.

15. Brincker H: Treatment of oral candidiasis in debilitated patients with miconazole-a new potent antifungal drug. Scand J Infect Dis 8:117–120, 1976.

16. Brugmans JP, van Cutsem JM, Heykants J et al: Systemic antifungal potential, safety, biotransport, and transformation of miconazole. Eur J Clin Pharmacol 5:93–99, 1972.

17. Brugmans JP, van Cutsem JM, Thienpont DC: Treatment of long-term tinea pedis with miconazole. Double-blind clinical evaluation. Arch Derm 102:428–432, 1970.

18. Burgess JL, Birchall R: Nephrotoxicity of amphotericin B, with emphasis on changes in tubular function. Am J Med 53:77–84, 1972.

19. Burgess MA, Bodey GP: Clotrimazole (Bay b 5097): in vitro and clinical pharmacological studies. Antimicrob Agents Chemother 2:423–426, 1972.

20. Busey JF: Blastomycosis. III. A comparative study of 2-hydroxystilbamidine and amphotericin B therapy. Am Rev Respir Dis 105:812–818, 1972.

21. Butler WT, Bennett JE, Hill GJH et al: Electrocardiographic and electrolyte abnormalities caused by amphotericin B in dog and man. Proc Soc Exp Biol Med 116:857–863, 1964.

22. Carter VH: A controlled study of haloprigin and tolnaftate in tinea pedis. Curr Ther Res 14:307–310, 1972.

23. Carter VH, Olansky S: Haloprigin and nystatin therapy for cutaneous candidiasis. Arch Derm 110:81–82, 1974.

24. Chernik NL, Armstrong D, Posner JB: Central nervous system infections in patients with cancer. Medicine 52:563–581, 1973.

25. Clayton YM: Antifungal drugs in current use: a review. Proc Roy Soc Med Suppl 4 70:15–17, 1977.

26. Codish SD, Tobias JS: Managing systemic mycoses in the compromised host. JAMA 235:2132–2134, 1976.

27. Collins MS, Pappagianis D: Inhibition of coccidioides immitis in vitro and enhancement of anticoccidioidal effects of amphotericin B by polymyxin B. Antimicrob Agents Chemother 7:781–787, 1977.

28. Cullen SI: Cutaneous candidiasis: treatment with miconazole nitrate. Cutis 19:126–129, 1977.

29. Cullen SI, Catalano PM: Griseofulvin-warfarin antagonism. JAMA 199:582–583, 1967.

30. Diamond RD, Bennett JE: A subcutaneous reservoir for intrathecal therapy for fungal meningitis. N Engl J Med 288:186–188, 1973.

31. Douglas JB, Healy JK: Nephrotoxic effects of amphotericin B, including renal tubular acidosis. Am J Med 46:154–162, 1969.

32. Drouhet E: Basic mechanisms of antifungal chemotherapy. Mod Treat 7:539–564, 1970.

33. Drutz DJ, Spickard A, Rogers DE et al: Treatment of disseminated mycotic infections: a new approach to amphotericin B therapy. Am J Med 45:405–418, 1968.

34. Edwards JE, Foos RY, Montgomerie JZ et al: Ocular manifestations of candida septicemia: review of seventy-six cases of hematogenous candida endophthalmitis. Medicine 53:47–75, 1974.

35. Elgart ML: Griseofulvin: a review of the literature and summary of present usage. Med Ann DC 36:331–334, 1967.

36. Feldman HA, Hamilton JD, Gutman RA: Amphotericin therapy in an anephric patient. Antimicrob Agents Chemother 4:402–405, 1973.

37. Fields BT, Bates JH, Abernathy RS: A rationale for pulse therapy with amphotericin B. Clin Res 20:51, 1972.

38. Fishman LS, Griffin JR, Sapico FL et al: Hematogenous candida endophthalmitis-a complicaton of candidemia. N Engl J Med 286:675–681, 1972.

39. Gadebusch HH, Pansy F, Klepner C: Amphotericin B and amphotericin B methyl ester ascorbate. I. Chemotherapeutic activity against candida albicans, cryptococcus neoformans, and blastomyces dermatitidis in mice. J Infect Dis 134:423–427, 1976.

40. Gellin GA, Maibach HI, Wachs GN: Contact allergy to tolnaftate. Arch Derm 106:715–716, 1972.

41. Goldman L: Griseofulvin. Med Clin N Am 54:1339–1345, 1970.

42. Goldman L, Lasser AE: Subtotal body inunction test for systemic toxicity of topical medication. In: Hobby GL (Ed): Antimicrobial Agents and Chemotherapy 1963. Ann Arbor, American Society for Microbiology, 1964.

43. Goldman L, Schwarz J, Preston RH et al: Current status of griseofulvin: report on one hundred seventy-five cases. JAMA 172:532–538, 1960.

44. Grin EI: Principles of mass treatment of tinea capitis. Dermatologia Internationalis 5:174–176, 1966.

45. Grunberg E, Titsworth E, Bennet M: Chemotherapeutic activity of 5-fluorocytosine. In: Hobby GL (Ed): Antimicrobial Agents and Chemotherapy 1962. Ann Arbor, American Society for Microbiology, 1963.

46. Harder EJ, Hermans PG: Treatment of fungal infections with flucytosine. Arch Intern Med 135:231–237, 1975.

47. Harrison EF, Zwadyk P, Jr, Bequette RJ et al: Haloprigin: a topical antifungal agent. Appl Microbiol 19:746–750, 1970.

48. Harrison EF, Zygmunt WA: Haloprigin: mode of action studies in candida albicans. Can J Microbiol 20:1241–1245, 1974.

49. Hellebusch AA, Salama F, Eadie E: The use of mannitol to reduce the nephrotoxicity of amphotericin B. Surg Gynecol Obstet 134:241–243, 1972.

50. Herman HW: Clinical evaluation of haloprigin. Toxicol Appl Pharmacol 23:598–605, 1972.

51. Herrell WE: Hamycin in the treatment of blastomycosis. Clin Med 75:19–20, 1968.

52. Hildick-Smith G, Blank H, Sarkany I: Fungus Diseases and Their Treatment. Boston, Little, Brown, 1964.

53. Hoeprich PD, Huston AC: Susceptibility of coccidioides immitis, candida albicans, and cryptococcus neoformans to amphotericin B, flucytosine, and clotrimazole. J Infect Dis 132:133–141, 1975.

54. Hoeprich PG, Goldstein E: Miconazole therapy for coccidoidomycosis. JAMA 230:1153–1157, 1974.
55. Huber FM, Gottlieb D: The mechanism of action of griseofulvin. Can J Microbiol 14:111–118, 1968.
56. Kauffman CA, Frame PT: Bone marrow toxicity associated with 5-fluorocytosine therapy. Antimicrob Agents Chemother 11:244–247, 1977.
57. Keczkes K, Leighten I, Good CS: Topical treatment of dermatophytoses and candidoses. Practitioner 214:412–417, 1975.
58. Kinsky SC: Nystatin binding of protoplasts and a particulate fraction of neurospora crassa, and a basis for the selective toxicity of polyene antifungal antibiotics. Proc Natl Acad Sci USA 48:1049–1056, 1962.
59. Kitahara M, Kobayashi GS, Medoff G: Enhanced efficacy of amphotericin B and rifampicin combined in treatment of murine histoplasmosis and blastomycosis. J Infect Dis 133:663–668, 1976.
60. Leikin S, Parrott R, Randolph J: Clotrimazole treatment of chronic mucocutaneous candidiasis. J Pediat 88:864–866, 1976.
61. Lockwood WR, Allison F, Jr, Batson BG et al: The treatment of North American blastomycosis: ten years' experience. Am Rev Respir Dis 100:314–320, 1969.
62. Marmion LC, Desser KB, Lilly RB et al: Reversible thrombocytosis and anemia due to miconazole therapy. Antimicrob Agents Chemother 10:447–449, 1976.
63. Masterton G, Napier IR, Henderson JN et al: Three-day clotrimazole treatment in candidal vulvovaginitis. Br J Vener Dis 53:126–128, 1977.
64. McCurdy DK, Frederic M, Elkinton JR: Renal tubular acidosis due to amphotericin B. N Engl J Med 278:124–131, 1968.
65. McKee LC, Jr, Koenig MG, Drutz DJ et al: Effect of amphotericin B on erythropoeisis. Clin Res 17:70, 1969.
66. Medoff G, Dismukes WE, Meade RH III et al: Therapeutic program for candida infection. *In*: Hobby, GL (Ed): Antimicrobial Agents and Chemotherapy 1970. Bethesda, American Society for Microbiology, 1971.
67. Meyer R, Axelrod JL: Fatal aplastic anemia resulting from flucytosine. JAMA 228:1573, 1974.
68. Meyers BR, Leiberman TW, Ferry AP: Candida endophthalmitis complicating candidemia. Ann Intern Med 79:647–653, 1973.
69. Montes LF: Oral amphotericin B on superficial candidiasis. Clin Med 78:14–17, 1971.
70. Montes LF, Soto TG, Parker JM et al: Clotrimazole troches: a new therapeutic approach to oral candidiasis. Cutis 17:277–280, 1976.
71. Moore TF: The headache associated with cisternal injections of amphotericin B. Headache 6:195–200, 1967.
72. Negroni R, Rubinstein P, Herrmann A et al: Results of miconazole therapy in twenty-eight patients with paracoccidioidomycosis (South American Blastomycosis). Proc Roy Soc Med Suppl I 70:24–28, 1977.
73. Normark S, Schonebeck J: In vitro studies of 5-fluorocytosine resistance in candida albicans and torulopsis glabrata. Antimicrob Agents Chemother 3:649–656, 1973.
74. Pansy FE, Basch H. Jamber NP et al: Hamycin: In vitro and in vivo studies. *In*: Hobby GL (Ed): Antimicrobial Agents and Chemotherapy, 1966. Ann Arbor, American Society for Microbiology, 1967.
75. Polak A, Scholer HJ: Fungistatic activity, uptake, and incorporation of 5-fluorocytosine in candida albicans, as influenced by pyrimidines and purines I. Reversal experiments. Pathol Microbiol (Basel) 39:148–159, 1973.

76. Polak A, Scholer HJ: Fungistatic activity, uptake, and incorporation of 5-fluorocytosine in candida albicans, as influenced by pyrimidines and purines II. Studies on distribution and incorporation. Pathol Microbiol (Basel) 39:334–347, 1973.

77. Powers SR, Jr, Boba A, Hastnik W: Prevention of postoperative acute renal failure with mannitol in 100 cases. Surgery 55:15–23, 1964.

78. Record CO, Skinner JM, Sleight P et al: Candida endocarditis treated with 5-fluorocytosine. Br Med J 1:262–264, 1971.

79. Remington JS, Anderson SE, Jr: Pneumocystis and fungal infection in patients with malignancies. Int J Radiation Oncol Biol Phys 1:313–315, 1976.

80. Roberts SAB, Champion RH: Treatment of ringworm infections with tolnaftate ointment. Practitioner 199:797–798, 1967.

81. Robinson HJ, Jr, Raskin J: Tolnaftate: a potent topical antifungal agent. Arch Derm 91:372–376, 1965.

82. Rollo IM: Miscellaneous drugs used in the treatment of protozoal infections. In: Goodman LS, Gilman A (Eds): The Pharmacological Basis of Therapeutics, ed 5. New York, Macmillan, 1975.

83. Rosch JM, Pazin GJ, Fireman P: Reduction of amphotericin B nephrotoxicity with mannitol. JAMA 235:1995–1996, 1976.

84. Rutherford AM: Gynodaktarin (Miconazole nitrate) for vulvovaginal candidiasis. NZ Med J 84:9–10, 1976.

85. Saladino AJ, Bently PJ, Trump BF: Ion movements in cell injury. Am J Pathol 54:421–466, 1969.

86. Scheef W, Symoens J, van Camp K et al: Chemotherapy of candidiasis. Br Med J 1:78, 1974.

87. Schonebeck J, Polak A, Fernex M et al: Pharmacokinetic studies on the oral antimycotic agent 5-fluorocytosine in individuals with normal and impaired kidney function. Chemotherapy 18:321–336, 1973.

88. Seki S, Nomiya B, Koeda T et al: Laboratory evaluation of M-1028 (2, 4, 5-trichlorophenyl—γ—Iodopropargyl ether), a new antimicrobial agent. In: Hobby GL (Ed): Antimicrobial Agents and Chemotherapy, 1963. Ann Arbor, American Society for Microbiology, 1964.

89. Shadomy S: In vitro studies with 5-fluorocytosine. Appl Microbiol 17:871–877, 1969.

90. Shadomy S: Further in vitro studies with 5-fluorocytosine. Infect Immun 2:484–488, 1970.

91. Singer C, Kaplan MH, Armstrong D: Bacteremia and fungemia complicating neoplastic disease. Am J Med 62:731–742, 1977.

92. Smith EB, Grahm JL, Ulrich JA: Topical clotrimazole in tinea pedis. South Med J 70:47–48, 1977.

93. Spickard A, Butler WT, Andriole V et al: The improved prognosis of cryptococcal meningitis with amphotericin-B therapy. Ann Intern Med 58:66–83, 1963.

94. Spiekermann, PH, Young MD: Clinical evaluation of clotrimazole. Arch Derm 112:350–352, 1976.

95. Steer PI, Marks MI, Klite PD et al: 5-fluorocytosine: an oral antifungal compound. A report on clinical and laboratory experience. Ann Intern Med 76:15–22, 1972.

96. Stevens DA, Levine HB, Deresinski SC: Miconazole in coccidioidomycosis II. Therapeutic and pharmacologic studies in men. Am J Med 60:191–202, 1976.

97. Sung JP: Treatment of disseminated coccidioidomycosis with miconazole. West J Med 124:61–64, 1976.

98. Sung JP, Grendahl JG, Levine HB: Intravenous and intrathecal miconazole therapy for systemic mycoses. West J Med 126:5–13, 1977.

99. Svejgaard E: Miconazole in the treatment of candidiasis of the digestive tract. Arch Dermatovener (Stockholm) 56:303–306, 1976.
100. Symmers W St C: Amphotericin pharmacophobia. Br Med J 4:460–463, 1973.
101. Thirumalachar MJ, Padhye AA: Experimental blastomycoses treated orally with hamycin. Sabouraudia 4:6–10, 1965.
102. Thirumalachar MJ, Sethna SB, Rahalkar PW: In vitro activity of hamycin with reference to its in vivo effect in treatment of systemic mycosis. Hindustan Antibiotics Bulletin 14:123–126, 1972.
103. Tosteson DC: Effect of macrocyclic compounds on the ionic permeability of artificial and natural membranes. Fed Proc 27:1269–1277, 1968.
104. Utz JP: Current and future chemotherapy of central nervous system fungal infections. Adv Neurol 6:127–132, 1974.
105. Utz JP: New drugs for the systemic mycoses: flucytosine and clotrimazole. Bull NY Acad Med 51:1103–1108, 1975.
106. Utz JP: Chemotherapy for the systemic mycoses. Br J Hosp Med 15:112–121, 1976.
107. Utz JP, Garriques IL, Sande MA et al: Therapy of cryptococcosis with a combination of flucytosine and amphotericin B. J Infect Dis 132:368–373, 1975.
108. Utz JP, Tynes BS, Shadomy JH et al: 5-fluorocytosine in human cryptococcosis. In: Hobby GL (Ed): Antimicrobial Agents and Chemotherapy, 1968. Ann Arbor, American Society for Microbiology, 1969.
109. Van Cutsem JM, Thienpont D: Miconazole, a broad-spectrum antimycotic agent with antibacterial activity. Chemotherapy 17:392–404, 1972.
110. Vandevelde AG, Mauceri A, Johnson JE III: 5-fluorocytosine in the treatment of mycotic infections. Ann Intern Med 77:43–51, 1972.
111. Watson CJ, Lynch F, Bossenmaier I et al: Griseofulvin and porphyrin metabolism. Arch Derm 98:451–468, 1968.
112. Weinstein L: Miscellaneous antibacterial agents. In: Goodman LS, Gilman A (Eds): The Pharmacological Basis of Therapeutics, ed 5. New York, Macmillan, 1973.
113. Weinstein L, Weinstein AJ: The pathophysiology and pathoanatomy of reactions to antimicrobial agents. Adv Intern Med 19:109–134, 1974.
114. Weissmann G, Hirschhorn R, Pras M et al: Studies of lysosomes VIII. The effect of polyene antibiotics on lysosomes. Biochem Pharm 16:1057–1069, 1967.
115. Weissman G, Sessa G: The action of polyene antibiotics on phospholipid-cholesterol structures. J Biol Chem 242:616–625, 1967.
116. Williams DM, Krick JA, Remington JS: Pulmonary infection in the compromised host. Part I. Am Rev Respir Dis 114:359–394, 1976.

CHAPTER 6

INFECTION IN THE COMPROMISED HOST
Recent Advances and Future Directions

James E. Pennington, M.D.

Introduction

The problem of infection in the immunocompromised host has grown in recent years to the extent that almost any practicing physician or surgeon can expect to have some encounter with such a patient. Since patients with all forms of neoplastic disease, patients with organ transplants, and an enlarging group of patients with collagen-vascular and immunologically mediated diseases, are all potential recipients of immunosuppressing medications, it is not surprising that interest in the clinical effects of immunosuppressing drugs has grown over the past decade. Although patients with certain congenital or acquired immunologic deficiencies also must be considered at risk for many of the infections to be described below, the present discussion will concentrate only upon patients who are rendered immunosuppressed by virtue of drug therapy. Many neoplastic diseases, especially hematologic malignancies, inherently lead to depressed immune function; however, drug-induced immunosuppression is almost always implicated when severe, life-threatening opportunistic infection occurs in these patients.

Although pharmacologic doses of glucocorticosteroids and immunosuppressing chemotherapy have been available for clinical usage for at least 25 years, it has been only during the past 10 to 15 years that widespread use of intensive immunosuppressing regimens have been employed. In fact, until the late 1960's, drug-induced thrombocytopenia and risk of fatal hemorrhage limited the amounts of antineoplastic chemotherapy which could be used. With the advent of modern platelet transfusion support facilities, more intense regimens of chemotherapy have been employed. Although risks of bleeding can now be minimized, these newer regimens often result in profound granulocytopenia as well

From the Infectious Diseases Division, Department of Medicine, Peter Bent Brigham Hospital, and the Department of Medicine, Harvard Medical School, Boston, Mass.

as suppression of immunologic responsiveness to infection. As bleeding deaths have decreased in these patients, infectious deaths have greatly increased. The risk of death from infection in acute leukemia patients now exceeds bleeding by four times [22], and for all hematologic malignancies by six times [60]. In fact, the single most important factor limiting further escalation of cancer chemotherapy is now infection.

In the 1960's, the rapid emergence of fatal infections in immunosuppressed patients with a wide and apparently unpredictable range of bacteria, fungi and even protozoal agents led to the belief that almost any microorganism could become pathogenic in the compromised host. Since these patients were seen to die within a short time when infection was inappropriately treated, it appeared necessary to begin prompt empiric broad-spectrum antimicrobial therapy for fever in the neutropenic patient. Unfortunately, little epidemiologic information was available to guide the choice of antimicrobial agents, and thus it was not uncommon to find a febrile, neutropenic patient receiving empiric cephalothin, kanamycin, polymyxin B, erythromycin, INH, amphotericin B, and perhaps even pentamidine. Needless to say, this approach was unnecessary and led to an unacceptable degree of drug toxicity. Besides fear of omitting the appropriate antimicrobial agent, there was also the fear of stopping broad-spectrum antibiotics when fever persisted but cultures remained negative. The author has witnessed innumerable neutropenic febrile (but clinically stable) patients with totally negative blood cultures and no apparent site for infection receive two, or even three or more, continuous weeks of such drugs as cephalothin and gentamicin, only eventually to die of disseminated candidiasis or invasive pulmonary aspergillus superinfections. Indeed, the knowledge of when to stop antibiotics in these patients is as crucial for their safety as when and what to start.

The past seven years have been ones of rapid accumulation of epidemiologic information concerning the problem of infection in the compromised host. A number of centers have reported large series of infections in various types of immunosuppressed patients [8,11,22,27,60,73,97] and patterns of infection have begun to emerge. Most helpful has been the evidence that certain infections, such as with gram-negative enteric bacilli and the staphylococcus, occur much more frequently than others. Also helpful is the understanding that patients with certain underlying conditions are particularly predisposed to specific infectious agents. For example, acute leukemia patients with severe granulocytopenia are prone to infection with enteric bacilli and aspergillus, while lymphoma and transplant patients are more susceptible to agents which depend upon cell-mediated immunity, such as cytomegaloinclusion virus (CMV), listeria, and cryptococcus. With this knowledge, empiric therapy can now be given in a much more organized fashion, generally beginning with a trial of antibacterials aimed at coverage for both staphylococcus and gram-negative rods, including *Pseudomonas aeruginosa*. Only when that fails are other empiric drugs, such as amphotericin B or antipneumocystis agents, used. Empiric antituberculous therapy is rarely used now, due to the low incidence of tuberculosis in these patients.

Presently, emphasis in this field is upon further dissemination of the epidemiologic information currently available so that appropriate choices for empiric therapy can be assured and so that risks of superinfection can be minimized. Clinicians have also become aware that conventional methods of diagnosis of infection in the compromised host are inadequate and that an aggressive diagnostic approach for such patients, often involving lung, skin or mucosal biopsies, is needed. Finally, newer methods for preventing or treating infection in these patients are under intensive investigation. Total sterile isolation and gut decontamination to prevent opportunistic infections during chemotherapy, as well as granulocyte transfusion therapy of infection, have both shown promising results and will be reviewed in detail below.

This paper will not attempt to provide details of the large number of past studies of infection in the compromised host, since several excellent reviews have appeared, dealing with these earlier studies [11,27,60]. The reader may wish to review some of these in order to place this paper in perspective. The purpose of the present report will be to describe the major advances in this field during the past three years (1974–1977), with an occasional reference to older studies when necessary.

Epidemiology and Immunology

The relationship of underlying disease, immunologic defects, chemotherapy, and predisposition to specific infections has been of interest to clinicians and investigators alike. An accidental experiment has been created by use of various immunosuppressing drugs. The most important host defense mechanisms for specific pathogens can now be discovered by correlating which immune defects render patients most susceptible to a given organism. For example, it is known that both a humoral and cell-mediated immune response is elicited by CMV infection, but patients with depressed cell-mediated immune systems appear to be more susceptible than patients with depressed humoral responses. The importance of adequate circulating granulocyte numbers for gram-negative infections has clearly been demonstrated. Also, humoral immune defects appear to predispose to infection with encapsulated bacteria, such as

Hemophilus influenzae and the pneumococcus. Until the recent era of intensive immunosuppression, most evidence for which immune function was most critical for which pathogen in man was indirect. Tattersall has recently reviewed the various mechanisms by which immunosuppressing agents depress specific immune functions [105]. Of greatest benefit to clinicians, however, is the ability to predict which infections are most likely to occur in which compromised hosts.

The central role of granulocytes in host defense from opportunistic infection continues to be stressed. Sickles et al. have described the clinical consequences of decreased granulocyte inflammatory response to local infections [98]. Lack of soft tissue erythema and fluctuance, decreased cough and sputum production in pneumonia, abscence of pharyngeal exudates, and decreased dysuria in urinary tract infections were all noted in granulocytopenic patients. In another article, Chang et al. have reviewed the causes of death in 315 adults with acute leukemia from 1966 to 1972 [22]. A direct correlation between numbers of circulating granulocytes and death from infection was found. As expected, infection was the leading cause of mortality (66%) in this series, with bacterial agents most prevalent and the respiratory tract the most common source for septicemia (64%).

The lung continues to be most prevalent as a site for infection in compromised hosts [22,108]. This is not surprising, considering the extensive exposure of alveolar surfaces to environmental microorganisms. The particular drug-induced pulmonary immune defects which contribute to lung susceptibility are not yet well defined, but recent evidence acquired in an animal model (guinea pigs) of immunosuppression has indicated that combined therapy with glucocorticosteroids plus cyclophosphamide decreases the number of alveolar macrophages available for phagocytosis [81]. In the same model, normal animals challenged with intrabronchial *Pseudomonas aeruginosa* had a prompt (2 hours) influx of polymorphonuclear leukocytes into the respiratory tract, while immunosuppressed and granulocytopenic animals failed in this response [82]. These drug-induced alterations in the kinetics of inflammatory cells in the lung have also been correlated with increased mortality from pseudomonas pneumonia [82a]. In another animal study, cyclophosphamide decreased humoral immune response in the lung secondary to viral infection [13]. It is likely that local host defenses in the lung are depressed in various ways by different drugs.

A recent review of gram-negative bacillary pneumonia in 189 cancer patients [108] was encouraging since a 61% over-all cure rate was reported. This is much improved over past series [85,99] and hopefully reflects more effective antibiotic utilization. Of interest in this series were a number of neutropenic patients who lacked early radiographic evidence of pneumonia. This is in contrast to an earlier study in which pulmonary infiltrates were seen as frequently in neutropenic patients as in patients with normal blood counts [99]. Another recent series has emphasized the high mortality for patients with the combination of hematologic malignancy, fever and lung infiltrates [84]. Mortality was 45% in 48 patients with this clinical presentation, while another group of clinically matched patients with fever but no pulmonary involvement experienced only a 9% mortality. In another recent series [101], pulmonary infections in patients with neoplastic disease were associated with a mortality of 76%, in contrast to generally lower mortalities associated with infections of other sites. These infections included both bacterial and fungal etiologies. Numerous advances in diagnosis of lung infection in the compromised host have been made and will be discussed below. Finally, the reader is referred to recent reviews of the clinical spectrum of lung infections in the compromised host [15,114]. Of special interest is the long list of noninfectious etiologies for fever and lung infiltrates in these patients, including drugs (e.g., bleomycin, busulfan), radiation pneumonitis, hemorrhage, tumor itself, or simply nonspecific interstitial pneumonitis, occasionally referred to as usual interstitial pneumonitis, or "U.I.P."

The role of splenectomy for the staging of Hodgkin's disease in predisposing patients to infection continues to be controversial. In the early 1970's, several reports of fulminant infection in such patients alerted clinicians that adults may experience the same infectious risks after splenectomy as previously described for children. However, an extensive series from Stanford University demonstrated no greater risk of infection among splenectomized lymphoma patients than among splenectomized non-lymphoma patients [25]. Similar results were recently reported by Edwards and Digioia [26]. Another series by Schimpff et al. revealed a remarkably low incidence of serious infection among 92 splenectomized patients with Hodgkin's disease, unless other predisposing factors, such as granulocytopenia, were associated [95]. However, a 24% incidence of local herpes zoster was reported in these patients. A recent report has described 20 serious infections among 200 splenectomized children (ages 1 to 15 years) with Hodgkin's disease [23]. Fifty per cent of these were with the pneumococcus and only 10 of 20 survived. In 14 of these cases, patients had received prior combined radiation and chemotherapy. In an additional series, 3 of 14 splenectomized patients (mostly adults) successfully treated for Hodgkin's disease with combined radio- and chemotherapy developed fulminant sepsis (2 fatalities) while in remission [110]. Similar cases were not observed among a larger group of 104 splenectomized patients who received less intense therapy. Weitzman et al. have documented that combined radio- and chemotherapy in Hodgkin's disease patients results in lower humoral antibody levels to *Hemophilus influenzae* and also lower IgM levels [111]. Splenectomy potentiated these effects but in itself did not lower antibody titers. Thus, it appears that more aggressive therapy of Hodgkin's disease renders patients less able to form antibody to encapsulated bacteria. Splenectomy in this setting likely presents increased risk for fulminant infection, and consideration of prophylactic penicillin or ampicillin plus pneumococcal vaccination for such patients must be given.

Bacterial Infections

Bacteria are the most common etiologic agents causing infection in the compromised host. As in past reports [60], enteric gram-negative bacilli, usually *E. coli* or Klebsiella, plus the common environmental or enteric colonizing bacteria such as *Pseudomonas aeruginosa* or *Serratia marcescens,* continue to be most prevalent in these patients [22,101,108]. Differences between medical centers in the frequency of isolation of specific gram-negative pathogens are common, and it is manditory that clinicians are kept aware of particular local trends in nosocomial infections, as well as patterns of antibiotic resistance. Two recent trends noted in several parts of the country have been an increasing number of serratia infections and also emergence of gentamicin-resistant gram negative pathogens. Infection with *Staphylococcus aureus* also continues to be common in the compromised host [19]. Staphylococci and enteric bacilli are commonly located at sites of cutaneous or mucosal breakdown, often secondary to cytotoxic chemotherapy, intravenous lines or minor skin or mucosal abrasions. The surprisingly low incidence of infection with the bacterial pathogens most commonly encountered in normal hosts, such as the pneumococcus or *Streptococcus pyogenes,* continues to be an interesting observation in leukopenic cancer patients [101].

Although bacterial sepsis in the compromised host continues to pose a difficult clinical problem, several recent studies have described lower mortality associated with bacterial infections in these patients [22,101,108]. A recent analysis [101] of 364 episodes of bacteremia and fungemia (all but 29 were bacteremias) in patients with hematologic malignancy (group 1) or solid tumor (group 2) described a mortality of 40.5% in group 1 and 27.8% in group 2. Although anaerobic infection was rare in leukemia and lymphoma patients, the solid tumor group in this study experienced 23 episodes of *Bacteroides species* sepsis.

Bacteroides was most frequently isolated in patients with genitourinary neoplasia and was notable for only a 4.3% mortality. As a rule, serious anaerobic infection has not been a major problem in compromised hosts.

Several new antibiotics have been introduced in the past few years which broaden the range of agents available for gram-negative infections. Tobramycin sulfate is an aminoglycoside with pharmacokinetics and bacterial spectrum similar to gentamicin. However, this agent has particular activity for *Pseudomonas aeruginosa* [7,19], often demonstrating minimal inhibitory concentrations several times lower than gentamicin for this organism. Since pseudomonas infection presents a particularly bad prognosis in the compromised host [60,85,101,104], any potential therapeutic advantage would be welcome. The observation that carbenicillin is synergistic with either gentamicin [9] or tobramycin [10] for pseudomonas is of importance and has led to routine combination therapy with these agents for pseudomonas infection. The benefits of using two drugs rather than one for gram-negative infections other than pseudomonas is less clear, but recent evidence indicates that mortality is significantly reduced in the compromised host when other gram-negative pathogens are treated with two synergistic antibiotics rather than a single agent [56].

The newest aminoglycoside to become available is amikacin [67,103]. This drug resembles kanamycin pharmacokinetically but broadens its spectrum to include most gram-negative rods, including those found to be resistant to gentamicin or tobramycin [72]. The increasing incidence of highly resistant gram-negative pathogens reported in several centers [51,68] makes this agent an important addition to aminoglycoside therapy. Although clinical studies show no superiority of amikacin over gentamicin [102] or tobramycin [31] for infections with organisms sensitive to either agent, it clearly is an effective agent for pathogens resistant to the other aminoglycosides [67,103]. A recent study has also confirmed the value of amikacin in the leukopenic compromised host [56]. Amikacin toxicity for the eighth cranial nerve, as well as nephrotoxicity, appears to be similar to that reported for gentamicin [102] and tobramycin [31]. Finally, the new carbenicillin analogue, ticarcillin, has now been approved for general use [77]. This drug offers the same gram-negative spectrum as carbenicillin but is used at about three-fifths the dose, thus decreasing the attendant sodium load. Whether this agent will alter platelet function to a lesser degree than carbenicillin is as yet uncertain.

The list of unusual bacterial pathogens infecting compromised hosts continues to enlarge. A number of cases of pneumonia with *Bacillus species* (non-anthrax), have recently been reported [32,58,83]. These patients have uniformly demonstrated hemorrhagic pneumonia at autopsy, with blood vessel invasion by the bacilli causing thrombosis and pulmonary infarction. Clinically, hemoptysis has been common, and this infection has been mistaken for acute pulmonary infarction in some cases. Microbiologists must beware of labeling *Bacillus species* isolates from blood or sputum as contaminants when dealing with these patients. These organisms are often resistant to multiple antibiotics and may require gentamicin for effective therapy. A recent report has described successful gentamicin therapy for a patient with acute leukemia and *B. cereus* pneumonia [58].

Listeria monocytogenes infection is not unique to the compromised host; however, Gantz et al. have emphasized the occult nature of listeria meningitis in renal transplant patients receiving immunosuppressive drugs [39]. Clinicians are thus advised to perform lumbar punctures on all compromised hosts with listeria sepsis, even in the abscence of neurologic signs or symptoms.

Nocardia pulmonary infection has continued to be a significant problem for compromised hosts, particularly those with organ transplants [54,76,114] or lymphoma [36,115]. Attention has been given to the value of early diagnosis, using percutaneous needle aspiration for culture [54]. Among seven cases of nocardia pneumonia in heart transplant patients, only one had nocardia isolated from sputum at the onset of infection, while in six patients (including the one with positive sputum) nocardia was isolated from lung needle aspirates. All six patients were treated with sulfisoxazole and survived. An interesting syndrome of fever and positive sputum cultures for nocardia in the abscence of radiographic chest infiltrates has been reported in the past [115] and recently reconfirmed [36]. Whether this represents mild infection or simply colonization of the tracheobronchial tree is uncertain. In one series, eight of nine such patients were followed without specific therapy for nocardia and failed to develop nocardia pneumonia [36]. Sulfonamide therapy continues to be the cornerstone of therapy for nocardia infection. However, synergism of sulfamethoxazole and trimethoprim for nocardia has recently been reported [63]. Convincing evidence of the superiority of two agents for this infection rather than sulfonamide alone is not yet available.

Tuberculosis continues to be a rare disease in the compromised host, likely reflecting the lower incidence of this disease in the general population. However, in patients with evidence of prior exposure to this organism, antineoplastic therapy appears to predispose to activation of the disease [53]. In a review of 201 cases of tuberculosis in cancer patients at Memorial Hospital in New York between 1950 and 1971, Kaplan et al. describe the greatest prevalence in patients with lung cancer (92 cases per 10,000) and Hodgkin's disease (96 cases per 10,000). Patients with leukemia had a much lower incidence of T.B. The over-all mortality for T.B. in this series was 17%, rising to 48% in patients with lymphoproliferative disorders. More severe tuberculosis was associated with adrenocorticosteroid therapy. Thus, while routine empiric use of antituberculous drugs for all compromised hosts with fever and pneumonia of uncertain etiology is not advocated, a past history of T.B. or suggestive radiographic findings (e.g., apical cavities, Ghon complex, etc.) would argue for T.B. coverage.

Fungus

Infections with fungi are less frequent than with bacteria in the compromised host but carry a much worse prognosis. Several recent series have indicated that candida and aspergillus continue to be the most frequent fungal species infecting the compromised host [22,101,119]. Patients with leukemia seem particularly predisposed to fungal infections [22]. In one series analyzing cause of death in a leukemia population, fungal infection accounted for 20% of all fatalities [22]. An increasing problem with disseminated candidiasis in patients with solid tumor was noted in another report [101]. In that series, candida accounted for 7 of 148 positive blood cultures in patients with hematologic malignancies, while candida occurred in 19 of 216 blood isolates in a solid tumor population. A frequent source for candidiasis in that study was intravenous parenteral nutrition catheters. Mortality from candidiasis was 71% in the hematologic malignancy group and 42% in the solid tumor group. In the same series, fungal superinfections were documented at autopsy in 52% of patients with leukemia or lymphoma, but in only 8% of the solid tumor group. In only six patients was an antemortem diagnosis of fungal superinfection made. Thus, the problem of diagnosing invasive fungal infection in the compromised host continues to plague clinicians.

One helpful study by Young et al. has analyzed 70 cases of fungemia in compromised hosts with neoplasia [119]. Forty-eight of the 70 cases had candida species fungemia. It was learned that even in the presence of an indwelling I.V. catheter, the compromised host should be treated for disseminated candidiasis if this organism is isolated from blood. If cultures are all negative after removal of a contaminated catheter, a shortened course of treatment with amphotericin B could be given. Also of interest was the rather prompt defervescence (4 to 6 days) of patients treated with amphotericin B for proven candidiasis. The implication of this finding is that clinicians using empiric amphotericin B for diagnostic trials in the febrile compromised host may learn quickly whether a response will occur.

Due to the relatively low incidence of positive blood cultures in disseminated candidiasis, various serologic tests for candida antibodies have been evaluated in this population. To date, the role of serology in diagnosing disseminated candidiasis in the compromised host is controversial and remains of limited practical value to the clinician. Although Gaines and Remington reported a useful role for the candida precipitin test, with only 2 false negatives and 5 false positives among 133 suspected cases, they concluded that serology alone could not dictate antifungal therapy [38]. A more recent study has failed to confirm the value of either candida precipitins or candida agglutination tests in patients with neoplastic disease, due to unacceptable rates of false positive and false negative reactions [35]. Until more conclusive proof is offered of the value for serology in diagnosing systemic candidiasis in compromised hosts, the diagnosis of candida infection will depend upon a combination of cultural data and clinical judgement.

Invasive pulmonary aspergillus infection continues to play a prominent role in compromised hosts [5,80]. Clustering of aspergillus infections has been reported, and this phenomenon may be associated with local environmental contamination [3]. Although the respiratory tract appears to be the usual portal of entry for aspergillus, four cases of cutaneous aspergillosis have recently been described [87]. In three of the four, skin infection preceded clinically evident visceral infection. As with systemic candidiasis, the clinical diagnosis of invasive aspergillosis in the compromised host is difficult. The sputum infrequently contains this isolate and blood cultures are almost never positive for aspergillus. Thus, attempts to utilize serology for diagnosis have been described. Although past studies have been unsuccessful in this effort [118], a recent paper reports a technic for an immunodiffusion assay of aspergillus precipitins in adult leukemia patients [93]. By using a microtemplate and concentrating serum specimens, seven of ten cases of invasive aspergillosis were shown to convert to a strongly positive test. Among 80 patients followed serially in this study, another six converted to a positive test but were not found to have aspergillosis. Thus, the test had 30% false negatives and 50% false positives. The potential role for this serologic test in the compromised host awaits further investigation. However, at this time, the clinical setting plus microbiologic evaluation of lung tissue appear to be the only reliable methods to assure diagnosis.

The most exciting development in recent years regarding invasive aspergillus pulmonary infection has been the increasing number of reports of clinical cures from this infection. Both renal transplant patients [20] and patients with acute leukemia [5,40] and lymphoma [78,80] have been successfully treated with amphotericin B. In one report, granulocyte transfusions were also employed [40]. This is in contrast to past series in which the mortality has been 99% [70] to 100% [120] for aspergillus infection. Two reasons account for the improved prognosis in this disease. First, clinicians are now more aggressive in utilizing invasive diagnostic procedures in the compromised host with fever and lung infiltrate but negative sputum cultures. Bronchial brushing, lung aspirates or lung biopsies have all been useful in allowing an earlier diagnosis of aspergillus pneumonia. One recent paper correlates early diagnosis and therapy of aspergillosis with better prognosis [5]. In another report [80], among nine cases of aspergillus pneumonia occurring in a one-year period, two patients were cured, five had a premortem microbiologic diagnosis, and all but one received a trial of amphotericin B therapy (three empirically). This illustrates the second reason for improved prognosis from this infection, i.e., that clinicians are now more aware of the setting in which it occurs and are more apt to utilize empiric amphotericin B therapy than in the past. Any granulocytopenic patient being treated for suspected (but culture-negative) bacterial pneumonia should be considered a candidate for aspergillus (or less commonly mucormycosis) pneumonia if they fail to respond to broad-spectrum antibiotics in two to three days. Every effort to obtain pulmonary specimens for culture and histology should be made in such cases, but if this is not possible, a trial of empiric amphotericin B is quite reasonable. Lack of any response after a week of amphotericin B is suggestive that fungal infection is not involved.

Less common fungal infections in the compromised host include pulmonary mucormycosis, which closely resembles aspergillosis, cryptococcal pneumonia and meningitis, usually seen in transplant or lymphoma patients, and *Torulopsis glabrata*. The latter organism is a yeast which was recently reported to cause 27 cases of infection in cancer patients over a four-year period [4]. The infection was usually in the lung and was diagnosed ante-mortem in only three patients. Further epidemiologic information on the relative importance of this fungus as an opportunistic pathogen will be needed.

Several interesting developments in antifungal therapy deserve mention. A number of centers are evaluating combined (synergistic) therapy for cryptococcal infection, using lower doses of amphotericin B with full doses of 5-fluorocytosine. This apparently results in less toxicity from amphotericin B and better therapeutic results. Also, low-dose (5 to 10 mg per day for 10 days) amphotericin B therapy for symptomatic candida esophagitis continues to be a valuable palliative measure in the compromised host [65]. Whether this can prevent dissemination of candida is as yet unknown. Finally, a new antifungal agent, miconazole, is undergoing trials in the compromised host with fungal infections [88]. These results are as yet unpublished but recent reports of failures in treating coccidioidomycosis [69] with this agent are disturbing.

Pneumocystis carinii

In contrast to fungal infection, pulmonary infection by the opportunistic parasite, *Pneumocystis carinii,* often occurs during periods of bone marrow recovery and after cessation of glucocorticoids and other immunosuppressing agents. Past studies have indicated an over-all mortality for this infection of greater than 60% [109]. Recent series, however, are reporting lower mortality [49,50,55]. Several other interesting new aspects of this disease deserve mention. The classic radiographic pattern of bilateral, interstitial infiltrates is not always present. In two recently reported cases, in renal transplant patients, one patient had hypoxia and fever but no infiltrates on chest radiographs, while the other had similar symptoms with only a focal lung infiltrate [37]. In both cases, bronchial brushing was positive for pneumocystis and the patients improved on pentamidine therapy. Numerous other examples of radiographically atypical pneumocystis infection have been seen at our center [84] and others. Another interesting finding has been clustering of cases of pneumocystis. Eleven cases occurred in a 3-month period at one cancer center [100]. Three of these patients had roomed together. Three other patients had contact with a physician found to have a positive serologic (immunofluorescent antibody) test for pneumocystis. The possibility of man-to-man spread of disease was raised and isolation of pneumocystis cases was recommended pending further data. In another study, the incidence of pneumocystis pneumonia in children with acute lymphocytic leukemia was found to rise with more intense chemotherapeutic regimens [48]. Children treated with maintenance regimens of one, two, three or four drugs had an incidence of pneumocystis of 5, 2.3, 2.2 and 22.4% respectively.

Diagnostically, the inability to demonstrate pneumocystis in sputum specimens has been a problem [57,109]. The lack of means to culture the organism continues to demand direct morphologic demonstration of pneumocystis by use of special stains. Thus, efforts to find the least invasive method to obtain the diagnosis are appropriate. In one report, eight cases of pneumocystis were diagnosed, using transtracheal aspirates, and only one false negative with this technic was found [57]. In another study

[2], transtracheal selective bronchial brushing was valuable to diagnose lung infection, including one case of pneumocystis. However, others have had more difficulty with these methods and required more invasive diagnostic procedures [24,42,84,90]. Several reports of transbronchial biopsy with the fiberoptic bronchoscope in the compromised host have appeared [24,28,33,84]. A diagnostic efficiency of 76% was obtained with this procedure in this population [33]. This technic obviates the need for thoracotomy and offers the advantage over lung aspirates of obtaining lung tissue for histologic studies. Since the etiology of interstitial pneumonitis includes a long list of possibilities, some of which (e.g., tumor, nonspecific interstitial pneumonitis, radiation pneumonitis, etc.) are noninfectious, there is a distinct advantage in obtaining lung tissue rather than simply lung or tracheal aspirates. Although several invasive methods now exist for making the diagnosis of pneumocystis as well as for diagnosing other pulmonary problems in the compromised host, the most reliable method continues to be open-lung biopsy.

Reports from Europe of useful serologic tests for pneumocystis infection [66] have not been confirmed in this country [75]. Although an indirect immunofluorescent pneumocystis antibody titer of 1:16 is now being labeled as significant [100], the incidence of false negatives with this test makes it less valuable for clinical use.

The most exciting recent news regarding pneumocystis infection is the promising data on therapy with the combination of trimethoprim (TMP)-sulfamethoxazole (SMX) [49,50,55]. By utilizing large doses (20 mg/kg/day of trimethoprim and 100 mg/kg/day of sulfamethoxazole), Hughes et al. were able to cure 12 of 14 children with proven pneumocystis pneumonia [50]. No adverse reactions to the drugs were reported, which contrasts dramatically with the high incidence of side effects with pentamidine [109]. This new combination was also successful in four of eight adults treated by Lau and Young [55]. The problem of poor gastrointestinal absorption of drug due to ileus has been documented by low serum drug levels [55]. Thus, parenteral use of this two-drug combination may be advised in seriously ill patients unless serial determinations of serum drug levels can be followed. A recent randomized clinical comparison between TMP-SMX and pentamidine in children with pneumocystis has been reported [49]. Of 18 patients treated with pentamidine, 11 recovered with this drug alone and six required cross-over to TMP-SMX. Of these six, three survived. Of 19 patients begun on TMP-SMX, 13 recovered with these agents and six required cross-over to pentamidine. Two of the latter survived. Thus, the survival was 78% for the pentamidine group and 79% in the TMP-SMX group. The high rate of survival with both agents, in contrast to past studies, is encouraging.

The lower toxicity for TMP-SMX makes this agent now appear to be the drug of choice for pneumocystis. Whether the combination of pentamidine plus TMP-SMX would further improve survival is yet unknown. Finally, a randomized double-blind study of placebo versus TMP-SMX (in lower dosage) for prophylaxis of pneumocystis in a high-risk pediatric leukemia population has been reported to show prophylactic efficacy [47].

Toxoplasmosis gondii

This parasite may cause infection in both normal and compromised hosts. In contrast to the pathogens discussed above, the exact frequency and importance of this organism in compromised hosts is unclear. Several reasons account for this. First, this is a difficult infection to diagnose since many humans have elevated antibody titers for toxoplasmosis without active infection. Second, it is difficult to demonstrate this organism on biopsy or even autopsy. Finally, some cases appear to regress spontaneously without specific therapy. Thus, clinical series in which serologic studies alone are used for diagnostic criteria must be carefully scrutinized.

That the compromised host may be infected with this organism is undeniable. One experience describes 24 cases at one hospital center [21]. In 10 patients, fever, adenopathy and positive serology were the diagnostic criteria. Most of these patients had been referred to rule out lymphoma. All improved, eight with, and two without, specific therapy. Fourteen other patients had associated neoplasia (9 Hodgkin's disease), plus serologic evidence of toxoplasmosis. A number of these patients also had the organism isolated at autopsy and from mice inoculated with infected tissue. Neurologic signs and frequent involvement of brain at autopsy were prominent features in this series. Of the five patients with neoplasia who received specific therapy, four survived.

A more recent review of 81 cases of toxoplasmosis in compromised hosts has appeared [91]. Again, frequency of encephalitis and neurologic signs was stressed, and brain biopsy was recommended for the compromised host with fever and unexplained neurologic deterioration. This series also found serologic studies helpful when ordered, but rather infrequently used in most centers. Only a small number of patients were diagnosed premortem, but of 20 patients specifically treated, 18 survived. Also of interest in this series was a high incidence of concomitant DNA virus infection. Although it would appear that toxoplasmosis is not a common cause of infectious morbidity or mortality in the compromised host, clinicians should be encouraged to order specific serologic tests more frequently and consider the diagnosis in patients with progressive neurologic disease of unexplained origin. The therapy for toxoplasmosis is pyrimethamine and sulfadimidine [21,91].

Viruses

Cytomegaloinclusion virus (CMV) and varicella-zoster virus, both members of the herpes virus group, continue to account for the majority of serious viral infections in the compromised host. The most common setting for CMV remains the post-organ transplant recipient receiving immunosuppressive therapy, although lymphoma, and occasionally leukemia patients may also have clinical evidence for CMV [1]. Infection with CMV can be manifest in protean ways, as noted in a paper by Fiala et al. [34]. In this study, 25 of 26 (96%) renal transplant patients developed clinical and virologic evidence of CMV after transplantation was carried out. The majority (42%) developed the infection within two months after surgery. Clinical illness included fever, arthralgias, pneumonitis, and leukopenia in the first few months, with hepatitis and retinitis seen in later periods. Viremia developed in 42% and lasted a mean period of 1.75 months. Chronic viruria was also common. Especially notable were long periods of fever (up to four weeks) in some patients. Mortality was low in this study and could not definitely be ascribed to CMV infection alone.

Although this study [34] indicates good correlation between increased CMV serologic titers or positive CMV cultures with clinical manifestations of infection, others have not found such a close correlation. In one study [46], 21 of 32 (66%) renal transplant patients developed serologic or culture evidence of CMV infection, while only 9 patients manifested clinical illness compatible with CMV. Of interest in this study was an excellent correlation between development of CMV in organ recipients who were seronegative prior to transplantation and received kidneys from seropositive donors. Whether CMV is passed by infected renal tissue is controversial but deserves strong consideration.

CMV must be strongly considered in the differential diagnosis of interstitial pneumonia in all compromised hosts [1] but appears to be a particularly malignant infection in patients receiving bone marrow transplants for acute leukemia therapy [71,74,107]. Although a high incidence of concomitant infections has been reported with CMV lung infection [1], CMV alone can clearly account for fatal pneumonia in bone marrow transplant recipients [74,107]. Two recent reports from bone marrow transplantation services have reviewed the problem of CMV lung infection [71,107]. In one series [71], 33 of 85 patients developed interstitial pneumonia and 23 died. In 17 of these cases, autopsy was done and

CMV was documented in 9. Four cases (two with concomitant CMV) of pneumocystis infection were also found. Among the "clinical" (nonfatal) cases, CMV viruria was documented in 40% but lung tissue was not available. In another series [107], among 15 leukemia patients undergoing marrow transplantation, six developed interstitial pneumonia. CMV was documented in three and suspected by positive serology in two others. One patient had pneumocystis. There were no survivors with interstitial pneumonia. Thus, CMV accounts for a considerable number of cases of fatal interstitial pneumonia in leukemia patients undergoing marrow transplantation. Recent trials of adenine arabinoside therapy for CMV infection have been unsuccessful [92]. However, more aggressive diagnostic procedures for interstitial lung infections in the compromised host [1] should allow earlier trials of antiviral agents for this infection.

Varicella-zoster infection continues to evidence a predilection for Hodgkin's disease patients. In one series [95], 24% of Hodgkin's disease patients developed local herpes zoster infection of the skin after radiotherapy which included the involved regions. Although progression to disseminated zoster is unusual [95], it is associated with considerable morbidity when it occurs. Of interest is the rather low mortality from disseminated zoster. In one study [112], among 87 cases of herpes zoster in immunosuppressed patients, about one-third had evidence for dissemination but only one fatality (pneumonia) could be ascribed to this infection. In the same study, a randomized trial of adenine arabinoside therapy was carried out. Patients who received this agent early in their infection showed accelerated clearance of virus from vesicles and earlier cessation of new vesicle formation when compared with the placebo treated group. In another report [52], adenine arabinoside seemed less effective, once dissemination had occurred.

Although disseminated infection with herpes simplex virus appears not to be a unique problem to the compromised host, encephalitis and meningoencephalitis [62] may occur. A recently completed randomized trial of adenine arabinoside therapy for type 1 herpes simplex encephalitis has demonstrated reduced mortality in patients receiving this agent [113]. The implications that adenine arabinoside, which appears to be relatively nontoxic [113], could be an effective agent for herpes-group virus infection mandates further investigation and trial of this agent in the immunosuppressed patient population.

Fever and Neutropenia

Despite the introduction of newer antibiotics and increased availability of granulocyte transfusions, the sense of urgency remains for clinicians dealing with the febrile, neutropenic patient, usually with an underlying hematologic malignancy. The question of whether or not to begin empiric antibiotic therapy before culture results are available is no longer an issue. The high incidence of bacterial sepsis in these patients, even without an obvious source, and the rapid deterioration and high mortality with inadequate therapy [96], illustrate the urgent nature of the clinical problem. Past studies have indicated that in greater than 50% of febrile episodes in neutropenic patients with hematologic malignancies a documented pathogen could eventually be isolated [12,14,96,106]. However, it has recently been demonstrated that, with earlier and more widespread use of empiric antibiotics, a majority of these patients (79%) must now be treated throughout their febrile course without the benefit of microbiologic documentation of infection [79]. Other recent series have confirmed the growing dependency on complete courses of empirically chosen antibiotics rather than being able to adjust drug choices when pathogens are later isolated [56,89]. Despite the inability to demonstrate a bacterial pathogen, a high percentage of patients will respond quickly to institution of empiric antibiotics [56,79]. Such "empiric responses" are associated with excellent prognosis [79]. An encouraging trend noted with this widespread early use of empiric antibiotic treatment is the low mortality now reported for patients with fever and neutropenia [29,56,79]. In one recent series [79], mortality was only 28% for such patients. Although past experience has shown that recovery of bone marrow function is important for survival in these patients, it is evident that persistently neutropenic patients also can survive bacterial infection [14,79]. More frequent use of granulocyte transfusion therapy may lead to further improvement in prognosis for the febrile neutropenic patient with infection.

The question of which empirically chosen antimicrobial agents would be most effective in this setting has been extensively studied, and past studies are reviewed elsewhere [60,79]. The spectrum of bacteria to be covered must include the aerobic gram-negative rods, including *Pseudomonas aeruginosa*. Local problems with highly resistant nosocomial gram-negative infections may alter the exact choice of agents. For example, if gentamicin resistance is a local problem, amikacin may be a safer empiric choice [56], or if a pseudomonas epidemic is occurring, tobramycin would be a reasonable aminoglycoside choice. Coverage for penicillinase-producing staphylococcus must also be included. Whether aminoglycosides such as gentamicin, tobramycin or amikacin are sufficient agents for staphylococcal coverage is unclear, but recent evidence [29,56] demonstrates that they are able to suppress staphylococcus effectively while cultures are pending. The largest comparative trial of various drug combinations is the recently completed, multicenter European Organization for Research on Treatment of Cancer (EORTC) study [29]. A total of 625 febrile neutropenic cancer patients were randomized to receive empiric coverage with either cephalothin plus gentamicin, cephalothin plus carbenicillin, or gentamicin plus carbenicillin. There was an excellent response (70% favorable) with all regimens, but increased nephrotoxicity with cephalothin plus gentamicin was noted (12%), when compared with the other combinations (2–4%). Thus, many have advocated such choices as carbenicillin plus gentamicin [29], or amikacin [56], since this combination appears to be less nephrotoxic than cephalothin plus gentamicin and has a broad two-drug spectrum against gram-negative rods, including pseudomonas. The question of need for synergistic coverage of gram-negative rods with two drugs rather than a single agent has been discussed above, and appears to be beneficial for the compromised host [56]. Therefore, coverage with only one anti-gram-negative agent (e.g., nafcillin plus gentamicin) appears hazardous. Finally, the question of using three versus two agents is of interest. One study reported an 82% survival for 33 neutropenic leukemia patients with documented infection, using cephalothin, gentamicin and carbenicillin [14]. Others, however, have utilized only two agents, with almost identical results (75% survival) [56]. Thus, there is no evidence that three agents are better than two.

One of the most critical questions facing the clinician using empiric antibiotics for fever and neutropenia is the proper duration of therapy. If cultures are negative initially but fever persists, the fear of missing an occult infection often induces continuation of antibiotics. The increasing risk of fungal superinfection as duration of treatment increases is also of concern. The question, then, is—when can antibiotics be safely discontinued in the culture-negative febrile patient with neutropenia? Rodriguez et al. have isolated bacteria after the initial four days of fever in 22 of 81 (21%) such patients [89]. Thus, empiric coverage should likely extend beyond four days. In another study [79], the incidence of superinfection rose after seven days of therapy, and if infection was not documented by four to seven days of fever, no patient deteriorated when antibiotics were stopped. Based upon our experience and others, a reasonable clinical approach for the febrile neutropenic patient would be as follows. In patients who defervesce on antibiotics within three to four days, a total of five afebrile days of therapy should be given if cultures are negative, and at least seven days if positive. In patients with no response to institution of empiric treatment, if cultures are positive a change of antibiotics to allow two-drug coverage is indicated, plus use of granulocyte transfusions, if available. In clinically stable but continuously febrile patients with negative cultures, empiric antibiotics should be given more than four but not more than seven days. If these patients continue to deteriorate over the first week of therapy, however, consideration of an empiric trial of amphotericin B is indicated, especially if fungus is isolated from three or more sites.

Future Directions

The attention of many investigators is focused upon better means to prevent or treat infection in the compromised host. Prevention of infection would be the ideal solution and several measures are under investigation. Work continues on vaccines or hyperimmune serum for gram-negative infections. A heptavalent lipopolysaccharide vaccine for *Pseudomonas aeruginosa* has been prepared, and trials in cancer patients have been carried out [43,86,116]. In one randomized trial, a significant decrease in pseudomonas-related deaths was noted in the vaccinated group [116]. Another study demonstrated improved antibody response to vaccine if leukemia patients were vaccinated while in remission from disease [86]. Of interest was the unexpected finding that leukemia patients who were vaccinated experienced longer remission rates. A study is now in progress to confirm this finding. Others have considered the possibility of vaccinating patients against gram-negative infection with a common "core" glycolipid antigen derived from *Salmonella minnesota*. This antigen has been shown in animals to cross-protect against a variety of gram-negative pathogens [64,117]. Another group has utilized cross-reacting antibody derived from *E. coli* 0:111 to immunize rabbits successfully against a wide range of gram-negative infections [18]. The potential for clinical use of cross-reacting hyperimmune serum, developed by immunizing volunteers, has yet to be studied in humans.

Other than the prophylactic use of trimethoprim-sulfamethoxazole for pneumocystis, there is no convincing evidence that parental or absorbable oral antibiotics can prevent infection in the neutropenic patient. However, the use of nonabsorbable antibiotics to decontaminate the gut has been found by Schimpff et al. to reduce the incidence of infection during periods of neutropenia [94]. In the same study, a protected sterile environment in combination with gut decontamination also reduced the incidence of infection. Of futher interest in this study, was an increased remission rate in patients on either the nonabsorbable antibiotic regimen alone or with the sterile environment. A separate but similarly designed study was able to demonstrate fewer infections only when gut decontamination plus sterile environment were used [61]. Remission rates were not improved in the latter study. Thus, the reduction in quantity of external and internal bacterial and fungal organisms appears to be beneficial for patients entering a period of neutropenia. However, it should be stressed that oral nonabsorbable antibiotics cause diarrhea and are distasteful. Patient rejection has been as high as 20% in some experiences. Also, these regimens reduce the "pathogen load" but do not truly sterilize the gut. A number of serious infections have occurred in such "protected" patients [16]. Finally, the cost of total sterile environments (e.g., laminar-air-flow rooms, "life islands," etc.) is high, and data conflict regarding the extent of benefits such systems offer [59]. Therefore, the future of this approach to prevention of infection is uncertain at this time.

One of the most promising areas for improving therapy of infection in neutropenic patients is the use of granulocyte transfusions. The potential value of granulocytes for gram-negative sepsis was illustrated in an early study by Graw et al. [41]. This was not a randomized trial, however, and only recently have well controlled studies of the effectiveness of granulocytes been made available. In one randomized trial [45], neutropenic patients with clinical or documented evidence of infection received either antibiotics alone or in combination with daily granulocyte transfusions for four straight days. Transfusions were begun only if two days of antibiotics failed to cause improvement. Five of 19 controls and 15 of 17 transfused patients survived. More recently, Herzig et al. have described a carefully randomized study of granulocyte therapy for neutropenic leukemia patients with proven gram-negative sepsis [44]. Five of 14 controls survived and 12 of 16 in the transfusion group survived infection. Improved survival with transfusion was most striking in the patients in whom marrow function did not improve by the 10th day of infection. Another randomized trial of granulocyte transfusions for neutropenic febrile patients with or without proved infection has been described [6]. In contrast to the Herzig et al. study, patients randomized to receive granulocytes began therapy as soon as antibiotics were started, rather than only after positive blood cultures were obtained. Again, those patients with proved infection had significantly greater survival with transfusions if bone marrow function did not return. If no infection was demonstrated, granulocytes did not affect over-all survival. Thus, it appears that granulocyte therapy is an effective adjunct to antibiotics for persistently neutropenic patients with gram-negative sepsis. However, whether over-all survival will be significantly improved by this therapy is not yet clear.

Boggs [17] has recently pointed out several problems which must be faced before granulocyte support therapy could become practical on a widespread basis. Included in this list are the need for more economically feasible cell collection systems, better methods to assure quality control of cell function, collection technics less hazardous for the donor, methods to decrease the risk of transfusion reactions to the recipient, and better evidence that the expense and effort will truly alter the natural history of the patient's illness. Also unanswered is whether prophylactic granulocyte administration could decrease the incidence of infection during periods of neutropenia. Despite the difficult and important questions above, granulocyte therapy appears to be of sufficient potential value to warrant the enthusiastic support of investigators in this field.

SUMMARY AND CONCLUSIONS

Progress is being made. Mortality is now lower for almost all infectious complications in immunosuppressed patients. More effective antibiotics and prompt empiric coverage for fever, plus granulocyte transfusions, have lowered mortality for gram-negative bacterial infection. More aggressive use of invasive diagnostic technics for lung infections has led to earlier treatment of aspergillus pneumonia and better survival rates. A less toxic drug to treat pneumocystis infection is now available, and survival rates in recent series are much improved over past reports of pneumocystis pneumonia. Recent reports of effectiveness of adenine arabinoside for herpes simplex infections, without drug toxicity, make further investigations of this agent for herpes group viral infections a promising enterprise. Finally, several encouraging reports of methods for prophylaxis for a variety of infections are noted above. It is anticipated that as more information becomes available regarding the basic immunopathology induced by various antineoplastic and immunosuppressing medications, more specific protective and therapeutic measures for infection can be devised.

REFERENCES

1. Abdallah PS, Mark JBD, Merigan TC: Diagnosis of cytomegalovirus pneumonia in compromised hosts. Am J Med 61:326–332, 1976.
2. Aisner J, Kvols LK, Sickles EA et al: Transtracheal selective bronchial brushing for pulmonary infiltrates in patients with cancer. Chest 69:367–371, 1976.
3. Aisner J, Schimpff SC, Bennett JE et al: Aspergillus infections in cancer patients: association with fireproofing materials in a new hospital. JAMA 235:411–412, 1976.
4. Aisner J, Schimpff SC, Sutherland JC et al: Torulopsis glabrata infections in patients with cancer. Am J Med 61:23–28, 1976.
5. Aisner J, Schimpff SC, Wiernik PH: Treatment of invasive aspergillosis: relation of early diagnosis and treatment to response. Ann Intern Med 86:539–543, 1977.
6. Alavi JB, Root RK, Djerassi I et al: A randomized clinical trial of granulocyte transfusions for infection in acute leukemia. N Engl J Med 296:706–711, 1977.

7. Anderson EL, Gramling PK, Vestal PR, Farrar WE: Susceptibility of pseudomonas aeruginosa to tobramycin or gentamicin alone and combined with carbenicillin. Antimicrob Ag Chemother 8:300–304, 1975.

8. Anderson RJ, Schafer LA, Olin DB, Eickhoff TC: Infectious risk factors in the immunosuppressed host. Am J Med 54:453–460, 1973.

9. Andriole VT: Synergy of carbenicillin and gentamicin in experimental infection with pseudomonas. J Infect Dis 124(Suppl):S46–S55, 1971.

10. Andriole VT: Antibiotic synergy in experimental infection with pseudomonas II. J Infect Dis 129:124–133, 1974.

11. Armstrong D, Young LS, Meyer RD, Blevins AH: Infectious complications of neoplastic disease. Med Clin N Am 55:729–745, 1971.

12. Atkinson K, Kay HEM, McElwain TJ: Fever in the neutropenic patient. Br Med J 3:160–161, 1974.

13. Blandford G, Charlton D: Studies of pulmonary and renal immunopathology after nonlethal primary sendai viral infection in normal and cyclophosphamide treated hamsters. Am Rev Respir Dis 115:305–314, 1977.

14. Bloomfield CD, Kennedy BJ: Cephalothin, carbenicillin and gentamicin therapy for febrile patients with acute non-lymphocytic leukemia. Cancer 34:431–437, 1974.

15. Bode FR, Paré AP, Fraser RG: Pulmonary diseases in the compromised host. Medicine (Baltimore) 53:255–293, 1974.

16. Bodey GR, Rodriguez V: Infections in cancer patients on a protected environment-prophylactic antibiotic program. Am J Med 59:497–504, 1975.

17. Boggs DR: Neutrophils in the blood bank. N Engl J Med 296:748–750, 1977.

18. Braude AI, Ziegler EJ, Douglas H, McCutchan JA: Antibody to cell wall glycolipid of gram-negative bacteria: induction of immunity to bacteremia and endotoxemia. J Infect Dis 136(Suppl):S167–S173, 1977.

19. Britt MR, Garibaldi RA, Wilfert JN, Smith CB: In vitro activity of tobramycin and gentamicin. Antimicrob Agents Chemother 2:236–241, 1972.

20. Burton JR, Zachery JB, Bessin R et al: Aspergillus in four renal transplant recipients. Diagnosis and effective treatment with amphotericin B. Ann Intern Med 77: 383–388, 1972.

21. Carey RM, Kimball AC, Armstrong D, Lieberman PH: Toxoplasmosis: clinical experiences in a cancer hospital. Am J Med 54:30–38, 1973.

22. Chang HY, Rodriguez V, Narboni G et al: Causes of death in adults with acute leukemia. Medicine (Baltimore) 55:259–268, 1976.

23. Chilcote RR, Baehner RL, Hammond D et al: Septicemia and meningitis in children splenectomized for Hodgkin's disease. N Engl J Med 295:798–800, 1976.

24. Cunningham JH, Zavala DC, Corry RJ, Keim LW: Trephine air drill, bronchial brush, and fiberoptic transbronchial lung biopsies in immunosuppressed patients. Am Rev Respir Dis 115:213–220, 1977.

25. Donaldson SS, Moore MR, Rosenberg SA, Vosti KL: Characterization of post-splenectomy bacteremia among patients with and without lymphoma. N Engl J Med 287:69–71, 1972.

26. Edwards LD, Digioia R: Infections in splenectomized patients: A study of 131 patients. Scand J Infect Dis 8:255–261, 1976.

27. Eickhoff TC, Olin DB, Anderson RJ, Schafer LA: Current problems and approaches to diagnosis of infection in renal transplant recipients. Transplant Proc 4:693–697, 1972.

28. Ellis JH: Transbronchial lung biopsy via the fiberoptic bronchoscope. Chest 68:524–532, 1975.

29. E.O.R.T.C. International Antimicrobial Therapy Group: Three antibiotic regimens in the treatment of infection in febrile granulocytopenic patients with cancer. J Infect Dis 137:14–29, 1978.

30. Feld R, Bodey GP, Rodriguez V, Luna M: Causes of death in patients with malignant lymphoma. Am J Med Sci 268:97–106, 1974.

31. Feld R, Valdivieso M, Bodey GP, Rodriguez V: Comparison of amikacin and tobramycin in the treatment of infection in patients with cancer. J Infect Dis 135:61–66, 1977.

32. Feldman S, Pearson TA: Fatal bacillus cereus pneumonia and sepsis in a child with cancer. Clin Pediatr 13:649–655, 1974.

33. Feldman NT, Pennington JE, Ehrie MG: Transbronchial lung biopsy in the compromised host. JAMA 238:1377–1379, 1977.

34. Fiala M, Payne JE, Berne TV et al: Epidemiology of cytomegalovirus infection after transplantation and immunosuppression. J Infect Dis 132:421–433, 1975.

35. Filice G, Yu B, Armstrong D: Immunodiffusion and agglutination tests for candida in patients with neoplastic disease: inconsistent correlation of results with invasive disease. J Infect Dis 135:349–357, 1977.

36. Frazier AR, Rosenow EC, Roberts GD: Nocardiosis: A review of 25 cases occurring during 24 months. Mayo Clin Proc 50:657–663, 1975.

37. Friedman BA, Wenglin BD, Hyland RN, Rifkind D: Roentgenographically atypical pneumocystis carinii pneumonia. Am Rev Respir Dis 111:89–96, 1975.

38. Gaines JD, Remington JS: Diagnosis of deep infection with candida: a study of candida precipitins. Arch Intern Med 132:699–702, 1973.

39. Gantz NM, Myerowitz RL, Medeiros AA et al: Listeriosis in immunosuppressed patients. Am J Med 58:637–643, 1975.

40. Gercovich FG, Richman SP, Rodriguez V et al: Successful control of systemic aspergillus niger infections in two patients with acute leukemia. Cancer 36:2271–2276, 1975.

41. Graw RG, Herzig G, Perry S, Henderson ES: Normal granulocyte transfusion therapy: treatment of septicemia due to gram-negative bacteria. N Engl J Med 287:367–371, 1972.

42. Greenman RL, Goodall PT, King D: Lung biopsy in immunocompromised hosts. Am J Med 59:488–496, 1975.

43. Haghbin M, Armstrong D, Murphy ML: Controlled prospective trial of pseudomonas aeruginosa vaccine in children with acute leukemia. Cancer 32:761–766, 1973.

44. Herzig RH, Herzig GP, Graw RG et al: Successful granulocyte transfusion therapy for gram-negative septicemia: a prospectively randomized controlled study. N Engl J Med 296:701–705, 1977.

45. Higby DJ, Yates JW, Henderson ES, Holland JF: Filtration leukapheresis for granulocyte transfusion therapy. N Engl J Med 292:761–766, 1975.

46. Ho M, Suwansirikul S, Dowling JN et al. The transplanted kidney as a source of cytomegalovirus infection. N Engl J Med 293:1109–1112, 1975.

47. Hughes WT, Kuhn S, Chaudhary S et al: Successful chemoprophylaxis for pneumocystis carinii pneumonitis. N Engl J Med 297:1419–1426, 1977.

48. Hughes WT, Feldman S, Aur RJA et al: Intensity of immunosuppressive therapy and the incidence of pneumocystis carinii pneumonitis. Cancer 36: 2004–2009, 1975.

49. Hughes WT, Feldman S, Chandhary S: Comparison of trimethoprim-sulfamethoxazole and pentamidine in the treatment of pneumocystis carinii pneumonitis. Pediatr Res 10:399A, 1976.

50. Hughes WT, Feldman S, Sanyal SK: Treatment of pneumocystis carinii pneumonitis with trimethoprim-sulfamethoxazole. Can Med Assoc J 112:47S–50S, 1975.

51. Jauregui L, Cushing RD, Lerner AM: Gentamcin-Amickacin-resistant gram-negative bacilli at Detroit general hospital, 1975–1976. Am J Med 62:882–888, 1977.

52. Johnson MT, Luby JP, Buchanan RA et al: Treatment of varicella-zoster virus infections with adenine arabinoside. J Infect Dis 131:225–229, 1975.

53. Kaplan MH, Armstrong D, Rosen P: Tuberculosis complicating neoplastic disease. Cancer 33:850–858, 1974.

54. Krick JA, Stinson EB, Remington JS: Nocardia infection in heart transplant patients. Ann Intern Med 82:18–26, 1975.

55. Lau WK, Young LS: Trimethoprim-sulfamethoxazole treatment of pneumocystis carinii pneumonia in adults. N Engl J Med 295:716–718, 1976.

56. Lau WK, Young LS, Black RE et al: Comparative efficacy and toxicity of amikacin/carbenicillin versus gentamicin/carbenicillin in leukopenic patients. Am J Med 62:959–966, 1977.

57. Lau WK, Young LS, Remington JS: Pneumocystis carinii pneumonia: diagnosis by examination of pulmonary secretions. JAMA 236:2399–2402, 1976.

58. Leff A, Jacobs R, Gooding V et al: Bacillus cereus pneumonia. Survival in a patient with cavitary disease treated with gentamicin. Am Rev Respir Dis 115:151–154, 1977.

59. Levine AS, Robinson RA, Hauser JM: Analysis of studies on protected environments and prophylactic antibiotics in adult acute leukemia. Eur J Cancer 11:Suppl 57–66, 1975.

60. Levine AS, Schimpff SC, Graw RG, Young RC: Hematologic malignancies and other marrow failure states: progress in the management of complicating infections. Semin Hematol 11:141–202, 1974.

61. Levine AS, Siegel SE, Schreiber AD et al: Protected environments and prophylactic antibiotics. A prospective controlled study of their utility in the therapy of acute leukemia. N Engl J Med 288:477–483, 1973.

62. Linnemann CC, First MR, Alvira MM et al: Herpesvirus hominis type 2 meningoencephalitis following renal transplantation. Am J Med 61:703–708, 1976.

63. Maderazo EG, Quintiliani R: Treatment of nocardial infection with trimethoprim and sulfamethoxazole. Am J Med 57:671–675, 1974.

64. McCabe WR, Bruins SC, Craven DE, Johns M: Cross-reactive antigens: their potential for immunization-induced immunity to gram-negative bacteria. J Infect Dis 136(Suppl):S161–S166, 1977.

65. Medoff G, Dismukes WE, Meade RH, Moses J: Therapeutic program for candida infection. In: Hobby GL (Ed): Antimicrob Agents Chemother, 1970. Bethesda, Md., Amer Soc Microbiol, 1971, pp 286–290.

66. Meuwissen JH, Leeuwenberg AD: A microcomplement fixation test applied to infection with pneumocystis carinii. Trop Geogr Med 24:282–291, 1972.

67. Meyer RD, Lewis RP, Carmalt ED, Finegold SM: Amikacin therapy for serious gram-negative bacillary infections. Ann Intern Med 83:790–800, 1975.

68. Meyer RD, Lewis RP, Halter J, White M: Gentamicin-resistant Pseudomonas aeruginosa and Serratia marcescens in a general hospital. Lancet 1:580–583, 1976.

69. Meyer RD, Ruskin J, Linne SR, Sattler FR: Miconazole therapy for disseminated coccidioidomycosis. 17th Interscience Conference on Antimicrobial Agents and Chemotherapy, No. 57, 1977.

70. Meyer RD, Young LS, Armstrong D et al: Aspergillosis complicating neoplastic disease. Am J Med 54:6–15, 1973.

71. Meyers JD, Spencer HC, Watts JC et al: Cytomegalovirus pneumonia after human marrow transplantation. Ann Intern Med 82:181–188, 1975.

72. Moellering RC, Wennersten C, Kunz LJ, Poitras JW: Resistance to gentamicin, tobramycin and amikacin among clinical isolates of bacteria. Am J Med 62:873–881, 1977.

73. Myerowitz RL, Medeiros AA, O'Brien TF: Bacterial infection in renal homotransplant recipients. Am J Med 53:308–314, 1972.

74. Neiman P, Wasserman PB, Wentworth BB et al: Interstitial pneumonia and cytomegalovirus infection as complications of human marrow transplantation. Transplantation 15:478–485, 1973.

75. Normal L, Kagan IG: Some observations on the serology of pneumocystis carinii infections in the United States. Infect Immun 8:317–321, 1973.

76. Palmer DL, Harvey RL Wheeler JK: Diagnostic and therapeutic considerations in Nocardia asteroides infection. Medicine (Baltimore) 53:391–401, 1974.

77. Parry MF, Neu HC: Ticarcillin for treatment of serious infections with gram-negative bacteria. J Infect Dis 134:476–485, 1976.

78. Pennington JE: Successful treatment of aspergillus pneumonia in hematologic neoplasia. N Engl J Med 295:426–427, 1976.

79. Pennington JE: Fever, neutropenia and malignancy: a clinical syndrome in evolution. Cancer 39:1345–1349, 1977.

80. Pennington JE: Aspergillus pneumonia in hematologic malignancy: improvements in diagnosis and therapy. Arch Intern Med 137:769–771, 1977.

81. Pennington JE: Quantitative effects of immunosuppression on bronchoalveolar cells. J Infect Dis 136:127–131, 1977.

82. Pennington JE: Bronchoalveolar cell response to bacterial challenge in the immunosuppressed lung. Amer Rev Respir Dis 116:885–893, 1977.

82a. Pennington JE, Ehrie MG: Pathogenesis of Pseudomonas aeruginosa pneumonia during immunosuppression. J Infect Dis (in press 1978).

83. Pennington JE, Gibbons ND, Strobeck JE et al: Bacillus species infection in patients with hematologic neoplasia. JAMA 235:1473–1474, 1976.

84. Pennington JE, Feldman NT: Pulmonary infiltrates and fever in patients with hematologic malignancy. Am J Med 62:581–587, 1977.

85. Pennington JE, Reynolds HY, Carbone PP: Pseudomonas pneumonia: a retrospective study of 36 cases. Am J Med 55:155–160, 1973.

86. Pennington JE, Reynolds HY, Wood RE et al: Use of a pseudomonas aeruginosa vaccine in patients with acute leukemia and cystic fibrosis. Am J Med 58:629–636, 1975.

87. Prystowski SD, Vogelstein B, Ettinger DS et al: Invasive aspergillosis. N Engl J Med 295:655–658, 1976.

88. Rodriguez V: Miconazole therapy of fungal infections in cancer patients. 17th Interscience Conference on Antimicrobial Agents and Chemotherapy, No. 407, 1977.

89. Rodriguez V, Burgess M, Bodey GP: Management of fever of unknown origin in patients with neoplasms and neutropenia. Cancer 32:1007–1012, 1973.

90. Rosen PP, Martini N, Armstrong D: Pneumocystis carinii pneumonia: diagnosis by lung biopsy. Am J Med 58:794–802, 1975.

91. Ruskin J, Remington JS: Toxoplasmosis in the compromised host. Ann Intern Med 84:193–199, 1976.

92. Rytel MW, Kauffman HM: Clinical efficacy of adenine arabinoside in therapy of cytomegalovirus infections in renal allograft recipients. J Infect Dis 133:202–205, 1976.

93. Schaefer JC, Yu B, Armstrong D: An aspergillus immunodiffusion test in the early diagnosis of aspergillosis in adult leukemia patients. Amer Rev Respir Dis 113:325–329, 1976.

94. Schimpff SC, Greene WH, Young VM et al: Infection prevention in acute nonlymphocytic leukemia: laminar air flow room reverse isolation with oral, nonabsorbable antibiotic prophylaxis. Ann Intern Med 82:351–358, 1975.

95. Schimpff SC, O'Connell MJ, Greene WH, Wiernik PH: Infections in 92 splenectomized patients with Hodgkin's disease. Am J Med 59:695–701, 1975.

96. Schimpff SC, Satterlee W, Young VM, Serpick A: Empiric therapy with carbenicillin and gentamicin for febrile patients with cancer and granulocytopenia. N Engl J Med 284:1061–1065, 1971.

97. Schimpff SC, Young VM, Greene WH et al: Origin of infection in acute nonlymphocytic leukemia. Ann Intern Med 77:707–714, 1972.

98. Sickles EA, Greene WH, Wiernik PH: Clinical presentation of infection in granulocytopenic patients. Arch Intern Med 135:715–719, 1975.

99. Sickles EA, Young VM, Greene WH et al: Pneumonia in acute leukemia. Ann Intern Med 79:528–534, 1973.

100. Singer C, Armstrong D, Rosen PP, Schottenfeld D: Pneumocystis carinii pneumonia: A cluster of eleven cases. Ann Intern Med 82:772–777, 1975.

101. Singer C, Kaplan MH, Armstrong D: Bacteremia and fungemia complicating neoplastic disease. Am J Med 62:731–742, 1977.

102. Smith CR, Baughman KL, Edwards CQ et al: Controlled comparison of amikacin and gentamicin. N Engl J Med 296:349–353, 1977.

103. Tally FP, Louie TJ, Weinstein WM et al: Amikacin therapy for severe gram-negative sepsis. Ann Intern Med 83:484–488, 1975.

104. Tapper ML, Armstrong D: Bacteremia due to Pseudomonas aeruginosa complicating neoplastic disease: a progress report, J Infect Dis 130(Suppl):S14–S23, 1974.

105. Tattersall MHN: Aggressive cancer treatment and its role in predisposing to infection. Eur J Cancer 11(Suppl):9–19, 1975.

106. Tattersall MHN, Spiers ASD, Darrell JH: Initial therapy with combination of five antibiotics in febrile patients with leukemia and neutropenia. Lancet 1:162–166, 1972.

107. UCLA Bone Marrow Transplantation Group: Bone marrow transplantation with intensive combination chemotherapy-radiation therapy in acute leukemia. Ann Intern Med 86:155–161, 1977.

108. Valdivieso M, Gil-Extremera B, Zornoza J et al: Gram-negative bacillary pneumonia in the compromised host. Medicine (Baltimore) 56:241–254, 1977.

109. Walzer PD, Perl DP, Krogstad DJ et al: Pneumocystis carinii pneumonia in the United States: epidemiologic, diagnostic, and clinical features. Ann Intern Med 80:83–93, 1974.

110. Weitzman S, Aisenberg AC: Fulminant sepsis after the successful treatment of Hodgkin's disease. Am J Med 62:47–50, 1977.

111. Weitzman SA, Aisenberg AC, Siber GR, Smith DH: Impaired humoral immunity in treated Hodgkin's disease. N Engl J Med 297:245–248, 1977.

112. Whitley RJ, Ch'ien LT, Dolin R et al: Adenine arabinoside therapy of herpes zoster in the immunosuppressed. N Engl J Med 294:1193–1199, 1976.

113. Whitley RJ, Soong SJ, Dolin R et al: Adenine arabinoside therapy of biopsy-proved herpes simplex encephalitis. N Engl J Med 297:289–294, 1977.

114. Williams DM, Krick JA, Remington JS: Pulmonary infection in the compromised host. Am Rev Respir Dis 114:359–394; 593–627, 1976.

115. Young LS, Armstrong D, Blevins A, Lieberman P: Nocardia asteroides infection complicating neoplastic disease. Am J Med 50:356–367, 1971.
116. Young LS, Meyer RD, Armstrong D: Pseudomonas aeruginosa vaccine in cancer patients. Ann Intern Med 79:518–527, 1973.
117. Young LS, Stevens P, Ingram J: Functional role of antibody against "core" glycolipid of enterobacteriaceae. J Clin Invest 56:850–861, 1975.
118. Young RC, Bennett JE: Invasive aspergillosis: absence of detectable antibody response. Am Rev Respir Dis 104:710–716, 1971.
119. Young RC, Bennett JE, Geelhoed GW, Levine AS: Fungemia with compromised host resistance. A study of 70 cases. Ann Intern Med 80:605–612, 1974.
120. Young RC, Bennett JE, Vogel CL et al: Aspergillosis: the spectrum of the disease in 98 patients. Medicine (Baltimore) 49:147–173, 1970.

CHAPTER 7

BABESIOSIS

Gustave J. Dammin, M.D.*

Human babesiosis was first reported in 1957 by Skrabalo [1]. The patient was a 33 year old man living near Zagreb who presented with anemia, fever and hemoglobinuria. Intraerythrocytic parasites, identified as *Babesia bovis*, were numerous in the peripheral blood and marrow. The patient died of renal insufficiency during the second week of illness. Because of having sustained a traumatic rupture of the spleen eleven years earlier, he had had a splenectomy. The considerable interest in this case stemmed from its being the first appearance in man of an infection already known in biblical times as a cause of devastating epizootics among cattle and other domestic animals [2,3]. The absence of the spleen was reported as a major factor in increasing susceptibility to the infection and its rapid progression to a fatal outcome.

The protozoan parasite in this case was one which Babes described in 1888 when he was seeking the cause of febrile hemoglobinuria occurring in epizootic form among cattle grazing in the Danube River region of Rumania [4]. He identified an intraerythrocytic agent which he interpreted to be a bacterium and which he termed "*Haematococcus bovis.*" The protozoan nature of the agent causing this disease in cattle in North America was established by Theobald Smith, who also demonstrated that it was transmitted by a tick. In 1893, he and Kilborne [5] reported that the cattle tick, *Boophilus annulatus,* served as the vector in the transmission of Texas cattle fever, terming the causal agent *Pyrosoma bigeminum,* later changed to *Babesia bigemina.* These were landmark studies, since they implicated, for the first time, a blood-sucking arthropod in the transmission of a pathogen to a vertebrate host, antedating the demonstration of the role of the mosquito in malaria [6].

Human babesiosis had to be regarded as an isolated phenomenon, but concern about it accelerated when, in 1968 and 1969, three additional cases were reported, all in individuals who had had splenectomies. Two of these three infections proved fatal. The protective role of the spleen

---

* Friedman Professor of Pathology, Harvard Medical School—Peter Bent Brigham Hospital, Boston, Mass.

thus became even more evident, as did the need to modify the concept of host specificity of the *Babesia spp.* The only case to survive, of the initial four reported, occurred in 1968 in California, with the patient suspected of having babesiosis of equine origin [7]. The second case to be reported in 1968 was caused by a *Babesia* of probable bovine origin, *B. divergens.* The patient was a fisherman, who contracted his infection in County Galway, Ireland [2,8,9]. In 1969, the third case of this group was reported from Zagreb and appeared also to be caused by *B. divergens* [10].

The first infection in a patient with an intact spleen was contracted in 1969 on Nantucket Island, Massachusetts, and was caused by *B. microti,* a *Babesia* found in mice and other small rodents [11]. Since then, there have been 19 additional clinical infections contracted on Nantucket, all in patients with intact spleens. Some had severe and prolonged illness, but there were no fatalities [12].

Other aspects of this relatively new human infection, caused by a protozoan and transmitted by a tick, are presented below. The purpose of this opening summary is to illustrate how flexible our thinking and how broad our approach must be when infectious agents like *Babesia spp.,* known worldwide as pathogens of domestic and wild animals, appear abruptly in epidemic form in man. The event precipitates a cascade of questions about (1) the nature of the defense against such infection in the human host and its occasional inadequacy, (2) the characteristics of the presumably new human pathogen, (3) the features of the tick vector, not formerly regarded as indiscriminate enough in its search for blood as to attack man, and (4) the settings in which human babesial infections have occurred. The answers to well formulated questions about the clinical and epidemiologic aspects of babesiosis should help to explain this array of events of the past two decades.

I. THE PARASITES

Taxonomy

The position of the presently recognized Genus *Babesia* in the Phylum Protozoa has been debated for decades. Newer methods of study have led to a sounder basis for the characterization and, therefore, classification of candidate members of the genus, with a consequent emergence of order out of taxonomic turmoil. The agent now designated as the type species for the genus, *Babesia bovis* (Starcovici, 1893) had been termed *Haematococcus bovis* by its discoverer, Babes, in 1888, because he believed the forms to be cocci. Although *Haematococcus* was inappropriate, because it had been employed already to designate a flagellate, *Haematococcus babes* was applied to the type species in 1889 but only until *Babesia bovis* was proposed and accepted in 1893. It was after the monumental discoveries of Theobald Smith on the protozoal nature of the erythrocyte-invading agent causing Texas cattle fever and its tick vector that Starcovici in 1893 defined the genus *Babesia*. Thus, the agent responsible for the devastating Texas cattle fever which Smith and Kilborne termed *Pyrosoma bigeminum* became *Babesia bigemina*. Indeed, "*Pyrosoma*" was not acceptable because it was already in use as a generic term. The term *Piroplasma* was proposed by Patton in 1895 for the genus, but Starcovici's designation, *Babesia*, had precedence. Patton's term was incorporated into the name of the class and order in later taxonomic classifications. The class Piroplasmea Levine, 1961, became a member of a new subphylum Apicomplexa Levine, 1970, which includes protozoa possessing a similarity of apical complexes which are definable only by electron microscopy. On this basis, plasmodids, coccidids, and toxoplasmids were also placed into this subphylum. The genus *Babesia*, with seventy-one species, has a worldwide distribution and affects innumerable mammals and birds. It belongs to the family Babesiidae Poche, 1913, the order Piroplasmorida, Wenyon, 1926, the class Piroplasmea Levine, 1961, and the subphylum Apicomplexa Levine, 1970.

The recognition of babesiosis as an infection widespread in the animal kingdom developed rapidly, but an orderly taxonomy did not. According to Levine [13], over a dozen generic names were or had been in use until *Babesia* was accepted as the term for a single genus that could encompass all of the agents meeting the criteria outlined by Starcovici in 1893. Of the 71 species in the genus *Babesia*, only the following infect domestic animals: *B. bigemina, B. bovis, B. divergens* and *B. major* in cattle, *B. caballi, B. equi* in horses, *B. foliata, B. motasi* and *B. ovis* in sheep, *B. motasi, B. ovis* and *B. taylori* in goats, *B. perroncitoi* and *B. trautmanni* in pigs, *B. canis, B. gibsoni* and *B. vogeli* in dogs, and *B. felis* in cats. Mahoney [27] regards *B. bovis, B. berbera* and *B. argentina* as identical. The term *B. bovis* has priority and identifies all three species.

Morphology

Characteristic of the genus *Babesia* is the presence of piriform, round or oval parasites in the erythrocytes of the infected vertebrate host. The *Babesia* species vary in size, with the group of larger members represented by *B. bigemina*, which is piriform in shape and measures 4–5 μ by 2–3 μ. Among the group of smaller members are (1) the type species, *B. bovis* (Babes, 1888) Starcovici, 1893, which measures 2.4 by 1.5 μ (2) *B. divergens*, also a *Babesia* of cattle (1.5 by 0.4 μ), and *B.*

microti, a rodent *Babesia,* (2.0 by 1.5 μ). All three in this group of smaller members have proved infectious for man. Because of their small size, usual ring conformation, and occasional peripheral position in the human erythrocyte, they have often been mistaken for *Plasmodium falciparum* (see Fig. 1). However, in the intraerythrocytic development of the *Babesia,* hemoglobin-derived pigment is not visible, since the hemoglobin is catabolized completely. The developing *Plasmodium* in the red cell contains the hemoglobin-derived brownish pigment, hemozoin. The trophozoites of the smaller members of the genus *Babesia* remain small as ring and oval forms, and divide by budding, rather than schizogeny, resulting in pairs and tetrads [59]. There are no filaments on infected erythrocytes and there is controversy about the existence of sexual forms.

Early reports on the identification of presumably new members of the genus *Babesia,* especially during the four decades after the discoveries of Babes and Smith and Kilborne, led to the belief that the *Babesia spp.* were strongly host-specific. Each identification in a new animal host prompted a new designation for the *Babesia* isolated. In developing his classification, Levine combined and reduced the number of species to be recognized as individual members of the genus, and stated, "Quite a few species of *Babesia* have been named from rodents, mostly because they were found in different hosts. However, their structural similarity and the modern knowledge that there is relatively little host specificity in the Babesiidae makes it desirable to trim this nomenclatural bush" [13]. The lack of host specificity is exemplified by human babesiosis, which in just two decades has had two *Babesia spp.* of bovine origin and one of rodent origin established as causal agents, and one equine and one canine species suspected of having this capability.

Development

In the vertebrate host, the *Babesia spp.* invade and propagate solely in erythrocytes and injure the host by causing fever and hemolysis and the release of a variety of pharmacologically active substances. Among them is a potent kallikrein activator, which, by the production of kallikrein, can cause circulatory stasis, shock and anoxia, an event which may precede the clinical hemolytic manifestations of the infection [14].

In the invertebrate host, the *Babesia spp.* follow a variable course of development, with the first studies in this field reported by Robert Koch in 1906 [15]. He had earlier established the cause of African East Coast cattle fever as *Theileria parva,* a member of the family Theileriidae. This family, with the Babesiidae and Dactylosomatidae, comprise the order Piroplasmorida, Wenyon, 1926. A landmark contribution to this aspect of parasitic acarology was made in 1964 by Riek, who documented the

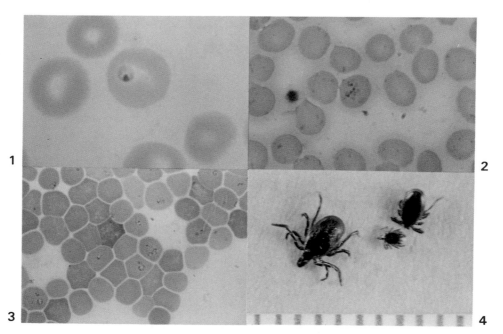

FIG. 1.   Human babesiosis on Nantucket. Giemsa-stained blood film of patient with *B. microti* infection. This ring form resembles that of *Plasmodium falciparum* and has been mistaken for it, leading to a diagnosis of malaria. This fully developed merozoite of *B. microti* contains no pigment, which helps to distinguish it from *P. falciparum*. (Courtesy of Dr. George R. Healy, National CDC, Atlanta and AFIP, Washington, D.C.)

FIG. 2.   Human babesiosis on Nantucket. Giemsa-stained blood film showing tetrad form of *B. microti* in erythrocyte near center of the field. The presence of this form permits a diagnosis of babesiosis.

FIG. 3.   *B. microti* infection in hamster. Giemsa-stained film shows a dozen erythrocytes manifesting various babesial forms, the protozoa showing some preference for immature erythrocytes. This film was made from blood of a hamster inoculated with blood from patient suspected of having babesiosis.

FIG. 4.   *Ixodes* sp. nr. *scapularis*. The female tick with bright reddish-colored body is on the left; the smaller male is on the right and has a dark brown body. The nymph has a tan-colored body, and, measured by the millimeter rule in the lower part of the field, is about 2 mm in length.

transovarial transmission of *B. bigemina* in *Boophilus microplus* [16]. Smith and Kilborne [5] had demonstrated that *B. bigemina* could be carried by the progeny of *Boophilus annulatus* which had matured on infected cattle, and could introduce the *Babesia* directly into the blood of other cattle. Riek detailed the sequential development of *B. bigemina* in *Boophilus microplus,* noting that all of the babesial forms present in bovine blood are found in the female tick's gut contents. In addition to intraerythrocytic and extraerythrocytic forms, there are degenerate forms present in shed epithelial cells of the gut wall. Variously shaped forms develop further in the gut epithelial cells through multiple fission, with ultimate liberation of the vermicule stage of the parasite from them into the gut lumen. The vermicules then penetrate the gut wall, enter the hemolymph and are distributed throughout the body. Oviposition begins by the fourth day, with vermicules present in the yolk material and multiplying as the larva develops. Once developed, the larva attaches to its vertebrate host, begins its blood meal, molts to become a nymph at 5–7 days after attachment, and molts again to become an adult about one week later. Transmission of *B. bigemina* begins during the nymph stage, upon completion of the parasite's further development and multiplication in the salivary glands [17].

Much less is known about the development of *B. microti* in its invertebrate hosts, which on Nantucket are *Ixodes* and *Dermacentor* species, hard ticks which belong to the family Ixodidae [18]. Spielman has demonstrated the dominant vector on Nantucket to be a deer tick, an *Ixodes* species currently designated *I.* sp. nr. *scapularis** because it differs from *I. scapularis* as defined by Cooley and Kohls [19]. Studies of the development of *B. microti* in these *Ixodid* ticks are under way, spurred by the report of additional cases of *B. microti* in man on Long Island and Shelter Island (N.Y.) and Nantucket and Martha's Vineyard (Mass.) [20–22,37,58], bringing the total number of clinical cases in humans to 33. Reexamination of the second reported case which occurred in California in 1966 suggests that the agent was *B. microti*. Attention is therefore directed toward *B. microti*, its reservoirs of infection and its vectors, since it may have been responsible for all of the clinical cases and subclinical infections observed in the United States and Mexico. The five clinical cases reported from Yugoslavia, Ireland and France were all instances of bovine babesiosis, four probably caused by *B. divergens* and one by *B. bovis*. It is noteworthy that all 5 cases had had splenectomies. (See Section IV, below.)

II. THE VECTORS

The epidemic appearance of babesiosis in man on Nantucket in recent years has accelerated studies of the vector(s) as well as the parasite for clues that would help to explain this outbreak of disease. With the causal

---

* *I.* sp. nr. *scapularis* = *I.* species near *scapularis*.

agent on Nantucket identified as *B. microti* and being responsible for clinical infections in nonsplenectomized patients, attention was directed to ticks because of their well established role in the transmission of animal babesiosis. The suspected ticks are "hard" ticks belonging to the family Ixodidae, which includes the medically important genera, *Ixodes* and *Dermacentor*, so termed because they bear a dorsal shield or scutum which persists throughout development. With respect to human babesiosis, we are concerned currently only with these two genera of the thirteen which comprise the family Ixodidae. Of the 250 or so members of the genus *Ixodes*, only the few economically important species have been studied in detail, leaving unsettled the taxonomic status of many species, including a large number of those in North America [23]. Members of the genus *Dermacentor* have received closer attention because of their well established roles in the transmission of viral and rickettsial agents of human disease.

Members of the genus *Ixodes* are "three-host" ticks in that, from larva to nymph to adult, a new host of the same or a different animal species, is required for each blood meal. After the first blood meal, that of the larva, transformation into the nymph occurs and search for a second host begins. After the blood meal from this host, the developing tick drops from the host, molts, and after several weeks becomes an adult. At this stage, the ticks are sexually differentiated, and, while the female is obtaining her blood meal, the male attaches to the female, accomplishing delivery of the sperm via his mouthparts. The engorged, replete female drops from the host, eggs mature, and several weeks later are extruded. Oviposition may continue for weeks, with up to 20,000 eggs being deposited.

It is still to be determined how frequently man is attacked by earlier stages as well as the adult stage of the deer tick, *Ixodes* sp. nr. *scapularis*, which is a known transmitter on Nantucket. Spielman [18] reports that all three stages of this tick commonly feed on man. The nymph has proved capable of transmitting infection experimentally and is active during the period of peak occurrence of human babesiosis on Nantucket, which is principally during the summer. Whereas all stages of *I*. sp. nr. *scapularis* are known to feed on man on Nantucket, only the adult stage of *D. variabilis* does so. Immature ticks can transmit piroplasms to man, but because of their small size, their presence may not be recognized. That is, attachment by the nymph for a blood meal may be overlooked, since the unengorged *I*. sp. nr. *scapularis* nymph measures only 2 mm. in its largest dimension (see Fig. 4). Thus, the history of tick bite does not have the same importance in the diagnosis of babesiosis as it does in Rocky Mountain spotted fever.

Spielman [18] found only two types of ticks, *Ixodes* sp. nr. *scapularis* and *Dermacentor variabilis*, on the white-footed mouse *Peromyscus leucopus*, which is the major reservoir of *B. microti* on Nantucket. The ratio of *I.* sp. nr. *scapularis* to *D. variabilis* on these animals was 10:1. His study of the competence of these ticks as vectors proved that a *Babesia* strain obtained from one of the Nantucket cases, when established in a hamster, could be acquired by *I.* sp. nr. *scapularis* larvae through a blood meal. Following the development of these infected larvae to the nymphal stage, these nymphs were capable of transmitting *B. microti* to noninfected hamsters. Thus, the capacity of the larval *I.* sp. nr. *scapularis* to become infected was demonstrated, as was the capacity of the next or nymphal stage to transmit this *B. microti* of human origin to another vertebrate host, the hamster. Spielman reported that *I.* sp. nr. *scapularis* collected on Nantucket is currently present also in Ontario, and that *I. scapularis* as defined by Cooley and Kohls in 1945 is found largely in the southeastern United States. Studies thus far suggest that *D. variabilis* is less important on Nantucket as a transmitter of babesial infection than is *I.* sp. nr. *scapularis*.

The recent occurrence of over 20 cases of clinical babesiosis in island communities of Massachusetts and New York prompts a consideration of the determinants of host preference and feeding behavior of candidate ticks. Factors which affect feeding patterns of ticks during their development are detailed in the encyclopedic monograph of Balashov [24]. The candidate vector in human babesiosis must be classified with ticks that have nonspecific host preference and which include primates in their selection of sources for blood meals, as observed by Hoogstraal and Theiler [25]. The history of the dissemination in the new world of the dog tick, *Rhipicephalus sanguineus*, illustrates the directions which host selection and questing behavior may take, depending upon particular ecologic circumstances. The selection of man as a host for this dog tick may relate to the development of a biologic race with a greater predilection for feeding on man or the existence of geographic variations for which we lack morphologic criteria [26].

III. BABESIOSIS IN DOMESTIC AND WILD ANIMALS

Background

The beginnings of animal babesiosis occurring in epizootic or enzootic form are not known. Presumptive recognition of the infection by microscopic examination of a blood film was discovered almost a century ago, and the worldwide distribution of the infection in the animal kingdom has been appreciated for decades. What was described in Exodus [3] as "the murrain of beasts" may have been an epizootic affecting cattle, horses, asses, camels, oxen and sheep, the animals listed in that order in Chapter 9, Verse 3. The term "murrain" can be traced to several ancient languages, deriving from words denoting pestilence, plague and death. "Murrain" today is still used in parts of Ireland to describe "redwater" in cattle, which is the febrile hemoglobinuria of babesiosis [8]. The reports of Babes [4] and Smith and Kilborne [5] created considerable interest and prompted broad investigation, especially in cattle-raising countries, because of the adverse economic impact that this disease was known to have.

In his address to the Association of American Physicians in 1893 [6], Theobald Smith summarized his previous reports on Texas cattle fever and extended his analysis of the disease to such aspects as the vertebrate host's immune response in relationship to the course of the infection and the pathogenesis of the visceral lesions. His research was to become a guide for future decades of work on animal babesiosis. Smith had shown that Texas cattle fever (1) was primarily "a disease of the blood characterized by the destruction of red corpuscles" by parasites which invaded them, (2) could be produced in susceptible cattle by inoculation of blood containing the pathogen, (3) could occur in enzootic form, with otherwise healthy cattle harboring the parasite, (4) was caused by a pathogen which was incapable of infecting sheep, rabbits, guinea pigs and pigeons, (5) was transmitted from cattle in an enzootic area to other cattle by the cattle tick, and (6) was transmissible "by the progeny of the ticks which matured on infected cattle" and which "introduced them directly into the blood" of the bovine provider of the next blood meal.

Smith remarked on the immaturity of the erythrocytes which appeared following an acute febrile attack, a consequence of the extensive hemolysis which occurs during the attack. Such an attack was characterized by a reduction in the number of parasitized erythrocytes in the peripheral blood. If the viscera were examined at the height of the febrile attack, however, blood in the myocardium was found to have 50% of the erythrocytes parasitized, the spleen, kidneys and liver would have 5 to 20% parasitized, and only 1–2% in the peripheral blood contained parasites. Because capillaries in various organs were distended, and at times filled only with parasitized erythrocytes, Smith speculated that "the infection of fresh corpuscles takes place in the capillaries, where the latter are wedged in by infected corpuscles."

Smith believed that in the enzootic region, immunity was at least in part acquired through infection. He believed also that there was a natural resistance in young calves, because very few died of an acute attack. This

resistance and that acquired through repeated mild attacks was thought
to account for the immunity of adults in enzootic regions. Smith thought
it remarkable that the agent "lingered indefinitely in the blood of
apparently healthy and insusceptible cattle from the enzootic territory."
"This symbiotic relation between an otherwise fatal micro-parasite and
an insusceptible host is, as far as I know, a new fact in the domain of the
infectious diseases. . . ." "The question of progressive immunity as a
possible modifier of these diseases has not been brought up heretofore, so
far as my information goes."

The anatomic findings in fatal cases which impressed Smith were the
"absence of any inflammatory phenomena," even in the viscera most
affected, i.e., the liver, spleen and kidneys. But he regarded the liver necrosis, the splenic congestion with marked erythrophagocytosis, and
extreme engorgement of the kidneys as an "inference that the reaction of
the body moves within physiological limits and that the pathological elements which enter into the mechanism of bacterial diseases are absent."
It might be added that one acute bacterial infection does act in the
manner of acute babesiosis, and that is cholera.

Clinical Course and Laboratory Findings

Babesiosis is characterized by fever, anemia, hemoglobinuria and jaundice, with morbidity and mortality varying with geographic location. Illness appears from 8 to 16 days after the tick has begun its blood meal.
Natural infection is usually mild early in life and protects animals
indigenous to an enzootic region. Protection may manifest itself for a
period as premunition, a state in which the animal lives in symbiosis with
the parasite and if challenged with that parasite, will not manifest overt
disease. This state, also termed "non-sterile" immunity, was described by
Theobald Smith, as mentioned above, and is one which occurs with regu-
larity in avian malaria. But premunition is a phenomenon and by no
means a major protective response. The host's defense is mediated by
cellular and humoral immunity.

In severe infection, fever parallels the level of parasitemia, and a
temperature of 41°C may be reached soon after the onset of illness.
Hemoglobinemia, hemoglobinuria and jaundice occur in that order.
Cerebral damage may be the dominant terminal sign in some *B. bovis*
and *B. canis* infections. Shortly before death after a brief but stormy
febrile course, body temperature may drop to subnormal levels. Principal
macroscopic findings at postmortem examination are jaundice, dark red
urine and marked congestion of the abdominal viscera, lungs and brain.
Microscopically, the plugging of cerebral capillaries by parasitized erythrocytes resembles that seen in *P. falciparum* infections. There is centri-

lobular and midzone hepatic necrosis, with hemosiderin in Kuppfer cells and prominent erythrophagocytosis by macrophages in the sinusoids. Capillaries in the kidneys have a high concentration of parasitized erythrocytes, and there is hemosiderosis and tubular necrosis. The lymphoid components of the spleen are depleted and there is hemosiderosis and erythrophagocytosis. The lesions may be explained in their entirety by the release of potent pharmacologically active substances and the destruction of erythrocytes by the parasite, in that order. Wright and Mahoney [14] ascribe the early alarming signs of hypotension, slow flow, vascular congestion and anoxia, as observed in cattle with acute babesiosis, to the activation of plasma kallikrein. This event occurs before tissue damage is evident or an immune response can be detected. If the animal survives a severe initial infection such as this, there may be extended protection against clinical babesiosis, as mentioned above.

Immunity

The relative insusceptibility of calves to severe clinical infection is a form of nonspecific resistance or immunity which Smith had recognized. He postulated that this resistance combined with the immunity contributed by infection accounted for the stability of cattle herds in enzootic regions. The nonspecific resistance early in life lasts longer than can be accounted for by the transfer of maternal antibody, which lasts approximately two months.

Although premunition may offer protection against challenge with the same *Babesia* strain, there are other forms of acquired immunity which protect against reinfection and clinical babesiosis. These other forms of acquired immunity are demonstrable in a variety of models but are difficult to define. Mahoney et al. [28] studied naturally acquired immunity to *B. bovis* and *B. bigemina* in cattle infected in calfhood in an enzootic region of Australia. During subsequent rearing in a tick-free area, tests for parasitemia in cattle with *B. bovis* infections were positive in all subjects after four years in this area, but with *B. bigemina* infections, only two of twenty-two cattle had parasitemia. When challenged, no cattle in either group developed clinical infection, showing the long duration of premunition in the cattle population with *B. bovis,* and that in the absence of premunition in the *B. bigemina* group, infection early in life conferred immunity that differed from premunition. In another model, Callow et al. [29] demonstrated immunity to *B. bovis* in cattle which had had drug termination of subclinical infection six months earlier. Presumably because of strain variation within a *Babesia* species, challenge of cattle manifesting subclinical infection (premunition) may result in clinical infection. Strain or antigenic variation within species of protozoan pathogens is a common phenomenon, first documented as an antibody-induced alteration in trypanosomes and later in *Babesia* species. Through such alteration, the parasite theoretically eludes the host's immune response and survives until challenged by the host's production of a new antibody [27].

Interest in the role of the spleen in protection against babesiosis was accelerated by the reports of the initial human infections, all of which occurred in splenectomized individuals. The increased susceptibility of splenectomized chimpanzees to infection with *B. divergens* was demonstrated by Garnham and Bray in 1959 [30]. Using the Gray strain of *B. microti* isolated from Nantucket's first case, the strain designation deriving from the patient's surname, Wolf [31] investigated in hamsters the effects of splenectomy and anti-lymphocyte serum (ALS). Splenectomy before induction of infection resulted in a high and persistent parasitemia; when performed during subclinical or latent infection, splenectomy caused return of parasitemia. ALS effects were more dramatic and, when given before induction of infection, ALS caused high parasitemia and death; when given during subclinical or latent infections, ALS caused relapse with patent infection and death. The action of ALS was thought to be mediated through suppression of T cells, with consequent reduction in T and B cell-mediated immunity.

Some experimental immunization procedures have consisted of the inoculation of infected blood and then control of the level of parasitemia by treatment with a babesiacidal drug. The aim is to provide protection by inducing subclinical infection.

Diagnostic Procedures

Prompt and detailed examination of a blood film well stained by the Giemsa method should be the first step in detecting and characterizing babesial infection. Following fatal infections, touch preparations should be made from the cut surface of the myocardium, kidney, spleen and liver as well as of the peripheral blood because of the higher concentration of the parasites in the capillaries of these tissues.

Serodiagnosis is valuable in testing the individual animal and in surveying an area for subclinical infection. Tests recommended by Mahoney for determining the enzootic status of herds and conducting epizootiologic surveys are the complement-fixation, indirect fluorescent antibody, indirect hemagglutination and rapid agglutination tests [27].

Chemotherapy and Chemoprophylaxis

Development of this aspect of babesiosis has been hampered by the absence of *in vitro* culture systems. Many of the drugs tested are cholinesterase inhibitors, and erythrocytes have a high cholinesterase content. Should bovine *Babesia* require this enzyme, then drug effects may be mediated through the inhibition of the enzyme [32]. That complement is required for the development of *B. rodhaini* in rats, and that in a test system employing human erythrocytes, *B. rodhaini* penetrate only when C3 and C5 with proteins of the alternate pathway are present, has been shown by Chapman and Ward [33]. This may offer new approaches to the development of therapeutic agents.

Drug use must be gauged to assure recovery from clinical infection and also to permit survival of sufficient numbers of parasites so that subclinical infection can ensue.

An effective chemoprophylactic regimen would be welcomed in cattle, horse and sheep-raising regions. Drugs with greater safety than those now available are needed, particularly because antibabesial effects might be required over long periods to permit development of immunity. Candidate drugs would have to have low toxicity and to be free of immunosuppressive effects.

Note: The above account of animal babesiosis is offered in some detail since selected aspects of this subject may have pertinence for human babesiosis. Cases in man are appearing in new sites and continue to appear in those already recognized as potentially endemic; thus the need for both epidemiologic and epizootiologic studies.

IV. BABESIOSIS IN MAN*

A. Clinical Features

Human babesiosis is now recognized as a protozoal infection which may present as (i) severe febrile illness with jaundice and hemoglobinuria observed in some of the initial 4 patients, 3 of whom died, (ii) the moderate to severe clinical infection noted in the 20 or more cases which occurred since 1969, when Nantucket's first case was identified, (iii) mild illness not suggestive of a specific infection, and (iv) subclinical infection

---

* In 1904, L. B. Wilson and W. M. Chowning reported their studies on *Pyroplasma hominis,* which they regarded as a cause of "spotted fever" or "tick fever" of the Rocky Mountains (J. Infect. Dis. 1:31–57, 1904). In a select few of a large number of cases, among whom the mortality rate was high, they identified intra- and extraerythrocytic forms which they classified with, but considered different from, the *Pyrosoma bigeminum* described by Smith and Kilborne in 1893. The observations are difficult to evaluate since there was no further study on this population for babesiosis.

detected through serologic surveys and retrospective study (see Section IV,B, Subclinical Infection).

The incubation period for man and the large domestic animals, estimated from the beginning of tick feeding to the onset of clinical manifestations of infection, ranges from 7 to 16 days [12,27].

(i) The course of the patients who had had splenectomies and whose infections were caused by bovine *Babesia spp.,* which includes all five European cases, was particularly severe. The first three cases proved fatal, each with a clinical course lasting about one week. High fever, hemoglobinemia, hemoglobinuria, anemia, jaundice, anuria, hypotension and coma were the dominant manifestations [1,2]. The remaining two cases in this group had fever, hemolytic anemia, jaundice and anuria with azotemia as principal signs. Serious illness lasted about one month and convalescence was prolonged [34,35]. The ages of the fatal cases were 27, 33 and 48 years, of the nonfatal cases 53 and 61 years. These cases illustrate the role of the spleen in containing babesial infection, and particularly in splenectomized man, the increase in susceptibility to infection with *B. bovis* and *B. divergens.*

The study of Garnham and Bray [30] showed that the chimpanzee and rhesus monkey, like man, were totally resistant to infection with these *Babesia spp.* However, inoculation of the chimpanzee with *B. divergens* after splenectomy resulted in a prolonged parasitemia, during which hemoglobinuria and proteinuria occurred. The parasitemia lasted three weeks, and when blood from the chimpanzee was inoculated three months later into a splenectomized calf, no infection resulted. Thus, the higher ape does not manifest premunition, as do cattle. Splenectomy in the lower African monkey can transform latent infection with *B. pitheci* into a fulminant patent infection which is usually fatal [30].

(ii) The age range of the 20 patients with moderate to severe illness who had intact spleens and had infections proved as, or suspected of being, *B. microti* infections was 37 to 86 years. Thirteen were 56 years old or older. The relatively greater susceptibility of older subjects is comparable to that observed in cattle. Furthermore, assuming exposure to infection being about the same for young and old people, there may be a lesser susceptibility of the young to clinical infection, as obtains among cattle. This is supported by the observations of Osorno et al., who detected asymptomatic infections due to *Babesia spp.* in Mexico in the course of a serologic survey for *Babesia* antibody [36]. In sera from 101 asymptomatic individuals, antibodies to *B. canis* were detected in 38 with titers of 1:10 to 1:80. Blood from 3 of the reactors inoculated into splenectomized hamsters resulted in patent babesial infection. The seropositives were Caucasian males aged 25, 31, and 49 years (see Section IV,B, Subclinical Infection).

Ruebush et al. [12] analyzed the clinical features of 5 cases of *B. microti* infection which occurred on Nantucket in 1975. This brought the number of Nantucket cases then to 7. Symptoms and signs presented by the first 7 cases were, in decreasing order of frequency, fever, fatigue, myalgia and arthralgia, mental depression, drenching sweats, shaking chills, nausea and vomiting, hyperesthesia and splenomegaly. Lymph node enlargement, rash and abnormal neurologic signs were not present. The average age of the patients in this group was 60.8 years. More recent cases on Nantucket and two cases from Martha's Vineyard [37,58] have presented a similar range of clinical features and have occurred in patients usually over 50 years of age.

Three cases of babesiosis occurring on Shelter Island and one in Montauk, Long Island, New York [20,22] involved patients aged 59, 54 and 64 and 57. The first patient was treated for Rocky Mountain spotted fever until plasmodia-like parasites were seen in the blood film, at which time chloroquine and primaquine were administered. The patient became afebrile in three days but had a long convalescence. Intraerythrocytic parasites were not typical of *B. microti* but serum was positive at 1:256 with *B. microti* antigen and negative with malaria antigens at the Center for Disease Control (C.D.C.), Atlanta. The second patient had fever of three weeks' duration, with chills, weakness and malaise. The spleen was palpable and there was pallor, with reduced hematocrit, 26%, hemoglobin 8.5 Gm/dl and red cell count 2.6 million/mm^3. Temperature rose from 104° on admission to 106° F, at which time blood films were made and found to contain malaria-like organisms. Given chloroquine, the patient's fever subsided slowly, but the hemoglobin and hematocrit levels declined further. Two units of blood were required and convalescence was prolonged. The C.D.C., Atlanta reported the blood films as showing *Babesia* species and a *Babesia* antibody titer of 1:1024. The third patient had a febrile episode of 4 days' duration, about 2 weeks following a tick bite. His temperature was 104°F, hemoglobin 8.8 Gm/dl, hematocrit 27.5% and red cell count, 2.45 million/mm^3. He had had a splenectomy the year before, during surgery for hiatus hernia. A long period of fever and lassitude followed. Almost two years after this illness, a serum specimen was sent to the C.D.C., Atlanta, where a *Babesia* antibody titer of 1:4096 was obtained.

The 57 year old patient who acquired *B. microti* infection in Montauk, Long Island, had a prolonged febrile episode with chills, easy fatiguability and anorexia. There was slight jaundice and pallor and no enlargement of the liver, spleen or lymph nodes. The peripheral blood film contained many intraerythrocytic parasites. The clinical response to chloroquine was good and the parasitemia subsided. A relapse occurred three weeks later, with fever and parasitemia. Chloroquine was given again, but the response was slow and convalescence prolonged. The presumptive diagnosis was confirmed by the demonstration of parasitemia in splenectomized hamsters inoculated with the patient's blood and a serum antibody titer of 1:1024 to *B. microti* antigen.

(iii) The presence of mild infection may be established by retrospective serologic study and/or microscopic examination of the stained blood film. Sensitivity is added to the search procedure for *B. microti* if blood from a high-titer seropositive individual is inoculated into a hamster. This has identified carriers who must be regarded as individuals with subpatent infections, since microscopic examination of stained slides for parasites is negative in this group.

Studies by Ruebush et al. [41] to detect self-limited and subclinical human babesiosis on Nantucket were rewarding and informative. Of 710 serum samples collected between August 1975 and July 1976, there were 21 specimens with *B. microti* antibody titers between 1:64 and 1:4096. Of 254 specimens obtained on Martha's Vineyard and on Cape Cod, all had titers of less than 1:16. The test for antibody to *B. microti* employed an indirect immunofluorescent technic. By this method, the seven Nantucket patients referred to above, had titers of 1:1024 or higher. In this serologic survey, individuals with titers of 1:64 or higher were considered seropositive. From seropositives, a medical history and blood film were obtained, as well as blood for inoculation into splenectomized hamsters.

Of the 21 seropositives mentioned above, 11 came from 577 samples collected from patients at the Nantucket Hospital for routine diagnostic tests and 10 from 133 specimens obtained from Nantucket residents and visitors who had a history of tick bite or fever. All of the samples obtained at the Martha's Vineyard and Cape Cod Hospitals came from blood specimens collected for routine diagnostic tests. Of the 19 seropositives who could be contacted, 6 had had a febrile illness in the previous 6 months and 3 had been hospitalized, but all were well at the time of the blood specimen collection and had no history of malaria. Of the hospitalized subjects, one had had a short febrile illness with temporary recovery, followed by a relapse with myalgia and arthralgia of six weeks' duration. Blood films were negative, but the *B. microti* antibody titer was 1:1024. Another hospitalized subject also had fever but with chills, sweating and fatigue. *B. microti* antibody titer was 1:1024. She was discharged within a week, but the blood films collected early in her course were re-stained and examined at the C.D.C., where *Babesia* were found in small numbers on both slides. The third hospitalized subject had a history of fever, chills, headache, malaise and myalgia. Blood films were negative for *Babesia* but the antibody titer was 1:1024. Convalescence required five weeks, and, four weeks after recovery, blood was collected for microscopic examination and was inoculated into two splenectomized hamsters. Blood films were negative for *Babesia,* but both hamsters developed *B. microti* infection. None of the remaining seropositives, even those with serum antibody titers of 1:4096, had blood films positive for *Babesia* during the survey study.

The important conclusions emerging from this study, as summarized by the authors, are as follows: (1) *B. microti* infection in man may range in severity from prolonged febrile illness to self-limited illness, (2) the carrier state may last for weeks to several months and may not be detectable by blood film examination but may be identified by inducing *B. microti* infection in hamsters, (3) the indirect immunofluorescent test for *B. microti* antibody is valuable as a survey tool to detect past infections in an endemic area like Nantucket, and (4) transfusion-induced babesiosis may have occurred but has not been documented. That it could occur can be appreciated from the account of the third hospitalized case, described above. This patient had circulating parasites nine weeks after hospital discharge, at a time when she was well, but the parasitemia could not be proved by blood film examination, only by inoculation of blood into the splenectomized hamster and demonstrating *B. microti* infection.

B. Subclinical Infection

Subclinical babesiosis in man could be expected because many types of human infection may go unrecognized until their identity is disclosed by laboratory tests, and because, in animal babesiosis, the ratio of subclinical to clinical infection is high. An episode of mild babesiosis may not be identified as such until evidence for it emerges from serologic testing and blood film examinations, and also from retrospective examination of blood films prepared during an episode of mild nonspecific illness.

Serologic surveys conducted by Osorno et al. in a Mexican gulf coast region detected as *Babesia* carriers 3 individuals of a group of 101 who had no history of illness. The *Babesia* were identified as probably of rodent origin, since hamsters inoculated with blood from the serologically positive individuals developed babesiosis. The survey covered residents of a Mexican gulf coast rural area known to have enzootic and epizootic bovine, equine, ovine and canine babesiosis [36].

In Nigeria, three populations living in areas known to be endemic for *P. falciparum* and enzootic for *B. bigemina* and *B. bovis* infections were surveyed for malaria and babesiosis [38]. All of the human blood films were negative for *Babesia* organisms. The range of films positive for *P. falciparum* in the three populations was 42%–48% and for *P. malariae,* 2%–12%. All of 173 serum specimens were positive for *Plasmodium* fluorescent antibodies, whereas 23/173 were positive for *B. bigemina* in low IFA (indirect fluorescent antibody) titer, 63/173 for *B. bovis* in higher titers, and 49/173 for *B. ratti* (probably identical to *B. microti*) in titers similar to those for *B. bovis.* Over a third of the sera reacted with more than one babesial antigen. The effect of the antibody response to *P. falciparum* on the titers to babesial antigens is difficult to determine because of cross-reactivity between these antigens [39]. Inoculation of blood from seropositive individuals into splenectomized calves and rats did not result in parasitemia. The results suggest that babesial infection, if indeed present in these Nigerian populations, was well handled by these groups, whose age range was 12 to 37 years. If *B. ratti* is synonymous with *B. microti,* then the hamster would be advised as a sensitive test animal. Some seropositive individuals on Nantucket with negative blood films have been shown to be carriers and have parasitemia on the basis of *B. microti* infection being inducible in hamsters by the inoculation of blood from such individuals.

In Georgia, Healy et al. [40] identified a case of asymptomatic babesiosis in the course of searching for the source of a presumptive *Plasmodium vivax* infection acquired by transfusion. One of five donors had intraerythrocytic organisms in low concentration, presenting features of the small variety of *Babesia.* Attempts to establish the infection in the hamster and monkey were unsuccessful. The donor found positive was a 51 year old black male Georgia resident who had not traveled outside of the United States and had no history of parenteral drug use.

C. Laboratory Diagnosis and Findings

A presumptive diagnosis of babesiosis can be made by identifying in the erythrocyte, one of the various forms which characterize this stage of the parasite's life cycle. In man, infection has been caused thus far only by the small *Babesia spp.,* i.e., *B. bovis, B. divergens* and *B. microti. B. microti* differs from the bovine *Babesia spp.* in that it varies more in size and shape, and forms tetrads. Prime requirements for proper identification in the red cell are (1) a thin blood film which is (2) well stained by the Giemsa method. The *Babesia spp.* will have a blue cytoplasm and a compact mass of red-staining chromatin. The small *Babesia spp.* are round, rod-shaped or ameboid organisms, measuring 20 × 2.5 microns. They contain no pigment, thus distinguishing them from the Plasmodia. They multiply to form 2, 4 or more merozoites, and in heavy infections are seen outside erythrocytes [27,42,43] (Figs. 1-3). Tetrad forms may be produced by budding of *B. microti.* The presence of these forms helps to distinguish *B. microti* and morphologically differentiate it from *Plasmodium spp.*

Steps in the penetration of the red cell by *B. microti* have been illustrated by electron micrography in the studies of Rudzinska, Trager, et al. [44]. Using the Gray strain of *B. microti,* isolated from Nantucket's first case, and hamster erythrocytes, it was observed that the *Babesia* merozoite first touches its anterior end to the erythrocyte and promptly becomes attached to it. At the point of attachment, the host cell membrane invaginates, forming a parasitophorous vacuole. The single membrane of the *Babesia* remains intact, the vacuolar space disappears, and parasite and host cell membranes are applied temporarily one to another. As the host cell membrane disintegrates, the parasite's single membrane becomes the interface between host cell and parasite during its life span in the cell (Figs. 5 and 6).

Serodiagnosis has become an important means of determining the extent of babesial infection in a population [27,41]. For animal populations, Mahoney states that serodiagnosis offers the only practical means of identifying subclinical infection, since blood film examination lacks sensitivity and subinoculation technics are prohibitively expensive [27]. He has outlined the serodiagnostic procedures of preference for the survey of infections in cattle, horses and dogs.

For the survey of *B. microti* in human population groups, Ruebush [41] has employed an indirect immunofluorescent (IIF) antibody test based on technics developed and evaluated at the CDC, Atlanta, by Sulzer et al. [45], Ludford et al. [39] and Chisholm et al. [46]. Required for the test are erythrocytes from hamsters heavily infected with the Gray strain of *B. microti* and goat anti-human immune-globulin labeled with fluorescein isothiocyanate. Test serums are set up in four-fold dilutions beginning with 1:16. With the method they have described, Chisholm et al. found that the IIF test for *B. microti* antibody proved to be sensitive, specific and reproducible. Nine patients with *B. microti* infection tested during their acute phase had antibody titers of ≥1:1024. Serum samples from these patients showed cross-reactivity with three species of *Babesia* (*B. argentina, B. bigemina* and *B. equi*) and three species of *Plasmodium* (*P. vivax, P. falciparum* and *P. brasilianum*), but

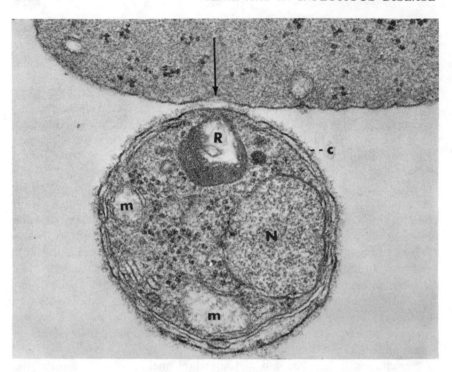

FIG. 5. Merozoite of *B. microti* with apical end touching portion of a hamster reticulocyte. Arrow indicates site of attenuation of the reticulocyte's membrane, with thinning of the coat (c) of the merozoite at the contact point. The area of low density in the rhoptery (R) suggests a release of enzymes from this structure to facilitate the entry of the merozoite. N, nucleus; m, mitochondria. (×59,000)

titers to *B. microti* were almost always higher than titers to other *Babesia* species and the *Plasmodium* species tested. However, serums from these patients had titers high enough to *Plasmodium* species antigens to make it advisable to seek evidence for the presence of both malaria and babesiosis. Also in endemic foci of *B. microti* infection, i.e., Nantucket [47], high serum titers to both *B. microti* and *Plasmodium* species should prompt a search for the presence of both infections (see Section B, above).

Laboratory findings in clinical babesiosis have been referred to above and will be summarized here. In the European cases, all five had had splenectomies and were infected with a bovine *Babesia;* rapid hemolysis occurred with anemia, hemoglobinuria, and hypotension. In the Belfast case [2], for example, the patient was moribund by the fourth day of illness, jaundice and oliguria followed, fever persisted at 103°F, and death came on the seventh day of illness. The hemoglobin level had fallen from

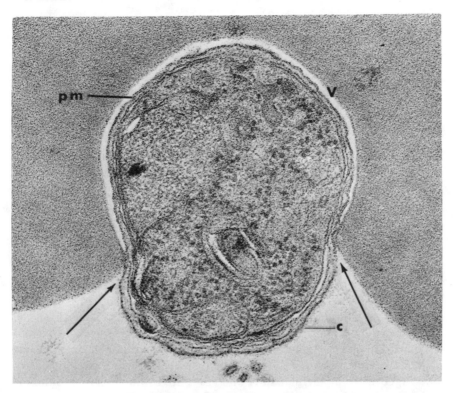

FIG. 6.   Merozoite entering erythrocyte, with the invaginated portion showing a smooth plasma membrane (pm), and outside portion, covered by a coat (c). Ends of the erythrocyte's invaginated membrane adhere closely to the entering merozoite (see arrows). Beginnings of the parasitophorous vacuole are seen at V. (×60,000) (Figs. 5 and 6 were generously provided by Dr. M. Rudzinska of the Rockefeller University [44].)

7.2 g/100 ml to 4.0 g/100 ml, the blood urea had risen from 273 mg/100 ml to 312 mg/100 ml, and reticulocytes peaked at 25%, leukocytes at 46,500 cu/mm. Erythrocytes numbered 1×10^6/cu mm and showed anisocytosis and polychromasia. Polymorphonuclears were 47%, metamyelocytes 19%, myelocytes 22%, and lymphocytes 12%, with 36 immature erythrocytes per 100 leukocytes. Total bilirubin was 5.4 mg/100 ml, with 1.1 direct. Working diagnoses were Weil's disease and then viral hepatitis, until the intraerythrocytic parasites were noted, identified initially as *P. falciparum,* later as *B. divergens.* The principal postmortem findings included (a) intense jaundice of the skin, mucous membranes, serosal surfaces and viscera, (b) a normal heart but lungs heavy because of advanced edema, (c) an enlarged smooth and uniformly yellow liver, and no spleen, (d) swelling of the pancreas with focal fat necrosis, (e) congestion and swelling of the kidneys, each weighing 225 g with red-brown pigment at the corticomedullary junction and with 30 ml of almost black urine in the bladder, and (f) swelling of the brain and bile-staining of the meninges. The blood vessels contained many immature red and white cells, and there was hemoglobinuric nephrosis with dark brown hemoglobin casts in the tubules. There was no malarial pigment, but bile distended the hepatocellular canaliculi. Cerebral vessels and perivascular spaces were distended and leukoerythroblastosis was marked.

In less severe cases of human babesiosis, namely those originating on Nantucket and due to *B. microti,* Ruebush et al. [12] reported (a) lesser degrees of anemia, the lowest level being 8.8 g/dl, (b) no leukocytosis, rather a leukopenia with one count of $3600/mm^3$ upon admission to the hospital, (c) moderately elevated LDH levels, and (d) high IIF titers, ranging between 1:1024 and 1:4096. Four of five patients had transient proteinuria, possibly on the basis suggested by the studies of Annable and Ward [48]. Using the rat and *B. rodhaini,* they demonstrated proteinuria between the 5th and 10th day following infection, with the peak on the 8th day. Onset occurred one day before the appearance of hemoglobinuria, which paralleled the parasitemia. Hypocomplementemia was noted between day 5 and 18, coinciding with the presence of complement and IgG in the glomerular tufts and associated with a transient immune complex type of proliferative glomerulonephritis. Babesial antigen was identified in the complexes eluted from the kidneys. By the 28th day, serum complement levels were normal and glomerular deposits no longer present.

D. Treatment

The first case of babesiosis to receive drug treatment occurred in California, the patient being given chloroquine because malaria was suspected [7]. He recovered, and, after discharge from the hospital, took 250 mg of chloroquine weekly for about two months. The patient had had a splenectomy for hereditary spherocytosis two years before this illness. After study of his blood films at the Center for Disease Control, Atlanta, he became the second recognized case of babesiosis, and was reported as such in 1968. The *Babesia* species was not identified, but microscopic appearance of the parasites was compatible with that of *B. microti,* and other laboratory tests and epidemiologic data also suggested that the *Babesia* could be of rodent origin.

The second patient to receive drug therapy was a Zagreb factory worker who had a *B. divergens* infection which ran a fulminating course to death on the fifth day after onset [10]. He had had a splenectomy in 1966, three years before his fatal illness. Because a bovine *Babesia* was identified on the third day, Berenil® (diminazene aceturate—Hoechst Pharmaceuticals) was given, 3 ml intramuscularly, but this did not affect his course. Berenil® has had wide use in veterinary medicine for treatment of trypanosomiasis, babesiosis and some bacterial infections and trials in human trypanosomiasis.

The next patient, Nantucket's first case, was treated with chloroquine because malaria was diagnosed [11]. Her spleen was intact. She had a remitting fever and appeared pale (hemoglobin 8.8 g/dl; hematocrit 25.5%). Presence of the spleen, which was normal in size, was proved by radioactive scan. Chloroquine phosphate was begun when the presumptive diagnosis of *P. falciparum* infection was made (1.5 g during first day, 0.5 g per day for 30 days). Babesiosis was diagnosed (at the CDC, Atlanta) on the third hospital day, and by the seventh day the patient was afebrile. This *Babesia,* consistent with *B. microti,* became the "Gray" strain, following its establishment in the hamster and splenectomized monkey. Despite the prolonged period of chloroquine therapy, peripheral blood smears contained parasites as late as four months after the onset of infection.

Human babesiosis was not reported again until the 6th documented case, described by Anderson, Cassaday and Healy, occurred on Nantucket in September 1973 [cited in reference 12]. She was given tetracycline upon hospital admission because of a history of recent tick bite, high intermittent fever and because Rocky Mountain spotted fever is endemic on Cape Cod and adjacent islands. Because the high fever continued, a blood film was searched for parasites. Forms resembling *Babesia* were found, tetracycline was discontinued and chloroquine treatment begun on the third hospital day. Although the temperature was elevated for another week, the patient felt definitely improved by the second day of chloroquine treatment. Despite symptomatic improvement on chloroquine, parasites were present for another week. A rapid decline of the hematocrit and slow recovery with hypotension, required administration of two units of blood. Following this, hematocrit and blood pressure stabilized.

The above summarizes the state of therapy for human babesiosis when the first case in Nantucket's small epidemic of 1975 occurred. The studies conducted by Ruebush et al. [12] that year demonstrated that chloroquine phosphate therapy (1.5 g initially and 0.5 g daily or every other day for 2 to 12 weeks) could result in symptomatic improvement and abatement of the fever in 3 to 7 days. However, the parasitemia persisted in 2 patients for 4 weeks and in one for 12 weeks, and convalescence was prolonged, with malaise matching the parasitemia in duration.

There has been no relationship noted between chloroquine treatment and parasitemia, and extended treatment is not advised since this by itself may carry its own risks. Chloroquine treatment should be limited to two weeks, and if no response is obtained, Berenil® [27], pentamidine isethionate or trimethoprim-sulfamethoxazole should be considered. The efficacy of Berenil® in some protozoal infections of animals and man is accepted, and although it is babesiacidal, the risk of its use in man is not known. Pentamidine isethionate (Lomidine®), also administered intramuscularly, has been used in human *Pneumocystis carinii* infections and African sleeping sickness due to *Trypanosoma gambiense* [49]. Because relatively high mortality and morbidity characterize these infections, moderate toxicity is acceptable. However, only drugs of lower toxicity would be acceptable for use in *B. microti* infections. Such a drug may be trimethoprim-sulfamethoxazole, which is given orally, with therapeutic results in *P. carinii* infections which compare favorably with those obtained with pentamidine, and which is free of significant adverse side effects [50]. In acute cases with hypotension, use of a kinin inhibitor, i.e., Trasylol (Bayer, Leverkusen) may be appropriate [27].

E. Epidemiology and Prevention

Man becomes infected with various *Babesia spp.* due to the nondiscriminatory questing behavior of certain vector ticks. In Europe, *Ixodes ricinus* is the major vector for the bovine *Babesia spp.* and in the United States, *Ixodes* sp. nr. *scapularis* has been identified as a major vector in the transmission of *B. microti* to man.

Man and the simian primates tested have a natural resistance to the bovine *Babesia spp.* mentioned above, as well as to *B. bigemina* and less common members of this group [30]. Only splenectomized man has developed clinical infection due to *B. bovis* and *B. divergens,* and these are the only bovine *Babesia spp.* known to have infected man. Man is susceptible to *B. microti* and, until recently, it was not clear why so few human cases have occurred on Nantucket, considering the enormous rodent reservoir of *B. microti* infection and the abundance of vector ticks [47]. The enigma was resolved in part by the recent epidemiologic studies of Ruebush on Nantucket [41] and the tick vector research of Spielman. Ruebush et al. reported that about 8% of 133 Nantucket residents and visitors who gave histories of tick bite or fever had IIF *B. microti* antibody titers of 1:64 or higher. Thus, babesiosis is more prevalent than previously recognized. This evidence, and the clinical features presented by patients with *B. microti* infections occurring on the other islands (Martha's Vineyard, Long Island and Shelter Island) further suggest that a *B. microti* of no unusual virulence has emerged recently in these new foci of human babesiosis.

Examining the tick vector component of the epidemiology of human babesiosis reveals that Nantucket's major vector also thrives on the other islands mentioned above, and in parts of the northern United States and Canada which have not yet seen clinical babesiosis [18]. Spielman and his associates have now delineated the features which remove this tick from the category defined by Cooley and Kohls [19] as *Ixodes scapularis*—thus, the designation *Ixodes* sp. nr. *scapularis,* used earlier in this chapter [51]. The tick vector on Nantucket has manifested an indiscriminate type of questing and feeding behavior in that both the larva and nymph may obtain blood for their development from the mouse (deer mouse and field vole) or the deer or man. The adult tick, however, obtains its blood meal only from larger mammals, primarily the deer. In enzootic murine babesiosis, infection appears to be maintained primarily by the nymph, having developed from a larva which has fed on an infected mouse (transstadial transmission).

During its next feeding in the usual cycle in nature, the nymph infects another mouse. Following the nymph's transformation into an adult, the tick usually feeds on the deer, but not on the mouse, and during this feeding, egg production and fertilization assure the propagation of the tick species. Transovarial transmission of babesiosis in this setting has not been demonstrated. Few adult ticks are infected, and those which may be, do not establish infection in the deer during their feeding because of the deer's natural resistance to *B. microti* infection [51]. The deer provides the adult stage with the blood meal required for completion of the tick's life cycle but has no direct role in maintaining this zoonosis. The nymph has such a role and a direct one, since this stage has emerged from the larva, which, if it has fed on an infected mouse, will transstadially transmit *Babesia* to the nymph, which may now feed on, and infect, a mouse or man. Field studies by Spielman and associates have established that the nymph obtains its blood meal during the late spring and summer [51], the months of the year when most human cases of *B. microti* infection occur. The adult feeds and propagates during the late fall months and into the early spring.

The origin of the *Babesia microti* responsible for the recent human infections is not known, but Tyzzer [52] described the isolation of

Babesia spp. while studying *Cytoecetes microti,* a new parasite of leukocytes of small rodents. Tyzzer's studies focused on field voles and deer mice captured on Martha's Vineyard by Dr. Marshall Hertig in the course of a tick eradication project there [55]. *Babesia spp.* were identified by Tyzzer in the blood of field voles which had been inoculated with a suspension of liver and spleen from field voles and a deer mouse. In a further investigation of field voles from Martha's Vineyard, Tyzzer and Weinman [53] reported *Babesia spp.* among the blood parasites of voles trapped between July 1937 and January 1939. Thus, the presence in this area of what was presumably *B. microti* was recorded over 40 years ago. The tick control work of Wolbach and his associates in 1927 led to the identification of *Ixodes scapularis* among the ticks which inhabited Naushon Island along with *D. variabilis,* these ticks comprising most of that island's tick population [54]. However, *Ixodes scapularis* was absent from Nantucket and Martha's Vineyard between 1937 and 1944, according to surveys cited by Spielman [18].

The remaining component of the epidemiologic picture, the deer, did not appear until the 1930s, when a deer buildup occurred on Nantucket. Deer had been eliminated by hunting pressure by 1880 and only after 1926, when deer from Michigan were brought to Nantucket, was there a return of a deer population [18]. Having accounted historically for the steps in the life cycle of a tick vector for murine babesiosis and presumably for perpetuation of this zoonosis, a question still remains regarding the relatively late appearance in this setting of human *B. microti* infection. The answer may lie in a search for and study of a vector new to this area, which only in recent years has reached a density critical to transmission of infection to man.

On the basis of the above epidemiologic data, efforts to prevent human infection should be concentrated on the control of transmission during the late spring and summer months. Terrain with foliage in which deer, ticks and mice (deer mice and field voles) are known to thrive, should be avoided. If such areas must be entered, then clothing covering the lower parts of the body should be sprayed or impregnated with diethyl toluamide or dimethyl phthalate. After a stay in such an area, the body should be searched carefully for nymphs and adult ticks (note the small size of unengorged nymphs and adults in Fig. 4). If embedded forms are found, it is advised that the entire tick be extracted from the skin, particularly the deeply penetrating hypostome. The application of alcohol, chloroform or comparable agents will not simplify removal.

Effective prevention and control of human infection hinges upon a better understanding of enzootic murine babesiosis. There are now no simple steps that would be effective, because the elimination of babesial infection and its vector involves a cycle that has been perpetuated in wild mammals [43]. A reduction in the numbers of (a) ticks below a disease-maintenance level, (b) mice which constitute the reservoir of infection, and (c) deer which provide the prime haven for the procreative activities of the disease vector, are aims which are logical but difficult to pursue. The most practical would be an effort to control the tick population. Past attempts include a biologic control project devised by Professor E. Brumpt of Paris and Professor S. B. Wolbach of Boston. Brumpt had discovered a chalcid wasp, *Ixodiphagus caucurtei* (akin to *Hunterellus hookeri*), to be a parasite of the important tick vector, *Ixodes ricinus,* with a capacity to destroy it. In a 1913 publication, Brumpt proposed the use of the parasitic wasp to control disease-bearing ticks and particularly *Dermacentor,* the transmitter of Rocky Mountain spotted fever. Brumpt sent parasitized nymphs of two tick species to Wolbach, who found that *D. variabilis* was easily parasitized by the chalcid wasp, as was *I. scapularis,* both common ticks on Naushon Island, where the test was to be conducted. Large numbers of the parasites were released in the fall of 1926 in locations heavily infested by both ticks. Tests conducted the next year suggested a notable decrease of ticks on Naushon, which was in marked contrast to the high density of tick populations in adjacent areas [54]. No further information is available on the project, but tick and tick parasite populations have persisted on the island.

Many of the medically important ticks are subject to infections which they may contract in nature, but whether study of these infections can lead to means of biologic control of these vectors must still be determined. Bacterial, fungal, rickettsial and viral agents have been identified as tick pathogens, some in field studies and others in the laboratory [56,57].

Increased knowledge about the vertebrate host's defense mechanisms against babesial infection may help to explain resistance to some *Babesia spp.,* susceptibility to others, and lead possibly to approaches to prophylaxis against infection. Clark, Wills, Richmond and Allison [60] have demonstrated the unusually effective prophylactic value of BCG against *B. microti* infection in the mouse. Their experiments show convincingly the high level of protection afforded by BCG, taking the form of a nonspecific immunity, when this is administered before the *B. microti* challenge. Parasitemia was short-lived in BCG-treated mice, with clear evidence by electronmicroscopy that intraerythrocytic death of the parasite was mediated by a soluble effector substance acting in the absence of a detectable humoral or phagocytic response. Immunity so induced was noted to protect against *B. microti* challenge for more than six months.

The future incidence of human babesiosis will be a major determinant in the application of possible control measures directed against the tick, the murine reservoir of infection, or the deer. Recurrent and expanding occurrence of human infection would stimulate attempts to provide (a) more effective chemicals for environmental control of ticks, (b) pheromones or pheromone-like chemicals which would impede the propagation of the tick, (c) synthetic hormones which might misdirect the usual propagational events in the tick life cycle, and (d) means to impair the mating and fertilization procedure, possibly through the induction of sterility in the male. Environmental control of ticks through the use of such chemicals as malathion has been effective in containing tick populations living in circumscribed and definable settings. This applies largely to *D. variabilis,* which seeks to feed on the dog, usually living in a domestic setting, and less often to *Ixodes* sp. nr. *scapularis,* which thrives where deer and field rodents abound.

Prevention against infection is currently a matter of personal attention to possible exposure to the vector of *B. microti* and the establishment of safeguards against the other mode of transmission, namely, blood transfusion.

ACKNOWLEDGMENTS

The author thanks Dr. Thomas H Weller for his helpful review of the manuscript, Dr. Andrew Spielman for his generous assistance with the preparation of the narrative and illustrations, Mr. Joseph Piesman for his advice on the selection of figures and references to the literature, and Ms. Ruth M Powers, Ms. Claire Butler and Ms. Nancy Rowan for their expert typing and organization of the manuscript.

REFERENCES

1. Skrabalo Z, Deanovic Z: Piroplasmosis in·man: report on a case. Doc Med Geogr Trop 9:11–16, 1957.
2. Fitzpatrick JEP, Kennedy CC, McGeown MG, et al: Human case of piroplasmosis (babesiosis). Nature 217:861–862, 1968.
3. Exodus, Chapter 9, verse 3; The Holy Bible, King James Version.
4. Babes V: Sur l'hemoglobinurie bacterienne boeuf. Compt Rend Acad Sci 107:692–694, 1888.
5. Smith T, Kilborne FL: Investigation into the nature, causation, and prevention of southern cattle fever. US Dept Agr Bur Anim Indust Bull 1:1–301, 1893.
6. Smith T: Some problems in the etiology and pathology of Texas cattle fever and their bearing on the comparative study of protozoan diseases. Trans Assoc Am Physicians 8:117–134, 1893.
7. Scholtens RG, Braff EK, Healy GR, Gleason N: A case of babesiosis in man in the United States. Am J Trop Med Hyg 17:810–813, 1968.

8. Fitzpatrick JEP, Kennedy CC, McGeown, MG. et al: Further details on third recorded case of redwater (babesiosis) in man. Br Med J 2:770–772, 1969.
9. Garnham PCC, Donelly J, Hoogstraal H, et al: Human babesiosis in Ireland: Further observations and the medical significance of this infection. Br Med J 2:768–770, 1969.
10. Skrabalo Z: Babesiosis. *In:* Marcial-Rojas RA (Ed): Pathology of Protozoal and Helminthic Diseases. Baltimore, Williams and Wilkins, 1971, pp 232–233.
11. Western KA, Benson GD, Gleason NN, et al: Babesiosis in a Massachusetts resident. N Engl J Med 283:854–856, 1970.
12. Ruebush TK II, Cassaday PB, Marsh HJ, et al: Human babesiosis on Nantucket Island. Clinical features. Ann Intern Med 86:6–9, 1977.
13. Levine ND: Taxonomy of the piroplasms. Trans Am Microsc Soc 90:2–33, 1971.
14. Wright IG, Mahoney DF: The activation of kallikrein in acute *Babesia argentina* infections of splenectomised calves. Z Parasitenkd 43:271–278, 1974.
15. Koch R: Beitrage zur Entwicklungsgeschichte der Piroplasmen. Z Hyg und Infektions-krankheiten 54:1–9, 1906.
16. Riek RF: The life cycle of *Babesia bigemina* (Smith and Kilborne, 1893) in the tick vector *Boophilus microplus* (Canestrini). Aust J Agr Res 15:802–821, 1964.
17. Riek RF: Babesiosis. *In:* Weinman D, Ristic M (Eds): Infectious Blood Diseases of Man and Animals. New York, Academic Press, 1968, pp 219–268.
18. Spielman A: Human babesiosis on Nantucket Island: transmission by nymphal *Ixodes* ticks. Am J Trop Med Hyg 25:784–787, 1976.
19. Cooley RA, Kohls GM: The genus *Ixodes* in North America NIH Bull 184:1–246, 1945.
20. Grunwaldt E: Babesiosis on Shelter Island. NY State J Med 77:1320–1321, 1977.
21. Scharfman WB, Taft EG: Nantucket Fever. An additional case of babesiosis. JAMA 238:1281–1282, 1977.
22. Parry MF, Fox M, Burka SA, Richar WJ: *Babesia microti* infection in man. JAMA 238:1282–1283, 1977.
23. Hoogstraal H: Acarina (ticks). *In:* Gibbs AJ (Ed): Viruses and Invertebrates. London, North-Holland Publishing Co., 1973, pp. 90–103.
24. Balashov, YS: Bloodsucking Ticks (Ixodoidea)—Vectors of Diseases of Man and Animals. Leningrad, Nauka Publishers, 1968, pp. 223–297. (Translated and published as No. 5, Miscellaneous Publications of the Entomological Society of America 8:161–376, 1972.)
25. Hoogstraal H, Theiler G.: Ticks (*Ixodoidea, Ixodidae*) parasitizing lower primates in Africa, Zanzibar and Madagascar. J Parasitol 45:217–222, 1959.
26. Philip, CB: Tick transmission of Indian tick typhus and some related rickettsioses. Exp Parasitol 1:129–142, 1952.
27. Mahoney DF: Babesiosis of domestic animals. *In:* Kreier JP (Ed): Parasitic protozoa, Vol IV. New York, Academic Press, 1977, pp 1–52.
28. Mahoney DF, Wright IG, Mirre GB: Bovine babesiasis: the persistance of immunity to *Babesia argentina* and *B. bigemina* in calves (*Bos taurus*) after naturally acquired infection. Ann Trop Med Parasitol 67:197–203, 1973.
29. Callow LL, McGregor W. Parker RJ, Dalgliesh RJ: The immunity of cattle to *Babesia argentina* after drug sterilisation of infections of varying duration. Aust Vet J 50:6–11, 1974.
30. Garnham PCC, Bray RS: The susceptibility of the higher primates to piroplasms. J Protozool 6:352–355, 1959.
31. Wolf RE: Effects of antilymphocyte serum and splenectomy on resistance to *Babesia microti* infection in hamsters. Clin Immunol Immunopath 2:381–394, 1974.

32. Eyre P: Some pharmacodynamic effects of the babesicidal agents quinuronium and amicarbalide. J Pharm Pharmacol 19:509–519, 1967.

33. Chapman WE, Ward PA: *Babesia rhodaini:* Requirement of complement for penetration of human erythrocytes. Science 196:67–70, 1977.

34. Gorenflot A, Piette M, Marchand A: Animal babesiosis and human health: Babesioses animales et santé humaine. First case of human babesiosis observed in France. Rec Med Vet 152:289–297, 1976.

35. Bazin C, Lamy C, Piette M, et al: A new case of human babesiosis. Nouv Presse Med 5:799–800, 1976.

36. Osorno BM, Vega C, Ristic M, et al: Isolation of *Babesia* spp. from asymptomatic human beings. Vet Parasitol 2:111–120, 1976.

37. Miller LH, Neva FA, Gill F: Failure of chloroquine in human babesiosis (*Babesia microti*). Ann Intern Med 88:200–202, 1978.

38. Leeflang P, Oomen JMV, Dwart D, Neuwissen HET: The prevalence of *Babesia* antibodies in Nigerians. Internat J Parasitol 6:159–161, 1976.

39. Ludford CG, Hall WTK, Sulzer AJ: *B. argentina, P. vivax,* and *P. falciparum:* antigenic cross-reactions. Exp Parasitol 32:317–326, 1972.

40. Healy GR, Walzer PD, Sulzer AJ: A case of asymptomatic babesiosis in Georgia. Am J Trop Med Hyg 25:376–378, 1976.

41. Ruebush, TK, Juranek DD, Chisholm ES, et al: Human babesiosis on Nantucket Island. Evidence for self-limited and subclinical infections. N Engl J Med 297:825–827, 1977.

42. Imes GD JR, Neafie RC: Babesiosis. *In:* Binford CH, Connor DH (Eds): Pathology of Tropical and Extraordinary Diseases. Washington, D.C., Armed Forces Institute of Pathology, 1976, pp. 301–302.

43. Ristic M, Lewis GE JR: Babesia in man and wild and laboratory-adapted mammals. *In:* Kreier JP (Ed): Parasitic Protozoa, Vol IV. New York, Academic Press, 1977, pp. 53–76.

44. Rudzinska MA, Trager W, Lewengrub SJ, Gubert E: An electron microscopic study of *Babesia microti* invading erythrocytes. Cell Tissue Res 169:323–334, 1976.

45. Sulzer AF, Wilson M, Hall EC: The use of thick smear antigen slides in the malarial indirect immunofluorescent antibody test. Am J Trop Med Hyg 18:199–205, 1969.

46. Chisholm ES, Ruebush TK II, Sulzer AJ, Healy GH: *Babesia microti* infection in man: evaluation of an indirect immunofluorescent antibody test. Am J Trop Med Hyg 27:14–19, 1978.

47. Healy GR, Spielman A, Gleason N: Human babesiosis: reservoir of infection on Nantucket Island. Science 192:479–480, 1976.

48. Annable CR, Ward PA: Immunopathology of the renal complications of babesiosis. J Immunol 112:1–8, 1974.

49. Western KA, Perera DR, Schultz MG: Pentamidine Isethionate in the treatment of *Pneumocystis carinii* pneumonia. Ann Intern Med 73:695–702, 1970.

50. Lau WK, Young LS: Trimethoprimsulfamethoxazole treatment of *Pneumocystis carinii* pneumonia in adults. New Engl J Med 295:716–718, 1976.

51. Spielman A, Piesman J, Etkind P: Personal communication.

52. Tyzzer EE: *Cytoecetes microti* ng nsp, a parasite developing in granulocytes and infective for small rodents. Parasitology 30:242–257, 1938.

53. Tyzzer EE, Weinman D: *Haemobartonella* ng, *H microti* nsp of the field vole, *Microtus pennsylvanicus.* Am J Hyg 30:141–157, 1939.

54. Larrouse F, King AG, Wolbach SB: Overwintering in Massachusetts of *Ixodiphagus caucurtei.* Science 67:351–353, 1928.

55. Hertig M, Smiley D: The problem of controlling woodticks on Martha's Vineyard. Vineyard Gazette, 15 January 1937.
56. Hoogstraal H: XXI Pathogens of Acarina (ticks). *In:* Roberts DW Strand MA (Eds): Pathogens of Medically Important Arthropods. Geneva, World Health Organization, 1977, pp 337–340.
57. Strand MA: Ibid, pp 341–342.
58. Younger LR: Personal communication, 1977.
59. Rudzinska MA, Trager W: Formation of merozoites in intraerythrocytic *Babesia microti:* an ultrastructural study. Can J Zool 55:928–938, 1977.
60. Clark IA, Wills EJ, Richmond JE, Allison AC: Suppression of babesiosis in BCG-infected mice and its correlation with tumor inhibition. Infect & Immun 17:430–438, 1977.

CHAPTER 8

ANTIVIRAL AGENTS

Douglas D. Richman, M.D. and
Michael N. Oxman, M.D.

In this review we shall discuss major problems encountered in the development and evaluation of antiviral agents, describe the process of virus replication and the sites of action of a number of current and prospective antiviral agents, and summarize the results of controlled trials of antiviral chemoprophylaxis and chemotherapy in man. We will not consider active or passive immunization. No attempt will be made to discuss all of the agents which inhibit virus replication in cell cultures or animals, or to summarize the voluminous uncontrolled experience with antiviral drugs in man. The reader may find much of this information in several published symposia and reviews [17,37,113,114,198,236,286a].

The impact of chemotherapy and chemoprophylaxis on viral diseases has been negligible in comparison with the impact of antibiotics on bacterial diseases. The lack of success with antiviral agents is due, in large part, to fundamental differences between viruses and bacteria. Bacteria are endowed with sufficient genetic information to specify all of the structures and metabolic pathways required for autonomous growth. Furthermore, as a result of their independent evolution, bacterial and animal cells exhibit great differences in structure, metabolism and mode of replication. These differences provide numerous targets for the selective inhibition of bacterial multiplication. Viruses, in contrast, have a much smaller endowment of genetic information than bacteria, far too little to specify all of the metabolic reactions, structural components and organelles required for virus replication. Consequently, viruses are obligate intracellular parasites dependent upon their host cells for the energy, nucleotide and amino acid building blocks, and metabolic

From the Departments of Medicine and Pathology, University of California, San Diego, Calif., and the San Diego Veterans Administration Hospital.

Acknowledgments: We are grateful for the excellent secretarial assistance of Mrs. Delfinia King, Mrs. Mary Beyers and Mrs. Virginia Hennings.

Research by the authors was supported by USPHS Research Grant AI-13872 from the National Institute of Allergy and Infectious Disease, National Science Foundation Grant PCM 76-22432, and by the Research Service of the Veterans Administration.

machinery required for replication. Since there are relatively few virus-specific metabolic reactions, there are relatively few potential targets for selective chemotherapy. The fact that all virus-associated metabolic activity takes place within the infected cell imposes the added restriction that, to be effective, an inhibitor of virus replication must traverse the host cell membrane and achieve an adequate intracellular concentration. In many cases, the cell membrane constitutes a formidable barrier to effective chemotherapy, a problem which has also complicated the antibiotic therapy of intracellular bacterial infections [123,242,276]. Finally the toxicity of an antibiotic is only rarely due to the mechanism by which it inhibits bacterial growth, whereas the same mechanism of action underlies the antiviral activity and the host cell toxicity of most antiviral drugs. As a consequence, the therapeutic index (the ratio of the minimum toxic dose to the minimum effective dose) of most currently available antiviral agents is low.

The viral chemotherapist must also contend with a frequent difference between viral and bacterial diseases. The signs and symptoms of bacterial disease generally develop in parallel with the growth of the bacterial population. This permits the establishment of a diagnosis and the initiation of therapy prior to maximal bacterial multiplication and dissemination. In contrast, virus multiplication and dissemination often peak during the incubation period and are diminishing during symptomatic illness. Consequently, by the time the viral disease is recognized, the extent of tissue involvement and the concentration of virus may be so great that chemotherapy is rendered relatively ineffective. The problem is further complicated by the frequent participation of host immune responses in the production of pathology. Thus, inhibition of virus multiplication may not always halt the progression of a virus-induced disease.

The capacity of the clinical bacteriology laboratory to rapidly, accurately and economically isolate and identify bacterial pathogens has facilitated the evaluation and rational use of antibiotics in bacterial infections. Diagnostic virology is more difficult, expensive, time-consuming and insecure. The paucity of rapid and reliable viral diagnostic procedures will make the rational choice of chemotherapeutic agents difficult, particularly if these agents are effective against a narrow spectrum of viruses. The problem of establishing a reliable viral diagnosis has already had an adverse effect upon the clinical evaluation of candidate antiviral agents in man. It is now apparent that the prognosis is quite different in cases of herpes simplex virus encephalitis diagnosed on clinical grounds and definitively diagnosed by isolation of virus from central nervous system tissue [25,322]. Much of the confusion as to the clinical efficacy of iododeoxyuridine in this disease can be traced to differences

TABLE 1. Animal Virus Genetic Systems[1]

Class[2]	Genome	mRNA Transcription	Virion-associated transcriptase for mRNA synthesis	Genome Replication	Necessary involvement of virus-specific replicase	Examples
I	+DNA	+DNA → +RNA	No (but present in poxviruses)	+DNA → +DNA	No[3]	DNA Viruses: Poxviruses Herpesviruses Adenoviruses Papovaviruses Hepatitis B virus
II	+RNA	+RNA → −RNA → +RNA	No	+RNA → −RNA → +RNA	Yes	Picornavirus Togaviruses Coronaviruses
III	−RNA	−RNA → +RNA	Yes	−RNA → +RNA → −RNA	Yes	Orthomyxoviruses Paramyxoviruses Arenaviruses Rhabdoviruses
IV	±RNA	±RNA → +RNA	Yes	±RNA → +RNA → ±RNA	Yes	Reoviruses Orbiviruses Rotaviruses
V	+RNA	+DNA → +RNA	No	$+RNA \to -DNA \to \pm DNA \to \dfrac{+RNA}{+RNA}$	Yes[4]	Oncornaviruses

[1] Modified from Baltimore [12].

[2] Single-stranded DNA viruses (parvoviruses) omitted from consideration.

[3] But present in some members (e.g., Herpesviruses, Poxviruses, Hepatitis B virus).

[4] RNA-dependent DNA polymerase.

between the diagnostic criteria applied to drug recipients and control patients. The bacterial chemotherapist has available rapid, inexpensive and well standardized *in vitro* antibiotic sensitivity tests, the results of which are highly predictive of *in vivo* efficacy. This facilitates the choice of antibiotics in clinical situations and provides a reliable and economical means for the detection and selection of new antibiotics. These *in vitro* tests have no parallel in viral chemotherapy. A major problem in the development and selection of drugs for the chemotherapy of viral diseases has been the poor correlation between *in vitro* and *in vivo* data obtained with the same virus-drug combinations [256].

The problems outlined above are formidable, but there is reason for some optimism. While the number of potential targets for selective metabolic inhibition is certainly much smaller for viral than for bacterial pathogens, biochemical and biophysical studies of viruses and of virus replication have revealed essential steps in the virus replication cycle which have no counterpart in animal cells. These studies have also demonstrated that the genomes of many viral pathogens differ fundamentally from the genome of the animal cell. These different viral genetic systems require modes of genome replication and transcription which differ from those of the host cell (Table 1), and the enzymes and intermediates involved offer potential targets for truly selective antiviral chemotherapy. Perhaps the most compelling evidence for the existence of fundamental differences between viral and cellular gene expression is the capacity of interferon, by an unknown mechanism, to inhibit the replication of a wide variety of DNA and RNA viruses in the absence of significant toxicity for host cells.

Many of the antiviral drugs which we have today were developed as cytotoxic agents for cancer chemotherapy. Thus their toxicity should not be surprising. Thorough exploration of the mechanism of their antiviral action and of their toxicity for host cells should provide information to guide the synthesis of more selective antiviral drugs. Thus the next generation of antiviral drugs, aimed at molecular events unique to virus replication and selected for the absence of host cell toxicity, should have much higher therapeutic indices that those which we have today.

THE VIRUS REPLICATION CYCLE AND SITES OF ACTION OF ANTIVIRAL AGENTS

The Initial Virus-Cell Interaction

The initial events in the virus replication cycle are *attachment* of the infecting virion to the host cell membrane, *penetration* of the virion into the host cell cytoplasm and *uncoating* of the viral nucleic acid. These viral processes would appear to have no counterpart in the uninfected mammalian cell. Thus they constitute a potential target for selective inhibition of virus replication. Attachment refers to the adsorption of the virus to the cell. Attached virus is not removed by ordinary washing procedures, but it remains on the external surface of the cell membrane, where it is still accessible to neutralization by specific antibody. When the virus has penetrated the cell membrane it is no longer accessible to neutralization by antibody, but the capsid is still intact and thus the viral nucleic acid is not accessible to nucleases. When uncoating occurs, the viral genome becomes susceptible to hydrolysis by nucleases.

Attachment is mediated by the interaction of a protein on the surface of the virus (a capsid protein in the case of nonenveloped viruses or an envelope glycoprotein in the case of enveloped viruses) with a specific site (*receptor*) on the cell membrane. This interaction is usually highly specific. Some receptors (e.g., those for ortho- and certain para-myxoviruses) are glycoproteins containing terminal N-acetylneuraminic acid (NANA), whereas others (e.g., the receptors for most picor-naviruses) appear to be lipoproteins. The presence or absence of recep-tors for a particular viruses, which is under host cell genetic control [93,192,201] is usually the major determinant of the susceptibility of the cell to infection. Thus, virus receptors play a key role in governing the species, organ and tissue tropism of viruses. Considering their importance, remarkably little is known of the structure and function of the cellular receptors for most viruses.

Since attachment involves the interaction of a viral surface protein with a cell surface receptor, agents which interfere with the function of either can prevent infection. For example, specific neutralizing antibodies are generally directed at viral surface proteins which mediate attach-ment. Similarly, NANA-containing glycoproteins found in mucous and serum may act as nonspecific inhibitors of the attachment of ortho- and paramyxoviruses by binding to their hemagglutinin subunits. Negatively charged polyanions, such as heparin, hyaluronic acid and sulfated agar polysaccharides, can interact with a variety of enveloped and nonen-veloped viruses, preventing their attachment to susceptible cells. The enzyme neuraminidase can destroy cell surface receptors for myxoviruses by removing NANA residues. Such treated cells are resistant to infection until new receptors are synthesized. Certain substances, such as concanavalin A, which bind to and alter cell surfaces, can block infection by a number of different viruses, also apparently by inhibiting attach-ment [221]. Prevention of virus attachment plays a central role in natural resistance to virus infection and, mediated by antiviral antibodies, is the major component of the resistance which develops following virus infection or immunization with killed or live attenuated virus vaccines. Furthermore, the efficacy of prophylactically administered immune globulins is dependent upon the capacity of passively acquired antiviral antibodies to prevent attachment by neutralizing extracellular virus. Unfortunately, this aspect of the virus replication cycle has yet to be effectively exploited for antiviral chemotherapy or chemoprophylaxis.

The processes of penetration and uncoating are poorly understood, mainly because of the limitations of methods by which they can be examined *in vitro*. These methods include electron microscopic examination of infected cells, and the biochemical and biophysical analysis of the fate of radiolabeled virions. Although the infection of a cell under natural conditions is probably initiated by only a few (and perhaps only one) infectious virions, both of these experimental approaches utilize high multiplicities of infection, as well as virus stocks which contain a large proportion of noninfectious virions. Since the results obtained are determined by the behavior of the majority of virions, they may not represent the fate of the small minority which actually initiate infection. Mechanisms described by which virions traverse the plasma membrane include direct penetration of intact virions, engulfment in vesicles formed at the cell surface by phagocytosis (viropexis) and, in the case of enveloped viruses, fusion of the viral envelope with the plasma membrane, which liberates the nucleocapsid directly into the cytoplasm. With some picornaviruses, the whole virion may fail to penetrate the plasma membrane, in which case uncoating takes place at the cell surface with the direct entry of the viral nucleic acid into the cytoplasm. In this situation, the distinction between penetration and uncoating may be artificial.

The process of uncoating, which results in the release of the viral nucleic acid from the viral capsid, varies in complexity with the size and complexity of the virus involved. With most viruses, uncoating is accomplished by the cell and does not involve virus-specific enzymes. However, in the case of the poxviruses, uncoating occurs in two stages. In the first, cellular enzymes degrade the outer viral membrane and convert the virus to a subviral particle called a "core," which contains the viral DNA and a DNA-dependent RNA polymerase. The virion polymerase then transcribes messenger RNA (mRNA) from a portion of the viral DNA within the core, and this mRNA is translated into early viral protein. The second stage, which results in the release of the viral genome, requires the participation of the early viral protein. The fact that, with most viruses, penetration and uncoating are accomplished by cellular processes might suggest that this portion of the virus replication cycle

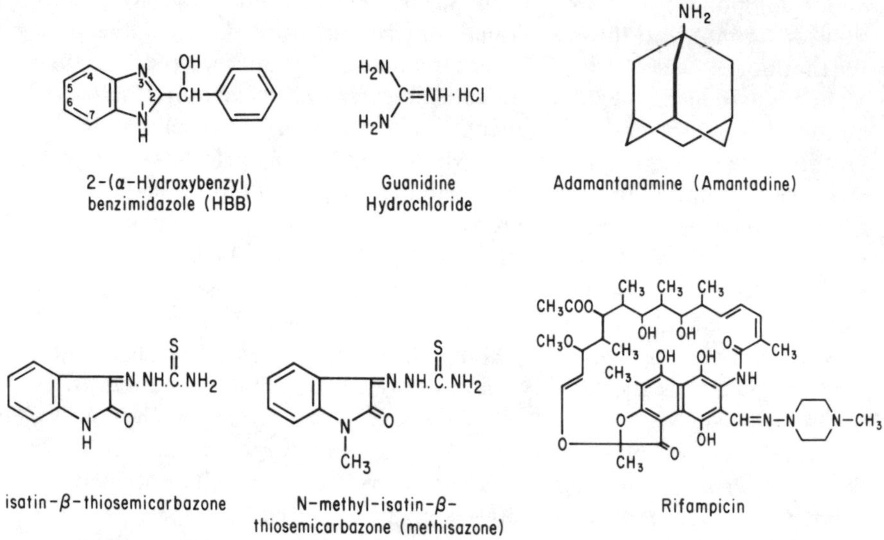

2-(α-Hydroxybenzyl)
benzimidazole (HBB)

Guanidine
Hydrochloride

Adamantanamine (Amantadine)

isatin-β-thiosemicarbazone

N-methyl-isatin-β-
thiosemicarbazone (methisazone)

Rifampicin

FIG. 1

is an unlikely target for selective inhibitors of virus multiplication. However, this is the site of action of amantadine hydrochloride
(l-adamantanamine hydrochloride, Symmetrel®, Fig. 1) a symmetrical
tricyclic amine that has proved to be a clinically effective and nontoxic
chemoprophylactic and chemotherapeutic agent. In fact, it is the only
drug for viral respiratory disease currently licensed in the United States.
Amantadine and its derivatives (e.g., α-methyl-l-adamantanemethyl-
amine hydrochloride [rimantadine hydrochloride] and N-methyladaman-
tanespiro-3'-pyrrolidine hydrochloride) have been reported to inhibit
strains of influenza A, arenaviruses, and certain other viruses in tissue
culture [120,213]. Amantadine and its derivatives prevent infection by
combining with the plasma membrane and inhibiting the penetration
[118,318] or uncoating [67,148] of infecting virions. Amantadine may
also inhibit the release of some enveloped viruses [318]. Cycloocytlamine
hydrochloride, another alicyclic amine, also inhibits infection by
influenza A and certain other enveloped viruses in tissue culture. Its
mode of action appears to be the same as that of amantadine.

Transcription of Parental Virus Genomes

Following uncoating, the sequence of events involved in virus replication varies greatly, depending upon the nature of the viral genome and its

site of replication. However, prior to genome replication, all viruses must synthesize mRNA, which serves as template for the synthesis of enzymes and other essential viral proteins [12]. Except for those viruses which, like mammalian cells, have double-stranded DNA genomes (Class I, Table 1) the pathway of viral mRNA synthesis will differ from that of the host cell and will require enzymes not ordinarily present in uninfected cells. In the case of RNA viruses with genomes which do not themselves function as mRNA, an RNA-dependent RNA polymerase is packaged within the virion (e.g., Class III, Table 1). Following uncoating, these virion polymerases transcribe mRNA, using the virion RNA as template. Most double-stranded DNA viruses replicate in the cell nucleus, where transcription of viral mRNA is carried out by cellular RNA polymerase II. Poxviruses are an exception. Their replication takes place in the cytoplasm and is independent of the cell nucleus. Perhaps for this reason they possess a virus-specific DNA-dependent RNA polymerase which is packaged in the virion. As noted above, this enzyme must transcribe the mRNA for the early viral protein required to complete the uncoating of the viral genome. Oncornaviruses (Class V, Table 1) are remarkable in that their replication requires a double-stranded DNA intermediate, the synthesis of which is accomplished by a unique enzyme, RNA-dependent DNA polymerase ("reverse transcriptase") which is present in the virion [11,303]. Although virion polymerases would appear to represent ideal targets for selective antiviral agents, there has been little progress in this area to date. A variety of compounds that chelate zinc are capable of inhibiting the virion RNA polymerase of influenza virus *in vitro* [223,225,226]. Rifampicin (Fig. 1) and its derivatives are antibiotics which bind to and inhibit bacterial but not animal cell RNA polymerases [316]. The virion RNA-dependent DNA polymerase of oncornaviruses is inhibited *in vitro* by some rifampicin derivatives, as well as by a variety of other compounds [22], and this may account, at least in part, for the capacity of these compounds to inhibit oncornavirus replication and oncornavirus-induced cell transformation [207].

Interferons, which will be discussed in more detail in the next section, have been reported to inhibit transcription of the parental viral genome by virion RNA polymerase in the case of vesicular stomatitis virus (a rhabdovirus) and influenza virus [15,185,187,188]. Interferon has also been shown to selectively inhibit the production of early viral mRNA in cells infected with simian virus 40, a papovavirus closely related to agents isolated from the brains of individuals with progressive multifocal leukoencephalopathy [200,227,328]. There are several reports of inhibition of viral mRNA synthesis in cells infected with other DNA viruses as well [88].

Other compounds, such as actinomycin D, which blocks DNA-directed RNA synthesis by binding to the DNA template, and α-amanitin, which selectively inhibits mammalian RNA polymerase II, are also capable of blocking the primary transcription of DNA virus genomes. In addition, where RNA virus replication requires host cell DNA function, as is the case for influenza virus, inhibitors of host cell DNA-dependent transcription can block virus replication. Although such inhibitors have proven useful for the study of virus replication in tissue culture, they have equivalent effects on host cell and virus mRNA synthesis, and thus have no therapeutic potential.

Synthesis of Viral Proteins

The synthesis of viral proteins is a vital step in the virus replication cycle and a prerequisite for viral genome replication. RNA viruses must synthesize RNA-dependent RNA polymerases, as well as structural proteins. With most DNA viruses, primary transcription of the incoming viral DNA results in the synthesis of mRNA corresponding to only a portion of the viral genome (the "early" genes). This early mRNA is translated to early viral proteins, which include the uncoating enzyme of the poxviruses, enzymes and other proteins which alter metabolic pathways in the host cell to facilitate viral DNA and protein synthesis, and enzymes concerned with DNA replication, such as the virus-specific DNA-dependent DNA polymerases of herpesviruses and poxviruses and the herpesvirus-induced deoxypyrimidine kinase. The viral DNA is then replicated, and it is the progeny viral DNA molecules which serve as templates for the transcription of mRNA from the remainder of the viral genome (from the "late" genes). The products of these late genes are mainly viral structural proteins. Although host cell ribosomes are utilized in the translation of viral mRNA, there is considerable evidence that viral mRNA differs in some fundamental way from cellular mRNA. For example, it is common during viral infection to observe the total cessation of cellular mRNA translation at a time when translation of viral mRNA is proceeding rapidly. This is presumably due to the synthesis of a virus-coded protein that specifically blocks the translation of cellular mRNA without adversely affecting the translation of viral mRNA. Even more compelling evidence for this fundamental difference is provided by the action of interferons [88,136].

Interferons are natural antiviral proteins produced by animal cells in response to virus infection or following exposure to certain nonviral inducers. They selectively inhibit the replication of a broad range of DNA and RNA viruses [88,118,199,308]. Although interferon preparations have been reported to inhibit cell multiplication *in vitro* and depress immune reponses in animals, cells generally exhibit no toxic effects when exposed to several hundred times the concentration of interferon required to render them resistant to virus infection. Thus, potentially, interferons have a very high therapeutic index. Interferons also exhibit a remarkably high specific activity. Assuming a molecular weight of 25,000, human interferon can protect cells against virus infection at a concentration of 10^{-12}M. Interferons also exhibit relative species specificity, probably because their activity requires the presence of a specific interferon receptor on the cell surface. For example, interferons produced by mouse or chicken cells will not protect human cells. The action of interferon is indirect. The attachment of interferon to the cell surface does not itself render the cell resistant to virus infection. Rather, it appears to result in the derepression of one or more cell genes, transcription of the corresponding mRNA(s) and synthesis of one or more proteins (antiviral proteins) which are actually responsible for the cell's resistance to virus infection. The exact mechanism by which virus replication is inhibited is still not clear. In fact, more than one step in the virus replication cycle may be affected. Interferon-induced inhibition of virus replication is characterized by the selective inhibition of viral protein synthesis. Although in some cases this may be due, at least in part, to inhibition of viral mRNA synthesis (see above) the major effect of interferon appears to be inhibition of translation of viral mRNA. The exact mechanism has yet to be fully elucidated, but it appears that an interferon-induced antiviral protein inhibits the capacity of cellular ribosomes to translate viral mRNA without reducing their capacity to translate host cell mRNA. Thus the interferon system is able to distinguish between viral and cellular mRNA. This capacity to selectively inhibit viral protein synthesis, and thereby selectively inhibit the replication of a broad range of DNA and RNA viruses, has encouraged attempts to use exogenous interferon for the chemotherapy of viral diseases.

Isatin-β-thiosemicarbazone (IBT) and its N-methyl derivative (methisazone, Marboran®, Fig. 1) interfere with viral protein synthesis and, as a consequence, are potent inhibitors of poxvirus multiplication in tissue culture [13,175,326]. Inhibition of adenovirus replication has also been reported, and some IBT derivatives inhibit the multiplication of certain picornaviruses [13,175]. At least in the case of poxviruses, these drugs act by selectively inhibiting the translation of late viral mRNA. This may be due to the induction of a cellular protein that blocks the association of late poxvirus mRNA with ribosomes.

Many other compounds, such as puromycin, cycloheximide and amino acid analogs like p-fluorophenylalanine, which interfere with host cell protein synthesis, also inhibit viral protein synthesis. However, they have no selective effect on viral protein synthesis and thus have no therapeutic potential.

Viral Genome Replication

The replication of RNA virus genomes requires an RNA-dependent RNA polymerase (replicase) which has no counterpart in the uninfected cell; however, few compounds have been described which selectively inhibit RNA genome replication. Two such agents, guanidine and 2-(α-hydroxybenzyl)-benzimidazole (HBB) (Fig. 1) are specific inhibitors of picornavirus replication in tissue culture [37]. These compounds inhibit the replication of viral RNA in cells, but have no effect on the activity of the replicase enzyme *in vitro*. They probably act by altering the function of a viral protein that regulates the process of viral RNA synthesis in the infected cell [53,54]. The rapid emergence of drug-resistant and drug-dependent mutants, and the relative lack of efficacy in animals, have discouraged further exploration of this important area. However, recent

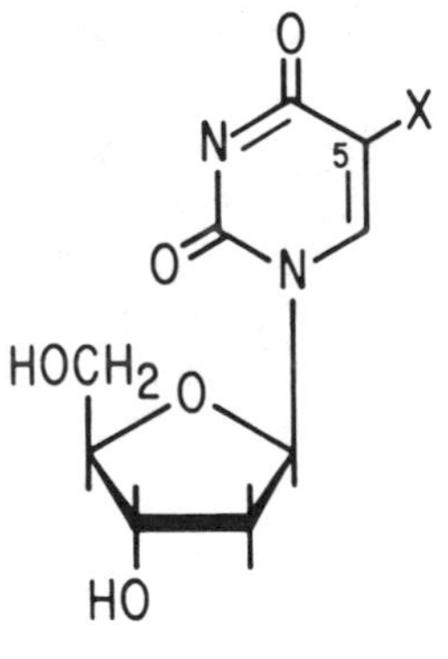

X	van der Waals' radii (A°)	Compound
H	1.2	UdR
F	1.35	FUdR
Cl	1.80	CUdR
Br	1.95	BUdR
CH₃	2.0	TdR
I	2.15	IUdR
CF₃	2.44	F₃TdR

5-substituted pyrimidine deoxyribosides

FIG. 2

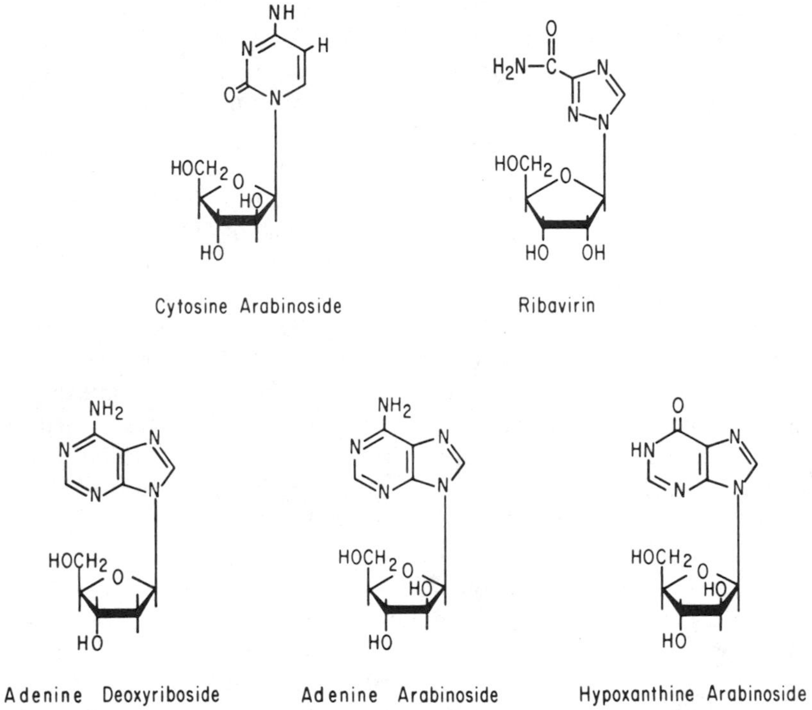

FIG. 3

studies indicating the efficacy of the combination of these two compounds in animals [76] suggest that further work with these and related compounds may be rewarding.

Ribavirin (1-β-D-ribofuranosyl-1,2,4-triazole-3-carboxamide, Virazole®, Fig. 3) is a synthetic nucleoside which has been reported to have antiviral activity in tissue culture against a variety of DNA and RNA viruses, including herpesviruses and influenza viruses [126,280]. It is an analog of guanosine [247,292], which is phosphorylated in mammalian cells and tissues to the mono-, di-, and triphosphate [202]. Ribavirin monophosphate is a potent competitive inhibitor of inosine-5′-phosphate (IMP) dehydrogenase. As a consequence, ribavirin interferes with the biosynthesis of guanine nucleotides and thus with nucleic acid synthesis. This mode of action does not, in itself, provide an explanation for any selective inhibition of viral replication. However, virus specificity might occur in nondividing cells because of the greater need for nucleic acid synthesis by the virus than by the cell. The drug might also exhibit greater toxicity for infected than uninfected cells if nucleoside kinases induced by virus infection facilitated the entry of ribavirin into the infected cells. Recently, ribavirin triphosphate has been shown to selectively inhibit the influenza virion RNA polymerase *in vitro* [79] and this may explain the selective inhibition of influenza virus RNA and protein synthesis observed in tissue culture [224,270].

A major problem encountered in attempting to inhibit the replication of DNA virus genomes is the similarity between host cell and viral DNA replication. Nevertheless, several purine and pyrimidine nucleoside analogs capable of inhibiting the replication of DNA viruses in tissue culture have already been employed in the treatment of human virus infections (Figs. 2 and 3) and others are currently being synthesized and evaluated in cell culture and animal systems. Their major clinical application has been in attempts to treat local and systemic infection by members of the herpesviruses group (herpes simplex virus, varicella-zoster virus and cytomegalovirus). Most of these agents inhibit cellular as well as viral nucleic acid synthesis and are incorporated, at least to some extent, into both cellular and viral DNA. Thus they are either proven or potentially mutagenic and teratogenic.

5-iodo-2′deoxyuridine (idoxuridine, IUdR) is a halogenated pyrimidine which has been licensed in the United States for the treatment of keratoconjunctivitis caused by herpes simplex virus and which has also been used experimentally for the treatment of other local and systemic infections my members of the herpesvirus group. It is one of several 5-halogenated pyrimidines which resemble thymidine because the Van der Waals radius of the halogen atom is similar to that of the methyl group of thymidine (Fig. 2). Consequently, it is handled by the cell as thymidine and phosphorylated to the mono-, di-, and triphosphate by thymidine kinase and thymidylate kinase. The triphosphate is incorporated into both viral and cellular DNA in place of thymidine. Since 5-iodouracil does not pair with adenine as faithfully as thymine, this results in mismatching during the replication and transcription of the substituted DNA. The capacity of IUdR to inhibit the replication of vaccinia and herpesviruses appears to be due primarily to the production of faulty viral DNA and proteins [248,294]. In addition, IUdR and its phosphorylated derivatives inhibit competitively DNA polymerase and the enzymes involved in the synthesis of thymidine triphosphate, including thymidylate synthetase, and this reduces the over-all rate of DNA synthesis. Detailed studies [248,294] have shown no significant differences between the effect of IUdR and its phosphorylated derivatives on the enzymes derived from uninfected cells and cells infected with herpes simplex virus. Thus it is not surprising that IUdR is toxic for rapidly dividing cells, both *in vitro* and *in vivo*. How, then, can IUdR have any therapeutic effect? There appear to be two probable explanations. IUdR has been accepted for clinical use only when applied topically in the therapy of ocular infections. The corneal cells involved have a very slow rate of division; thus, most of the DNA which is undergoing replication (and which is thus vulnerable to IUdR) is viral rather than cellular. The other possible explanation for the capacity of IUdR to inhibit virus replication at concentrations not obviously toxic for uninfected cells is the selective concentration of drug by infected cells. This is likely because vaccinia and herpes simplex viruses induce the synthesis of thymidine kinase, the enzyme responsible for the uptake and phosphorylation of IUdR [131,132,159]. Thus, levels of thymidine kinase are markedly increased in cells infected with these viruses. The effect of the increased levels of drug on cellular DNA synthesis in the infected cells is of no consequence, since they are already destined to die as a result of the virus infection.

5-trifluoromethyl-2'-deoxyuridine (trifluorothymidine, F_3TdR) is another halogenated analog of thymidine (Fig. 2). Its metabolism is similar to that of IUdR and it is incorporated into cellular and viral DNA. However, it is much more soluble than IUdR and, perhaps for this reason, appears to be somewhat more effective for the topical therapy of herpes simplex corneal ulcers [317].

The use of 5-halogenated pyrimidines as antiviral agents has a disadvantage, namely, the potential activation of latent viral genomes. IUdR and BUdR have been shown to induce the production of murine leukemia virus in mouse cells in tissue culture [179], to cause the appearance of Epstein-Barr virus particles and antigens in certain human lymphoid cells [94,108], to enhance the susceptibility of cells to transformation by simian virus 40 [304] and to enhance the replication of adenoviruses and cytomegalovirus in relatively nonpermissive cells [262,286].

1-β-D-arabinofuranosylcytosine (cytosine arabinoside, Ara-C) an analog of cytosine deoxyriboside, (Fig. 3) is a potent inhibitor of both cellular and viral DNA replication [17,44,87,248]. Ara-C inhibits the replication of all DNA viruses in tissue culture at concentrations of 10 μg/ml or less, but this inhibition is not virus-specific. In fact, DNA synthesis in uninfected cells appears to be more sensitive to inhibition by Ara-C than herpes simplex virus DNA synthesis [69]. The drug is phosphorylated by the cell to Ara-C mono-, di- and triphosphate, and is incorporated into both cellular and viral DNA. Its activity appears to be due, primarily, to the capacity of Ara-C triphosphate (Ara-CTP) to inhibit DNA polymerase. Ara-C is rapidly deaminated *in vivo* by 2'-deoxycytidine deaminase to uracil arabinoside, a metabolite without antiviral activity. In accordance with the lack of virus-specificity of Ara-C induced inhibition of DNA replication is the recent observation that *in vitro,* Ara-CTP inhibits cellular DNA polymerases to a greater extent than herpes simplex virus DNA polymerase [211]. The earlier acquisition and appreciation of such data might have prevented the unfortunate use of Ara-C in uncontrolled attempts to treat human virus infections.

9-β-D-arabinofuranosyladenine (adenine arabinoside, Ara-A, Vidarabine), an analog of adenine deoxyriboside (Fig. 3), inhibits the replication of human and animal herpesviruses and poxviruses, but exhibits less toxicity for uninfected cells than Ara-C [44,48,69,277]. The replication of rhabdoviruses and oncornaviruses is also inhibited by levels of Ara-A that do not appear to be cytotoxic. Ara-A is phosphorylated in the cell to the triphosphate (Ara-ATP) and this compound inhibits both cellular and herpes simplex virus DNA polymerase *in vitro* [211]. However, in contrast to Ara-CTP, Ara-ATP inhibits the viral enzyme to a much greater extent than the cellular enzymes. This selective inhibition of herpesvirus DNA polymerase provides a plausible explanation for the observation that in cell cultures, Ara-A inhibits herpes simplex virus DNA synthesis to a significantly greater extent than DNA synthesis in uninfected cells [69]. The apparent failure of Ara-A to inhibit selectively the replication of adenoviruses and papovaviruses, which lack their own DNA polymerases, may be due to the obligatory use of the host cell enzymes by these viruses. As is the case with other nucleoside analogs, Ara-A is incorporated into cellular and viral DNA. In cell cultures and *in vivo,* Ara-A is rapidly deaminated to hypoxanthine arabinoside (Ara-Hx) by adenosine deaminases present in cells and in serum (Fig. 3). Ara-Hx retains some antiviral activity, but it is 40 to 50 times less active than Ara-A [27]. Its inhibitory activity for uninfected cells is proportionately reduced and thus Ara-Hx appears to have a similar therapeutic index to Ara-A in cell culture [69]. While the activity of this relatively stable metabolite may make an important contribution to the efficacy of Ara-A *in vivo,* the rapid conversion of the parent compound to a less active metabolite has made the measurement of the *in vitro* susceptibility of virus strains to Ara-A unreliable and has confused *in vivo* pharmacologic studies [28]. The use of adenine deaminase inhibitors, such as Co-vidarabine [283], have led to more reliable estimates of virus sensitivity to Ara-A *in vitro* [27,28,50,51,180]. It now appears that replication of vaccinia virus is inhibited by Ara-A at a concentration of 0.5 μg/ml or less, and most herpes simplex and varicella-zoster virus strains by less than 3 μg/ml. It remains to be seen whether deaminase inhibitors will increase the therapeutic index of Ara-A or merely reduce the dosage required to obtain the same effects. Another problem with the clinical application of Ara-A its very poor solubility. Ara-A monophosphate (Ara-AMP) is currently being evaluated in an attempt to overcome this problem. Its mechanism of action is unlikely to differ significantly from that of Ara-A.

Phosphonoacetic acid (PAA) is a highly specific inhibitor of the replication of herpesviruses, including herpes simplex type 1 and type 2, varicella-zoster virus, cytomegalovirus and Epstein-Barr virus [18,186,222]. It has significantly less activity against poxvirus replication and is not inhibitory for members of other virus groups. PAA acts by specifically inhibiting the herpesvirus DNA polymerase, apparently by binding to the viral enzyme, and it has little activity against the corresponding host cell enzymes. PAA-resistant mutants, which synthesize a polymerase resistant to the drug, occur quite frequently *in vitro* [18]. Unfortunately, deposition in bone and toxic manifestations in animals make it unlikely that PAA itself will be suitable for use in man. However, detailed analysis of its mode of action should permit the synthesis of similar compounds without these adverse properties.

None of the nucleoside analogs discussed above appear to have a very high therapeutic index. This is because they affect the metabolism of uninfected as well as infected cells. The recognition that herpesviruses code for virus-specific deoxypyrimidine kinases with different properties than the corresponding host cell enzymes [131,132,159,220] has led to an important new development, namely the synthesis of nucleoside analogs that can be phosphorylated by the viral enzymes but not by the enzymes in uninfected cells [41,52,131,132,159,249,250]. Such compounds as 5'-amino-2',5'-dideoxy-5-iodouridine (AIU), 1-β-D-arabinofuranosyl-thymine (thymine arabinoside, Ara-T), 5-bromodeoxycytidine (BCdR) and 5-iododeoxycytidine (ICdR) appear to fulfill these criteria. Experiments in tissue culture indicate that these compounds markedly inhibit the replication of herpesviruses (herpes simplex and varicella-zoster) without affecting the metabolism of uninfected cells [9,42,64,135, 204,250]. The development of these and similar "second generation" antiviral agents, specifically designed to take advantage of virus-specific reactions, provides reason for optimism with respect to the future of antiviral chemotherapy.

Assembly and Maturation

Following the replication of the viral genome and the synthesis of viral structural proteins, these components must be assembled into a precisely ordered structure—the viral nucleocapsid. Subsequently, the nucleocapsids of enveloped viruses must acquire their envelope by budding through cellular membrane which has previously been altered by the addition of viral glycoproteins. Anything that reduces the fidelity of genome replication or viral protein synthesis is likely to interfere with this complex and poorly understood process. Many viral capsid proteins are now known to be synthesized in the form of larger precursors that must be cleaved, presumably by host cell proteases, to furnish the actual polypeptides found in mature infectious virions [122,130,165,295]. Inhibition of this cleavage process by protease inhibitors can prevent virus replication in cell culture by interfering with the process of virus assembly and maturation [165,296].

Rifampicin at concentrations below 100 μg/ml inhibits the replication of poxviruses in cell culture. Surprisingly, this is not due to an effect of the drug on viral DNA or RNA synthesis, but to inhibition of viral morphogenesis. This occurs because the cleavage of the precursor of one of the two major poxvirus capsid polypeptides is inhibited in rifampicin-treated cells [208,209].

Glycoproteins are essential components of the envelopes of all enveloped viruses. Thus it is not surprising that inhibition of the glycosylation of proteins with compounds such as 2-deoxy-D-glucose and D-glucosamine inhibits the replication of a broad range of enveloped viruses, including herpesviruses, orthomyxoviruses, paramyxoviruses, rhabdoviruses and togaviruses. These inhibitors interfere with virus maturation by preventing the glycosylation of viral polypeptides destined to become envelope glycoproteins [59,119,146,161,269,271]. Glycoprotein synthesis is also essential for the function of normal cells. Since the glycosylation of viral proteins appears to be carried out by cellular enzymes, there would seem to be some question as to the therapeutic potential of compounds that inhibit glycosylation. Thus it is interesting that topically applied 2-deoxy-D-glucose has been reported to be effective and nontoxic in the treatment of experimental herpes simplex keratitis in the rabbit eye [254].

Interferon has recently been found to inhibit the production of oncornaviruses by acutely and chronically infected cells. Surprisingly, there is no inhibition of virus protein or nucleic acid synthesis. Instead, interferon appears to be inhibiting virus release [88]. It is not clear whether this phenomenon represents still another effect of interferon-induced antiviral proteins or is the direct result of some change in the cell membrane caused by the interaction of interferon with its receptor.

The infectivity of paramyxoviruses requires the activity of two surface glycoproteins. One of these, designated HN, has both hemagglutinating and neuraminidase activity, and appears to be primarily responsible for the attachment of virions to susceptible cells and the efficient release of newly synthesized virions from infected cells. The other, designated F, is responsible for the hemolytic and cell-fusing capacities of these viruses.

Its function appears to be essential for penetration and uncoating [265,266]. The F glycoprotein is formed by cleavage of a larger (and inactive) precursor, and this is ordinarily accomplished by cell proteases. Some cells which lack the appropriate protease produce noninfectious virions which can be converted to infectious virions by cleavage of the precursor glycoprotein *in vitro* by trypsin [265,266]. Conversely, it may be possible to inhibit the formation of infectious virus by the use of appropriate protease inhibitors.

The neuraminidase of myxoviruses and paramyxoviruses is essential for the efficient release of virions from infected cells [30]. This is because removal of neuraminic acid from the envelope of newly synthesized virions by the enzyme appears to be necessary to prevent their extensive aggregation at the cell surface. Thus, as one might have predicted, the neuramidase inhibitor 2-deoxy-2,3-dehydro-N-trifluoroacetylneuraminic acid (FANA) has been found to inhibit the muticycle replication of influenza virus in cell culture [233]. This represents another instance in which inhibitors specifically directed at viral enzymes may selectively inhibit virus replication.

Many compounds will be found which appear to selectively inhibit virus replication *in vitro*. However, their utility *in vivo* will depend upon a number of factors which cannot be fully assessed in tissue culture systems, such as their capacity to reach infected tissues in concentrations adequate to inhibit virus replication, their stability in serum and other body fluids, their rate of absorption and excretion, and their toxicity for rapidly dividing cells in such organs as the bone marrow and gastrointestinal tract. It is the assessment of these factors and the estimation of the *in vivo* therapeutic index that constitutes the next step in the development of a clinically useful antiviral agent.

ESTIMATING THE THERAPEUTIC INDEX OF ANTIVIRAL DRUGS PRIOR TO HUMAN USE

Both ethical and practical considerations demand that a reasonable estimate of the therapeutic index of any drug be developed before human use. Many compounds found to inhibit viruses in cell culture act by inhibiting cellular functions essential for virus replication, and are therefore likely to have a low therapeutic index *in vivo*. Well standardized *in vitro* assays measuring the effects of antiviral compounds on both the metabolism of uninfected cells and the replication of viruses would permit a reasonable estimate of therapeutic index in cell culture. The eventual applicability of that estimate to the *in vivo* situation would be enhanced by the use of multiple cell types, including primary human cells and diploid human cell strains, and by the use of virus strains freshly isolated from man, in addition to well characterized laboratory strains. It is also important that toxicity be tested in rapidly dividing cells, which more closely resemble the rapidly dividing cells of the bone marrow and gastrointestinal tract than do the confluent stationary cell cultures which have been used in most antiviral assays. Other factors, including the multiplicity of virus infection, the tissue culture medium employed, the technique used to estimate the antiviral effect (e.g., inhibition of virus-induced cytopathology, virus plaque inhibition, single or multiple cycle virus yield reduction) and the criteria of inhibition (e.g., 50%, 99%, etc.) must also be considered. The *in vitro* therapeutic index should be determined against a wide variety of DNA and RNA viruses. Finally, analysis of the metabolism of the drug in tissue culture, and of the mechanism by which it affects virus replication and host cell metabolism can provide important data for subsequent *in vivo* studies. Unfortunately, this sort of thorough *in vitro* evaluation has rarely preceded the use of antiviral drugs in man.

Drugs which have a high therapeutic index in cell culture must still be evaluated *in vivo*. This is especially true because compounds that appear to be nontoxic in cell cultures may still cause significant toxicity to critical organs *in vivo*. Once again, ethical and practical considerations demand that candidate antiviral agents be tested in animal models prior to use in man. Animal models provide several advantages over human trials in the evaluation of a new antiviral agent. The numbers of subjects and the conditions of the model can be more readily manipulated so that a given therapeutic intervention can be reliably interpreted as successful or not. The animal model can more easily provide a true control population. Extremes of drug dosages can be administered to animals to assess toxicity, and one can freely obtain serum and other tissue specimens to examine for the presence of virus, drug, drug metabolites and manifestations of toxicity. Finally, animal studies are substantially less expensive than human trials.

The advantages of the animal model may be counterbalanced by significant disadvantages [95]. The pathogenesis of the disease in the animal model may be quite different from that in the human infection, as when herpes simplex virus encephalitis is induced in the mouse by intracerebral inoculation of virus. The immune responses of the animal may differ from those of the human. Many human viruses must be adapted to the animal by multiple passages before they can produce disease, as in the case of influenza in mice. Some animal models may employ a related non-human virus, like murine cytomegalovirus, whose drug sensitivities and pathogenic properties may not be equivalent to those of the human virus. In some cases—for example, varicella-zoster virus—no valid animal model may be available. Clearly, the choice of appropriate animal models requires a great deal of knowledge of the pathogenesis of both the human disease in question and the infection in the animal models. However, even when a compound exhibits a satisfactory therapeutic index in an appropriately chosen animal model, it may fail to do so in man. This is because significant species differences may exist with respect to drug pharmacology and toxicology. Absorption, distribution, metabolism and sensitivity to toxic effects may manifest relative or absolute species differences. Some interferon inducers work well in the mouse but poorly or not at all in man [62,84,85]. The major routes of metabolism of Ara-A differ between primates and rodents [97]. Both Ara-A and amantadine are well tolerated in doses 10 to 100-fold higher in rodents than primates [97,309]. Clearly, harmful effects observed in animal models caution against the use of an antiviral drug in man, but the lack of harmful effects in animals is no guarantee of safety. The ultimate test of the safety and efficacy of an antiviral agent must take place in humans.

Finally, clinical studies of efficacy in man should be preceded by precise and extensive pharmacokinetic studies, first in animals and then in humans. These are essential in order to find out how much drug should be given, how often and by what route, to establish its mode of excretion or detoxification, to discover its metabolic by-products and learn whether they are useful or harmful, and to determine its half-life, tissue distribution, sites of accumulation and penetration into such important areas as the brain, cerebrospinal fluid and aqueous humor. Unfortunately, clinical studies with most of the drugs discussed below were begun without the prior acquisition of this critical information.

CLINICAL EXPERIENCE WITH ANTIVIRAL THERAPY

In this section we will review the pharmacology and toxicity of antiviral agents that have been used clinically and summarize the results of controlled trials in man. The therapy of systemic infections will be considered first; this will include the use of aerosolized drugs for respiratory virus infections. Superficial infections can be treated topically with drugs or concentrations of drugs which would be toxic systemically. Thus, the antiviral therapy of cutaneous and ocular infections will be considered separately, although systemic chemotherapy has also been attempted for both zoster and uveitis.

Antiviral Agents Used for Systemic Infections

Amantadine Hydrochloride and its Congeners

In 1966, amantadine hydrochloride became the first antiviral agent for systemic use licensed in the United States by the Food and Drug Administration. The limited pharmacologic studies in man to date are consistent with the detailed findings in several animal species [23]. Almost complete absorption from the gastrointestinal tract follows oral administration. Peak blood levels of 0.3 to 0.6 μg/ml are attained 1–4 hours following the standard oral adult dose of 200 mg (6 mg/kg to a maximum of 150 mg in children 1 to 9 years of age). Amantadine is excreted unmetabolized in the urine, with a half-life in man ranging from 12 to 24 hours [23]. The drug is apparently concentrated in certain tissues of experimental animals [23]. In the mouse lung, concentrations exceed blood concentrations by approximately 10-fold. No information is available to assess the relevance of this drug distribution to human respiratory infection.

Adverse effects in man appear to be dose-related and to be limited, with a few exceptions, to central nervous system symptomatology. One large placebo-controlled therapeutic trial of 709 patients, most of whom were young and not receiving additional medications, demonstrated that the frequency of various complaints and symptoms was either lower or unchanged in the treated group [160]. Amantadine is well tolerated by children, including children with cystic fibrosis [327]. A sizeable experience has accumulated with the use of amantadine in patients with Parkinson's disease [272,273]. Such elderly patients are probably more representative of the population which is most susceptible to the complications of influenza, and for which chemoprophylaxis and therapy would thus be more strongly indicated. Twenty per cent of 430 patients receiving 200 mg amantadine daily for Parkinson's disease complained of a drug reaction, with confusion, nervousness, dizziness and insomnia representing the most frequent complaints [273]. A small proportion of these patients also developed livedo reticularis [273,278]. Patients receiving large doses of anticholinergics, and antihistamine derivatives such as trihexphenidyl hydrochloride (Artane®) or benztropine mesylate (Congentin®) appear to be especially susceptible to reactions to amantadine [273]. In Schwab's study of 430 patients, almost half of the total group took the drug for over one year; 6% discontinued the drug or reduced the dosage. No significant laboratory abnormalities were observed [273].

Patients with impaired renal function receiving full doses of amantadine have experienced nervousness, confusion and hallucinations, while concomitant blood levels of the drug ranged between 2.5 and

4.4 μg/ml, 10 times the normal peak blood level [5,128]. In several elderly depressed patients, 300 mg per day resulted in aggressive behavior and excitability after several weeks, at which time serum levels had reached 0.7–1.0 μg/ml [258]. In animals, adverse effects are not seen until the LD_{50} is approached [309]. The acute LD_{50} for most animals is approximately 100-fold greater than the therapeutic dose. These doses produce hyperexcitability, anorexia, emesis and convulsions. Ingestion of 2800 mg in a suicide attempt produced acute toxic psychosis and urinary retention, which was followed by complete recovery [80]. Teratogenicity has been described in rats receiving 50 mg/kg, thus contraindicating the use of the drug in pregnancy [170]. No other adverse effects have been documented with chronic administration of sublethal doses in rats, dogs, or nonhuman primates [309].

Amantadine has been evaluated both as a prophylactic and therapeutic drug for influenza A infections in humans. Over 40 placebo controlled studies have been reported [47,89,91,120,177,210,219,314,315]. The 31 studies performed through 1971 have been tabulated by Hoffman [120]. Of the nine placebo controlled studies of the prophylactic effect of amantadine administered prior to influenza A inoculation of volunteers, only one study has failed to demonstrate an effect [120]. These studies all utilized an antigenic variant of either the H2N2 or H3N2 subtypes of influenza A. Except for the negative study, amantadine produced at least a 50% reduction in the incidence of disease. In addition, treatment reduced the severity of disease that did occur. As a corollary, amantadine diminished the antibody responses to influenza in six of seven positive studies. It should be emphasized that these reduced antibody responses are the result of diminished virus multiplication and thus reduced antigenic stimulation. Amantadine is not immunosuppressive.

The prophylactic efficacy of amantadine has also been examined in naturally occurring epidemics due to H2N2 and H3N2 subtypes of influenza A virus [120,210,219]. Of 15 such studies utilizing placebo controls, 12 reported significant reduction of symptomatology. The absolute morbidity was reduced in some, only the relative severity of symptoms in others. In addition, 8 of 12 studies showed a parallel reduction in antibody rises in the treated group, indicating reduced viral multiplication. The earlier the intervention, the more effective was the drug. This general pharmacologic principle has been confirmed with amantadine in the murine influenza model [102].

Two studies using infected volunteers demonstrated little or no therapeutic efficacy of amantadine under conditions in which pretreatment was effective [284,288]. Nevertheless, 15 other placebo-controlled trials of amantadine initiated after the onset of the symptoms of naturally occurring influenza A have demonstrated a therapeutic effect [89,91,120,177,314,315]. Most therapeutic trials report a shorter duration of symptoms and fever and a lower peak fever in the treated group. A reduction in virus shedding is usually not seen. Because nasopharyngeal virus shedding in influenza A attains maximal levels at the onset of symptomatology [257], it is unlikely that chemotherapy will produce a dramatic reduction in virus shedding, even when given within 24–48 hours after the onset of symptoms. The impact of amantadine on severe viral pneumonitis will be difficult to evaluate in a controlled manner because of the relative infrequency of this syndrome. However, even natural influenza without radiologic evidence of pneumonitis regularly produces abnormalities in pulmonary mechanics [107]. Therapeutic administration of amantadine accelerates the resolution of restricted maximal helium-oxygen flow rates, a measure of resistance in peripheral airways [177]. Thus, despite initial skepticism about the efficacy of amantadine [261], controlled studies have consistently demonstrated both prophylactic and therapeutic efficacy of the same order of magnitude as that achieved with inactivated influenza vaccines. When possible, a single immunization would appear to be a more practical prophylactic measure than the prolonged administration of amantadine. Immunization offers the additional advantage of affording protection against influenza B. However, the additive effect of prior immunity and prophylactic amantadine [90] suggests that the use of both prophylactic modalities may be warranted in certain high risk individuals Amantidine also provides the only approach to the control of influenza caused by a new subtype during the period prior to the availability of a suitable vaccine.

Several potential areas of future application of amantadine are being investigated. Additional strains of influenza A are being examined for *in vitro* and animal model sensitivity to the drug. To date, newly emerging strains of the H3N2 subtype as well as A/New Jersey/76 ($H_{swine}N_2$) and A/FM/47 (H_1N_1) appear to be at least as sensitive as the Asian and Hong Kong strains [101]. A novel approach is the use of aerosolized amantadine, which is more efficacious than the intraperitoneal drug in a mouse model [311]. Pharmacologic studies in normal volunteers indicate that nebulization of a 25 mg/ml solution can be irritating but that a 10–15 mg/ml solution is well tolerated [110]. The drug is largely absorbed and excreted in the urine when administered via this route. After the aerosol administration of 10 mg over a 30 minute interval, drug concentrations in the nasopharyngeal secretion are 100 μg/ml in one hour and 30 μg/ml in two hours (G. Douglas, personal communication). The therapeutic efficacy of such high local concentrations, obtained with only one-tenth of the usual oral dose, will be of great interest.

A number of congeners of amantadine have been synthesized in the hope of discovering a more effective drug. Two such agents, rimantadine (α-methyl-1-adamantanemethylamine) hydrochloride (120,324) and 1'-methyl-spiro (adamantane-2,3'-pyrrolidine) maleate [6,16] have been evaluated in man. In both prophylactic and therapeutic trials with influenza A, these drugs appear to be at least as well tolerated and at least as effective as amantadine. Further comparative studies of amantadine and these two congeners will be helpful in assessing relative efficacy and toxicity.

Although some *in vitro* activity of amantadine has been demonstrated against several other viruses, including pseudorabies (a herpesvirus), rubella, and members of the parainfluenza, arenavirus and oncornavirus groups, no impact has been demonstrable in therapeutic trials against non-influenza A respiratory infections [190,241] measles [63], or rubella [261]. The lack of *in vitro* efficacy of amantadine against influenza B viruses has been supported by the negative results obtained in a prophylactic trial in volunteers challenged with influenza B virus [284]. An especially interesting study designed to examine the efficacy of amantadine for the therapy of influenza in a general practice setting was fortuitously able to compare the drug with a placebo during separate outbreaks of both influenza A and B [89]. Amantadine reduced the duration of fever and days in bed for the influenza A victims; however, there was no effect on patients with influenza B.

Thiosemicarbazones

The pharmacology of the thiosemicarbazones has not been systematically studied in man or animals. The appearance of a compound, as measured by a colorimetric assay which can detect the drug *in vitro,* has been reported in the serum of three patients after oral administration of methisazone, the N-methyl derivative of isatin-β-thiosemicarbizone [153a,307]. The drug has been administered orally in doses of 40–200 mg/kg/day, a route and dosage which appear to be efficacious in rodents with poxvirus infections [13,175]. Because of low solubility, methisazone is administered as a micronized suspension in a sucrose syrup [13]. With some variation from study to study, approximately one-half of patients so treated experience nausea, vomiting or diarrhea.

It appears to have been a matter of faith that the success with thiosemicarbazones in rodents could be transposed to man. The absorption, metabolism and excretion of these drugs have not been studied in humans, and serum levels of antiviral activity have not been documented. Methisazone has been the agent used for most of the antiviral studies in man. These studies have been restricted to infections by members of the poxvirus group. Two double-blind, placebo-controlled therapeutic trials for smallpox failed to document therapeutic benefits with either met- hisazone or isothiazole thiosemicarbazone [252,253]. Difficulty in docu- menting therapeutic efficacy in poxvirus infections might be expected, since viral multiplication is terminating by the time cutaneous lesions are becoming pustular. Levinson lists a dozen publications reporting thera- peutic trials for cutaneous complications of vaccinia [175]. A beneficial effect is perceived in most, but not all, of these uncontrolled anecdotal reports.

One nonrandomized, nonblinded study examined the prophylactic value of methisazone for close contacts of patients with alastrim [68]. In this Brazilian study involving 904 contact subjects, alastrim developed in 2% of the treated contacts and 8% of the untreated contacts. A similarly designed prophylactic trial, which allocated smallpox contacts into treat- ment on non-treatment groups, was performed with 5320 subjects in India [14]. The treated contacts experienced a 6-fold reduction in inci- dence of smallpox and a similar reduction in mortality. Another prophylactic study which allocated smallpox contacts alternately into drug and placebo groups demonstrated a 4-fold reduction in incidence, but this failed to attain statistical significance [251]. The second randomized, placebo-controlled study of the prophylactic efficacy of methisazone failed to demonstrate a statistically significant effect on smallpox inci- dence, morbidity, mortality or antibody responses, although a suggestion of a benefit was observed in previously unvaccinated contacts [112]. The inconsistency of results in these studies cannot be attributed to dosage dif- ferences and must reside with differences in study design or patient popu- lations.

The vague understanding of thiosemicarbazone pharmacology and the inconclusive results of these clinical trials will probably be rendered moot concerns if the present smallpox eradication program succeeds in relegat- ing life threatening poxvirus infections to history.

Idoxuridine (IUdR)

IUdR is relatively stable for months in solution at 37°C or below [78]; however, it is rapidly degraded to iodouracil and uracil by heating or in the body [34]. These breakdown products neither possess antiviral activity nor do they inhibit the activity of IUdR [78]. The half-life of IUdR in the plasma of man is approximately 30 minutes [35]. At infu- sion rates of 4 mg per minute, IUdR is inactivated rapidly enough to render drug concentrations undetectable (< 2.5 μg/ml) [173]. At an infu- sion rate of 50 mg per minute in one patient, serum drug levels gradually accumulated to 36 μg/ml after 60 minutes, at which time three grams had been administered. Approximately 10 μg/ml will reduce herpes simplex virus plaque formation *in vitro* by 10 to 100-fold (173). IUdR is generally not detectable in the cerebrospinal fluid of patients with encephalitis receiving large doses of intravenous IUdR [173].

Because IUdR interferes with DNA synthetic mechanisms common to both viruses and host cells, cells with a rapid turnover are the primary targets for drug toxicity. IUdR thus produces alopecia, leukopenia, thrombocytopenia, anorexia and stomatitis [25,34,215]. Three grams administered over one hour twice daily for five days results in significant bone marrow depression. This regimen has produced sufficient myelosuppression to result in infectious and hemorrhagic complications of therapy [25,215].

The initial use of IUdR for systemic viral infections comprised uncontrolled trials for vaccinia infections in immunosuppressed patients [33] and for herpes simplex encephalitis [26,105,127,215]. Much of the enthusiasm for the efficacy of IUdR in herpes encephalitis was based on a comparison of the outcome in treated patients with the grim results which had been observed in previously untreated patients. The inability to demonstrate a favorable effect of IUdR on experimental herpes simplex encephalitis in many animal models was disconcerting [4,45,154,189,229,282,289]. A double-blinded, randomized examination of IUdR therapy for herpes simplex virus encephalitis failed to demonstrate reduced mortality or diminution of the amount of virus present in the brain, but it did document unacceptable myelosuppression [25]. This report reinforced several important principles of antiviral chemotherapy which merit reiteration [3]: (1) because inhibition of viral replication by currently available drugs is usually accompanied by an effect on host cells, carefully controlled studies are required to determine a therapeutic index; (2) the unknown natural history of many viral infections, especially with the agents of the herpes group, undermines the value of historical controls; (3) specifically regarding viral encephalitis, those cases which cannot be documented by brain biopsy or serology to be unequivocally due to herpes simplex have a more benign prognosis [25,322]. Thus, the apparent results of therapy can depend upon the validity of the diagnostic criteria employed.

Cytosine Arabinoside (Ara-C)

The human pharmacology of Ara-C has been investigated only in a small number of cancer patients. The drug is poorly absorbed from the gastrointestinal tract [115]. Following intravenous infusion, the drug is rapidly deaminated and excreted in the urine as uracil arabinoside [60,117,301]. The serum half-life is only 5–12 minutes [60,117,301] with a prolonged second phase decay curve which is apparent after the first hour

[117]. Regardless of the precise rate of disappearance, a standard daily dose of 3 mg/kg given in a short intravenous infusion results in serum levels of approximately 1 µg/ml after one hour [117]. *In vitro,* 99% reduction in the infectivity of herpes simplex virus or of cytomegalovirus requires 5–10 µg/ml [182,216,277]. Following a loading dose of approximately 1 mg/kg, a two hour infusion of 112 mg/m^2 of Ara-C maintained a plasma level during the infusion of 0.06 µg/ml; 400 mg/m^2 maintained a plasma level of only 0.5 µg/ml [117]. The drug has been demonstrated in the cerebrospinal fluid in concentrations lower than in the serum [117]; however, transport into the central nervous system has not been studied systematically.

Bone marrow suppression with leukopenia, thrombocytopenia and megaloblastosis are the most prominent toxic manifestations of Ara-C [291,301], and a high incidence of chromosomal aberrations has been described [19]. Ara-C also produces significant aberrations in chick embryogenesis [147] and in neural and retinal morphogenesis in neonatal rodents [8,86]. Perhaps the best documentation of its toxicity was in the controlled therapeutic trials of Stevens et al. and Monsur et al., in which immunosuppression was also described [205,291].

Therapeutic studies with Ara-C for systemic viral infections have been limited because of the more promising efficacy and toxicity data with Ara-A both *in vitro* and in animal models. Uncontrolled case reports have been enumerated by Ch'ien et al. [44]. Analogous to IUdR, optimistic experience in the therapy of herpes simplex virus encephalitis in humans [46] could not be confirmed in animal models [100,189]. However, a slight reduction in mortality was discerned in one mouse model [4]. A controlled study of Ara-C for biopsy-proven herpes simplex encephalitis revealed no benefit [191]. Ara-C does appear to diminish urinary virus excretion in infants with congenital cytomegalovirus infection [166,182,243]. This effect, although generally consistent, required administration of sufficiently toxic doses (5–15 mg/kg/day) to produce serious marrow suppression. Although uncontrolled, these reports noted no other impact on the infection; moreover, pretherapeutic levels of urinary virus excretion resumed with the cessation of drug therapy.

Two randomized, placebo-controlled, double-blind studies of parenteral Ara-C therapy for herpes zoster in immunosuppressed oncology patients have been performed. One study involved immunosuppressed patients with disseminated herpes zoster [291]. The administration of 100 mg/m^2/day of Ara-C not only failed to curtail dissemination, but it delayed the appearance of vesicle interferon, induced bone marrow suppression, depressed antibody formation to herpes zoster virus, and prolonged the length of hospitalization [291]. These negative results, in the face of the usual optimism based on anecdotal experience, reinforces the principles of drug evaluation which concluded the analysis of the experience with IUdR. In the second study, cancer patients who presented with localized herpes zoster received $30/mg/m^2/day$ or placebo [267]. The treatment group experienced no obvious drug toxicity, but there was also no therapeutic benefit with regard to further development of local lesions, reduction of local pain or prevention of dissemination. A controlled study of Ara-C for herpes-zoster involving only eight immunosuppressed patients also failed to demonstrate efficacy [60a].

A controlled therapeutic study for smallpox, using 3 mg/kg daily of Ara-C, was discontinued after all nine treated patients died, while only four of eleven placebo recipients died [205]. Granulocytopenia and persistence of viremia in the treated group suggested to the investigators that the Ara-C had more impact on the host immune system than on viral replication. These controlled studies, and the introduction of Ara-A, appear to have terminated further consideration of Ara-C for the therapy of systemic viral infections.

Adenine Arabinoside (Ara-A)

Ara-A is poorly soluble in aqueous solution (0.5 mg/ml). The oral drug is ineffective in animal models, and intramuscular administration is both irritating and unreliable [97,167]. Thus, a liter or more of fluid is required for intravenous infusion of adult therapeutic doses (10–20 mg/kg) of Ara-A. This fluid volume is often an important consideration for the many herpes virus infected patients with renal impairment (patients with malignancies or organ transplants) or with elevated intracranial pressure (patients with encephalitis). Infusions are usually administered over an 8–12 hour period. The monophosphate (Ara-AMP) appears to have similar antiviral activity and greater solubility [227]. With the recent availability of practical production technics, Ara-AMP will be undergoing further clinical studies.

Much of the pharmacologic data of Ara-A is derived from studies using the tritium-labeled drug [97,158]. Studies with radiolabeled Ara-A have explained the greater susceptibility of primates to drug toxicity as a consequence of differences in drug metabolism [97]. Primates, including man, deaminate Ara-A to hypoxanthine arabinoside (Ara-Hx) [158,319], but only 15% of labeled Ara-A can be recovered as Ara-Hx in lower animals [97]. Dogs, rabbits and rodents rapidly oxidize Ara-A to xanthine and water [97]. Xanthine has no antiviral activity, while the antiviral activity of Ara-Hx, though considerably less than that of Ara-A, may be important. Unfortunately, the distribution and excretion of nonvolatile tritium fails to identify the distribution and duration of antiviral activity in the body.

Serum, many animal tissues, and cell cultures contain adenosine deaminase, which readily converts Ara-A to Ara-Hx [97,158,299]. Consequently, levels of Ara-A rapidly diminish in blood specimens obtained for drug assay and in most assay systems used either for determining viral sensitivity to the drug or for measuring drug concentrations [299]. One solution is the addition of adenine deaminase inhibitors to serum samples and to tissue culture assay systems to stabilize the Ara-A levels. The reliability of this technic depends upon the inhibitor being both effective and noninterfering (i.e., inhibiting neither virus replication nor the antiviral activity of Ara-A).

Viruses of the herpes group have been reported to be inhibited by 5–100 μg/ml in cell cultures [51,277]; however, using adenosine deaminase inhibitors to prevent degradation of the drug by tissue culture cells and by the serum in their growth media, this estimate of effective drug levels can probably be reduced at least 10-fold [27,28,50,51,180]. Thus, 90% plaque inhibition of herpes simplex viruses requires 1–2 μg/ml of Ara-A [51,180]. Connor has also pointed out that the usually quoted 10:1 ratio of antiviral activity of Ara-A to Ara-Hx may be artifactual. Initial preparations of Ara-Hx were probably contaminated by Ara-A. In addition, the relative activity of Ara-A has been underestimated because of deamination of the drug during microbiologic assays. Thus the ratio of Ara-A to Ara-Hx antiviral potency is close to 50:1 for varicella-zoster, herpes simplex and vaccinia viruses [27,51].

Many aspects of Ara-A pharmacology in man are as indefinite as its mechanism of action. The drug or its metabolites appear to be concentrated in tissues and red blood cells [319]. However, many important questions remain unanswered. What compounds are intracellular and what is their relative therapeutic and toxic impact? The serum concentration of Ara-Hx is usually 10 to 1000-fold greater than the Ara-A concentration. Since Ara-Hx appears to possess about 2% of the antiviral activity of Ara-A, what is the relative importance of these two compounds in the body? Finally, the rapid renal excretion of Ara-A and its metabolites indicate the requirement for dosage adjustments in the many infected patients with impaired renal function. At present there are no data on which to base a rational adjustment of dosage.

It is unclear why Ara-A fails to produce toxic manifestations similar to those produced by other nucleoside analogues which inhibit DNA synthesis [164,321,322], although it does appear unique in its capacity to inhibit selectively herpesvirus DNA synthesis [69] and the DNA polymerase [211] of herpes simplex virus. Rather than the marrow suppression, mucositis and alopecia which are typical toxic manifestations of therapy with IUdR and Ara-C, Ara-A has been reported to produce encephalopathy [172,260] and gastrointestinal disturbances (nausea, vomiting and weight loss) [1,24,153,244,260,321]. Megaloblastosis, leukopenia and thrombocytopenia are seen in man, but usually in hosts with preexisting marrow disease [24]. The encephalopathy, which is characterized by tremors, confusion and an abnormal EEG, was seen at dosage levels of 20 mg/kg in one study [260]. CNS aberrations have been seen in rhesus monkeys receiving 25 mg/kg but not in rodents receiving several times that dosage [167]. The limitations of animal models are well exemplified by the fact that acute toxicity is not seen in rodents or rabbits at doses 100-fold greater than these [167]. Neither Ara-A nor Ara-Hx produce aberrations in rat neurologic morphogenesis as does Ara-C [86]. Nevertheless, chromosomal breakage occurs in human leukocytes either exposed to Ara-A *in vitro* [214] or taken from patients receiving the drug [323].

Controlled therapeutic studies in man with Ara-A have been directed against smallpox and infections due to herpesviruses. No therapeutic benefit was derived from Ara-A in a double-blind controlled therapeutic trial for smallpox [164], but this still represents a distinct improvement over the adverse results obtained with Ara-C [205]. An uncontrolled trial of Ara-A for cytomegalovirus infection strongly suggested that the drug suppresses urinary excretion of virus in patients with congenital infection and mononucleosis, but not in renal transplant patients requiring immunosuppression [43]. As with Ara-C, virus excretion resumes with cessation of therapy.

Two collaborative studies of the therapeutic efficacy of Ara-A in herpes virus infections have been undertaken. In a randomized, double-blind, placebo-controlled study, immunosuppressed patients with herpes zoster, one third of whom had disseminated from the primary dermatome, were treated for five days with 10 mg/kg daily of Ara-A or placebo and then switched for the next five days to the alternate regimen [321]. During the first five days of the study, the recipients of Ara-A more promptly cleared virus from vesicles, ceased new vesicle formation and developed complete pustulation. Because of the cross-over study design, conclusions regarding therapeutic benefits after day five were impossible. The second placebo-controlled study indicated the value of 15 mg/kg Ara-A daily for 10 days in biopsy-proved herpes simplex virus encephalitis [322]. In 28 cases in which the diagnosis was proven by isolation of Type 1 virus from tissue obtained by brain biopsy, treatment reduced mortality from 70 to 28%. Those treated prior to the development of coma fared better. The brain biopsies also demonstrated that many cases diagnosed as herpes simplex virus encephalitis on clinical grounds are actually caused by unknown agents not responsive to Ara-A or by known agents responsive to standard antibiotic or antifungal chemotherapy. A third controlled cooperative study of the efficacy of Ara-A for disseminated neonatal herpes simplex virus infection is in progress [320]. No significant drug toxicity has been recognized in these controlled studies at dosages of 10–15 mg/kg daily.

Ribavirin (Virazole®)

The pharmacology of ribavirin has been examined in the rat [202]. The drug has an initial half-life in the serum of less than an hour. Using tritiated ribavirin, the drug or its metabolites are concentrated in the liver, where histopathologic signs of toxicity are first seen in animals [202]. Two-thirds of the tritium is recoverable in the urine in eight hours. No data on the pharmacology in man are readily available.

A 10- to 100-fold reduction [8] in infectivity and in virus yield is produced by 1–32 μg/ml of ribavirin in tissue cultures infected with herpes simplex, parainfluenza and influenza viruses [279–281, 305]. Ribavirin has also shown some efficacy in animal models of virus infections, most often influenza, when administered orally, intraperitoneally or by small particle aerosol [73,83,171,246,268,280,281,290]. Parenteral administration of 50–100 mg/kg will ameliorate viral infections in most animal models [83,246,268,281]. The delivery of 16 mg/kg by small particle aerosol has also proved therapeutically effective against influenza A virus in mice [290,311]. Animal efficacy has not been demonstrated at any dose below 15 mg/kg except in one study. However, that study is puzzling in that it also demonstrated a mortality of only 10% after a 1600 mg/kg oral dose in mice [73].

Studies of the toxicity of ribavirin have demonstrated an acute LD_{50} in rabbits and rodents of 150 mg/kg (137,281). Rabbit skin graft survival is prolonged by doses of 50–100 mg/kg, indicating ribavirin's immunosuppressive potential [137]. A single 2–4 mg/kg intraperitoneal dose on day eight of gestation is teratogenic in hamsters [157]. The pharmacologic and toxicity data available from animal models do not indicate a comfortable margin of safety between the therapeutic and the toxic, or even lethal, doses. Information regarding the pharmacology and toxicity in man is at present limited to the description of bilirubin elevations in patients receiving daily doses in the range of 4–15 mg/kg [184,305].

Most controlled studies in humans have been for the treatment of influenza. Three studies have examined the prophylactic efficacy of ribavirin against influenza virus challenge. In one, 600 mg daily for 10 days, beginning two days prior to challenge, marginally reduced signs and symptoms produced by influenza B virus [305]. This same regimen failed to affect an influenza A challenge in a second study [47], whereas 100 mg of amantadine twice daily for 10 days reduced virus shedding, fever and antibody responses [47]. A third study reported a statistically significant but minimal benefit against an influenza A challenge in a group of students receiving 1000 mg of ribavirin daily for five days beginning on the day of virus challenge. However, 4 of 14 of these students also experienced transient bilirubin elevations [184]. Surprisingly, a dose of only 300 mg daily for five days had a distinct therapeutic impact on a natural influenza outbreak in a Mexican boarding school [263]. A controlled study against acute viral hepatitis has also been reported [10]. Sixty-six patients with acute hepatitis were randomized to receive placebo or 100 mg of ribavirin every six hours for several days. Both groups improved but we see no statistically significant difference between the drug and placebo recipients. The authors, however, claimed a beneficial effect of the drug on the basis of their analysis of the data; they employed a novel statistical methodology that avoided a direct comparison between drug and placebo recipients.

In summary, although ribavirin has been administered to hundreds of patients in uncontrolled trials for various viral infections (330), the drug appears to have an unsure future as a useful antiviral agent because of its unknown human pharmacology, its potential toxicity and its borderline efficacy.

Inosiplex (Isoprinosine®)
Inosiplex, the paracetamidobenzoic acid salt of inosine dimethylaminoisopropanol [40], has been ineffective in several animal models of virus infections [96] and in prophylactic trials against rhinovirus and influenza A virus challenges in adult volunteers [155,178,228,285,306]. However, two controlled therapeutic trials, one each against rhinovirus 21 and influenza A, demonstrated a moderate reduction in symptoms as compared with results obtained with a placebo [155,310]. "Immunopotentiation," rather than direct antiviral activity, has been invoked as the mechanism of action of inosiplex [106,310]. The status of the drug must await further studies of its effects on the immune system and viral replication, and further controlled clinical trials.

Vitamin C
Pauling's book, "Vitamin C and the Common Cold" [234], stimulated great interest by a public which desires relief from this common affliction and which practices extensive self-medication. Two careful reviews of the controlled studies of the prophylactic and therapeutic efficacy of ascorbic acid on the common cold were published in 1975 [38,74]; two

additional studies were published subsequently [58,203]. No benefits have been sufficiently discernable to merit the cost, effort, and potential risk of the administration of ascorbic acid in large doses.

Interferon and Its Inducers

The potential of interferon as a nontoxic, highly selective antiviral agent effective against a broad range of DNA and RNA viruses has intrigued virologists for twenty years. The adequate assessment of interferon's promising clinical potential has been hampered largely by the technical difficulties in producing adequate quantities of pure material. Tyrrell has recently published a very thorough, lucid and succinct account of interferon from discovery to clinical utilization [308]. Merigan has also critically reviewed the theoretical problems, the pharmacology and the clinical experience with interferon [196].

Exogenous human leukocyte interferon when administered parenterally in the range of 10^8 units per day produces serum interferon levels above 100 units per ml [141]. (One unit is defined as the minimal quantity required to inhibit the infectivity of a test virus by 50%.) With these doses (which because of the very high specific activity of interferon correspond to less than 0.1 μg of pure interferon) the serum half life is approximately three hours after intravenous administration and five hours after intramuscular administration [141]. In contrast to Ara-C, these doses of interferon do not appear to inhibit antibody responses to varicella-zoster virus [141]. Many patients experience a mild febrile response to these high doses, but it is presently unclear whether this is due to the interferon itself or impurities in the preparation [7,20,141]. Other toxicity that has been suggested includes elevated serum transaminase and mild bone marrow suppression [7,99].

The prophylactic benefits of exogenous interferon for systemic infections have been examined in several double-blind, controlled studies. Infections with several respiratory viruses were not prophylactically affected by interferon (monkey interferon) delivered locally to the respiratory tract in doses of 10,000 units per patient [275] or 180,000 units per patient (reference in [195]). A total of 800,000 units of intranasal human leukocyte interferon administered one day prior to inoculation with influenza B appeared to delay the onset of a normal course of infection by one day [195]. However, an intensive course of 14,000,000 units of human leukocyte interferon administered in 39 intranasal sprayings did prevent clinical symptoms and virus shedding after challenge of volunteers with rhinovirus 4 [195]. Although this study provides hope; obtaining these quantities of interferon is currently a major endeavor and the regimen of 39 intranasal sprayings approaches the nuisance level of a common cold. In a single small study, the administration of 650,000 units of human leukocyte interferon in two intramuscular injections prior to RA27/3 live attenuated rubella vaccine virus challenge delayed virus excretion and antibody production [20].

No controlled therapeutic trials of interferon for systemic infections in humans have been completed, although a study in immunosuppressed patients with varicella-zoster infections is in progress (T. C. Merigan, personal communication). Nevertheless several trials are of interest. In several patients with chronic active hepatitis who had stable serum levels of hepatitis B antigens and DNA polymerase, parenteral courses of human leukocyte interferon resulted in the diminution or disappearance of these hepatitis B virus markers from their serum and the absence of viral antigens from subsequent liver biopsies [99]. The intramuscular and intrathecal administration of human leukocyte interferon following challenge of cynomolgus monkeys with rabies street virus appears to reduce mortality [115]. A transient suppression of cytomegaloviruria in congenitally infected infants can be produced by large parenteral doses of human leukocyte interferon [7,77].

Because of the real difficulties involved in producing and purifying large quantities of interferon and the potential problems which might arise from therapy with exogenous proteins, inducers of endogenous interferon have been explored as potential chemotherapeutic agents. These inducers can include other viruses, polynucleotides, or a diverse array of nonpolynucleotides [62,84,194]. Several inducers have been administered intravenously, providing information regarding pharmacology and toxicity [85,87a,104,151,194,197]. No controlled studies with parenteral interferon inducers in humans have yet been published. The bulk of induction studies have evaluated the efficacy of intranasal drug against respiratory virus infections [65,66,92,116,230,255, 287]. Although some of the trials have documented an effect, the benefits have not been dramatic. A poly-L-lysine and carboxymethylcellulose stabilized polyriboinosinic-polyribocytodylic acid (Poly I:C) appears to be an effective inducer in lower primates; however, tachyphylaxis develops by the third injection [176,264,293].

Cutaneous Infections

Primary Vaccinia

Exogenous interferon [274] and rifampicin [205] have been tested for their ability to prevent the take of a primary vaccination. In both studies, volunteers were vaccinated in two sites, one site receiving treatment, the other placebo. The interferon study represented the first study of the clinical applicability of that compound. An unknown quantity of impure monkey interferon inoculated subcutaneously at the site prior to vaccination prevented takes in most vaccinees. A 10–15% preparation of rifampicin applied locally prevented one-half of vaccination takes, while 12 mg/kg rifampicin administered orally had no definite effect. The failure of oral drug to affect vaccinia is not surprising, since the levels of rifampicin required to inhibit poxviruses (100 μg/ml) are 5–10 times the maximum attainable peak serum levels with nontoxic doses of the drug [207].

Mucocutaneous Herpes Simplex

0.1–0.5% IUdR in an aqueous solution failed to ameliorate cutaneous herpes simplex infections in four double-blinded, placebo-controlled studies [31,129,143,156]. A regimen of 0.1% IUdR in 1.4% polyvinyl alcohol, which involved several dozen applications on the first day alone, was alleged to hasten healing; however, neither the primary data nor statistics are available in this report [55]. Moreover, the regimen is clearly an impractical one. The same IUdR-polyvinyl alcohol preparation proved ineffective in a subsequent controlled trial [156]. Intradermal injection of 0.1% IUdR with an airjet spraygun did shorten the time to scabbing and the duration of pain [144]. Interestingly, many recipients of this novel therapy developed recurrent lesions in new sites [181], an unusual occurrence in the natural history of cutaneous herpetic disease and presumably a consequence of trauma. Dimethyl sulfoxide (DMSO) is an excellent solvent for IUdR and is itself highly soluble in the cutis [162,163]. A 5% solution of IUdR in DMSO reduced the interval to complete healing from 8.9 to 3.5 days; however, DMSO alone reduced this interval to 5.4 days [181]. Recurrences were not prevented, and this is not surprising considering the ganglionic residence of herpes simplex virus during periods of latency.

Neither 0.5% IUdR nor 3% Ara-A applied locally altered the course of primary or recurrent genital herpes in double-blinded, placebo-controlled studies [2,98,302]. However, duration of virus shedding and interval to healing were shortened in patients with recurrent genital herpes using IUdR in DMSO [231]. Twenty per cent IUdR was superior to 5% drug, and both were superior to DMSO control.

When certain viruses (including herpes simplex virus) are propagated in the presence of photoactive dyes, such as neutral red, proflavine, acridine orange and methylene blue, their infectivity is destroyed by subsequent exposure to light [312,313]. This process, called photodynamic inactivation, has been utilized to treat recurrent orolabial and genital herpes simplex virus infections. Initial enthusiasm for this form of therapy, based upon uncontrolled and anecdotal experience, was reinforced by a placebo-controlled study which claimed that photodynamic inactivation with neutral red and light hastened healing and decreased the recurrence rate in patients with recurrent mucocutaneous herpes simplex infections [81]. However, while this study employed a placebo, improvement was measured in each patient by comparison with pretreatment history of disease. Four subsequent double-blind, placebo-controlled studies employing neutral red or proflavine have failed to document any benefits of photodynamic inactivation in patients with orolabial or genital herpes simplex virus infection [212,259,302; McCarty, J. R. and Jarratt, M., personal communication]. Photodynamic inactivation neither shortened the duration of the treated episode nor reduced the frequency of recurrence. In view of this lack of efficacy, as well as the potential oncogenicity of photodynamically inactivated herpes simplex virus [72], treatment of mucocutaneous herpes simplex virus infections by photodynamic inactivation should be abandoned.

Levamisole, like inosiplex, has been suggested as an "immuno-potentiating" agent [105]; however, much room remains for precise definition of its activity. The drug had no effect in two controlled studies on recurrent herpes simplex [39,193]. Adverse reactions, including aberrant taste and smell, urticaria and granulocytopenia [39,193], raise concern about the therapeutic index of levamisole.

A recent controlled trial has also failed to document the therapeutic efficacy of the local application of ether in patients with herpes genitalis [56]. The failure to document the efficacy of these clinically popular modes of therapy should serve to emphasize that the highly variable and unpredictable natural history of many viral diseases, as well as the potential influence of patient and physician bias on the assessment of the therapeutic response, necessitates the use of prospective, double-blind, placebo-controlled clinical trials for the evaluation of the efficacy of any treatment regimen.

Localized Herpes Zoster

Herpes zoster can occasionally disseminate, especially in immunosuppressed patients, but in most victims it represents a significant nuisance which can lead to a prolonged, severely distracting neuralgia [145]. Repeated local application of an interferon inducer, poly I:C, failed to ameliorate localized herpes zoster in children with cancer [82]. Subcutaneous administration of Ara-C around the lesions, which resulted in systemic absorption sufficient to produce some nausea, vomiting and bone marrow suppression, was of no benefit in the resolution of localized zoster [21]. This trial had been preceded by an optimistic demonstration that this regimen produced systemic Ara-C concentrations which exceeded the *in vitro* inhibitory levels for varicella-zoster virus [329]; nevertheless, the Ara-C recipients tended to experience more prolonged neurologic symptoms than the placebo recipients. As already mentioned, intravenous Ara-C has also proved to be of no benefit [267].

Juel-Jensen reported some amelioration of pain and acceleration of healing in zoster lesions treated with 5 to 40% IUdR in DMSO [142], a result reminiscent of his success with cutaneous herpes simplex infections [181]. These results have since been expanded and confirmed [61,145]; however, the significant expense of this quantity of drug and the undefined long-term toxicity of such high concentrations of drug and solvent remain a concern. A small controlled trial reported the efficacy of 48 mg per day of the oral corticosteroid, triamcinolone. Steroid-treated patients who were older than 60 years experienced a diminished duration of postherpetic neuralgia [75]. No effect was seen on the rate of healing of the lesions. Considering the high dose of oral corticosteroid involved, a larger controlled study would be desirable to confirm these results.

Five per cent ribavirin in a topical ointment has been reported to ameliorate herpes zoster in a double-blind, placebo-controlled trial; however, only 14 patients were included in the study and the results would have been reversed had one placebo recipient been eliminated from the study [330].

Viral Infections of the Eye

Kaufman has succinctly reviewed the unique problems and current status of ocular antiviral therapy [149]. Epithelial infection is uniquely amenable to both therapy and its evaluation. Therapy is facilitated by the ease with which infection can be recognized at an early stage and by the ability to apply locally high concentrations of drugs which are poorly absorbed through the cornea. Evaluation of efficacy is made easier by the direct visibility of the disease, paired organs permitting controlled studies and animal models which to date have accurately predicted results in humans [149]. For these reasons, herpes keratitis represented the first infection for which antiviral chemotherapy was established as effective. The treatment of epithelial herpetic ocular infection is now a standard clinical practice of proven merit. Several well controlled studies have demonstrated that local instillation of 0.5% IUdR promotes more rapid clearing of local virus and more rapid healing of corneal ulcers than does placebo [32,109,133,134,169,232]. Therapy does not affect the incidence of recurrences.

There is some room for improvement over IUdR in the treatment of herpes keratitis. IUdR appears capable of inducing a true allergic reaction, toxic keratoconjunctivitis and clinical resistance [124,133,218,235]. A small proportion of clinical failures may also be due to the development of true drug resistance by the virus [49,133]. Thus other agents are now being examined, using IUdR as the standard for comparison. Ara-C and photodynamic inactivation have produced excessive toxicity [150,217]. Controlled human studies demonstrate both 1% trifluorothymidine (F_3TdR) and 3% Ara-A to be as effective, if not superior to IUdR, as measured by interval to healing and percentage of ulcers healed [57,70,124,139,168,183,235,317]. Ara-A also appears to be effective where IUdR was clinically unsuccessful [140,218,235]. However, in one controlled study, which also analyzed toxic reactions, IUdR and Ara-A appeared comparable [70].

Although Kaufman and others have documented the benefits of interferon and its inducers for herpetic keratitis in the animal model, 6000 units/ml were no better than placebo in recurrent human disease [152] and inferior to thermocautery [297]. However, in two separate encouraging followup studies, the use of $3\text{-}31 \times 10^6$ units/ml of human leukocyte interferon applied locally following thermocautery or debridment accelerated healing and inhibited virus shedding [138,298]. In a small nonrandomized, placebo-controlled trial, the interferon inducer poly I:C produced better results than did IUdR [103]; however, to our knowledge, followup studies have not been published.

Stromal disease and iritis are not as amenable to therapy as epithelial infection [149]. Several explanations have been invoked to explain this difficulty. Kaufman has presented evidence suggesting that much stromal pathology may be a consequence of an immunologically mediated inflammation evoked by viral antigens, rather than the direct result of cytolytic virus replication [300]. Furthermore, IUdR and Ara-A fail to penetrate into the aqueous humor prior to degradation by host enzymes [238]. Ara-A is almost invariably absent from the aqueous humor following topical application to the eye [238,245]. Thus, uveitis has only rarely appeared to respond to local antiviral therapy and then only when an unhealthy disrupted epithelium was present [238]. The failure of topical IUdR or Ara-A in patients with herpetic keratouveitis prompted a controlled study using 20 mg/kg Ara-A daily for seven days by intravenous infusion [1]. This high dose of Ara-A, which caused a moderate amount of gastrointestinal toxicity and some leukopenia, produced definite benefit in the treatment group. Single aqueous humor specimens were obtained from four patients. Ara-A levels ranged from 0.1 to 3 μg/ml and Ara-Hx levels ranged from 3.2 to 11.2 $\mu g/ml$. A recent study in rabbits using parenteral Ara-AMP, the highly soluble monophosphate of Ara-A, suggests that much higher levels of intraocular drug can be attained with the monophosphate [240].

Superficial corneal disease in the rabbit is equally responsive to 3% Ara-A, 15% Ara-Hx and 0.5% IUdR [239]. Assuming the Ara-Hx preparation was free of Ara-A, the Ara-Hx effect is of particular interest because of its good solubility and its capacity to penetrate into the aqueous humor [239]. Using an Ara-Hx cream, intraocular titers of 100 $\mu g/ml$ are attained [239]. These are effective antiviral levels *in vitro* [51,180]. If these results can be confirmed, further examination of Ara-Hx (as well as Ara-AMP) for intraocular infections is merited.

Therapy for nonherpetic ocular virus infections has also been studied. Adenoviral keratoconjunctivitis does not appear to respond to topical IUdR or Ara-A [71,111,237]. Controlled human trials with vaccinia keratitis have not been performed; however, in a rabbit model, 5% Ara-A is superior to 0.1% IUdR and both are superior to placebo in resolving that disease [125].

CONCLUSION

Clinical efficacy in a practical sense has now been documented for certain antiviral agents: amantadine for the prophylaxis and therapy of influenza A infections, Ara-A for the therapy of herpes zoster in immunosuppressed patients and of herpes simplex virus encephalitis, and topical drugs for the therapy of herpetic keratoconjunctivitis. Amantadine and topical drugs for herpetic keratitis (IUdR and Ara-A) have been licensed for use by the FDA; systemic Ara-A remains an investigational drug as of early 1978. Unfortunately, the array of untreatable viral afflictions and the imperfect results attainable with currently available modalities leave much room for improvement. Superior drugs are obviously needed. Many of the antiviral drugs which we have today were developed as cytotoxic agents for cancer chemotherapy. Thus, their toxicity should not be surprising. Moreover, their availability (as anticancer agents) facilitated their uncontrolled use in individual cases of virus infection thought to have very high mortality. This anecdotal experience lead to false optimism with respect to the efficacy of such agents as Ara-C and IUdR.

Analysis of the mechanisms responsible for the antiviral activity and host cell toxicity of currently available drugs is leading to the syntheses of new agents which are more active and less cytotoxic [41,42,249,250].

More virus-specific functions and enzymes are being recognized [131,132,159,220] which differ from those of the host cell and thus provide targets for truly selective inhibitors of virus replication. We can therefore expect that the next generation of antiviral drugs, aimed at molecular events unique to virus replication and selected for the absence of host cell toxicity, will have much higher therapeutic indices than currently available drugs. Combined therapy with two or more antiviral agents is also being explored in an effort to achieve additive antiviral activity without additive toxicity, and to reduce the emergence of drug-resistant mutants [29,76,174,325].

A number of important lessons have been learned with respect to the application of chemotherapeutic agents to virus infections in man. The requirement for more refined *in vitro* and animal model studies to evaluate the therapeutic index of an agent prior to any human use is now apparent, as is the need for detailed information on pharmacokinetics. No antiviral agent should be used in the absence of published knowledge of its absorption, distribution, metabolism and excretion. The uncontrolled phase II studies which assess feasibility, pharmacology and toxicity in man should not be followed by *uncontrolled* therapeutic trials. We now recognize the need for definitive laboratory diagnosis, the importance of knowledge of the pathogenesis and natural history of viral diseases, and the critical role played by host factors in determining the outcome of infection (and thus the apparent response to antiviral therapy). Finally, we seem at last to have learned that in evaluating the efficacy and toxicity of a given antiviral agent there is no substitute for a randomized double-blind placebo-controlled study involving proven cases of the disease. For less common infections such as encephalitis, the multi-hospital cooperative studies have set an excellent example and should be encouraged. Thus, there is reason to be optimistic that the next decade will be one in which the use of antiviral agents will have a major impact upon the morbidity and mortality of viral diseases.

REFERENCES

1. Abel R Jr, Kaufman HE, Sugar J: Intravenous adenine arabinoside against herpes simplex keratouveitis in humans. Am J Ophthalmol 79:659–664, 1975.
2. Adams HG, Benson EA, Alexander ER, et al: Genital herpetic infection in men and women: Clinical course and effect of topical application of adenine arabinoside. J Infect Dis 133:A151–A159, 1976.
3. Alford CA Jr, Whitley RJ: Treatment of infections due to *Herpesvirus* in humans: A critical review of the state of the art. J Infect Dis 133:A101–A108, 1976.
4. Allen LB, Sidwell RW: Target-organ treatment of neurotropic virus diseases: Efficacy

as a chemotherapy tool and comparison of activity of adenine arabinoside, cytosine arabinoside, idoxuridine, and trifluorothymidine Antimicrob Agents Chemother 2:229–233, 1972.

5. Armbruster KFW, Rahn AC, Ing TS, et al: Amantadine toxicity in a patient with renal insufficiency. Nephron 13:183–186, 1974.

6. Arroyo M, Beare AS, Reed SE, et al: A therapeutic study of an adamantane spiro compound in experimental influenza A infection in man. J Antimicrob Chemother 1:87–93, 1975.

7. Arvin AM, Yeager AS, Merigan TC: Effect of leukocyte interferon in urinary excretion of cytomegalovirus by infants. J Infect Dis 133:A205–A210, 1976.

8. Ashwal S, Finegold M, Fish I, et al: Effect of the antiviral drug, cytosine arabinoside, on the developing nervous system. Pediatr Res 8:945–950, 1974.

9. Aswell JF, Allen GP, Jamieson AT, et al: Antiviral activity of arabinosylthymine in herpesviral replication: Mechanism of action in vivo and in vitro. Antimicrob Agents Chemother 12:243–254, 1977.

10. Ayrosa-Galvao PA, Castro IO: The effect of 1-8-D-ribofuranosyl-1,2,4-triazole-3-carboxamide on acute viral hepatitis. Ann NY Acad Sci 284:278–283, 1977.

11. Baltimore D: RNA-dependent DNA polymerase in virions of RNA tumor viruses. Nature 226:1209–1211, 1970.

12. Baltimore D: Expression of animal virus genomes. Bacteriol Rev 35:235–241, 1971.

13. Bauer DJ: Thiosemicarbazones. In: Radouco-Thomas C, Bauer DJ (Eds): International Encyclopedia of Pharmacology and Therapeutics. Chemotherapy of Virus Diseases, Sec 61, Vol I. Oxford, Pergamon Press, 1972.

14. Bauer DJ, St Vincent L, Kempe CH, et al: Prophylaxis of smallpox with methisazone. Am J Epidemiol 90:130–145, 1969.

15. Bean WJ Jr, Simpson RW: Primary transcription of the influenza virus genome in permissive cells. Virology 56:646–651, 1973.

16. Beare AS, Hall TS, Tyrrell DAJ: Protection of volunteers against challenge with A/ Hong Kong/68 influenza virus by a new adamantane compound. Lancet 1:1039–1040, 1972.

17. Becker Y: Antiviral drugs. Mode of action and chemotherapy of viral infections of man. Monographs in Virology, Vol 11. Melnick JL (Ed). Karger, Basel, 1976.

18. Becker Y, Asher Y, Cohen Y, et al: Phosphonoacetic acid-resistant mutants of herpes simplex virus: Effect of phosphonoacetic acid on virus replication and in vitro deoxyribonucleic acid synthesis in isolated nuclei. Antimicrob Agents Chemother 11:919–922, 1977.

19. Bell WR, Whang JJ, Carbone PP, et al: Cytogenetic and morphologic abnormalities in human bone marrow cells during cytosine arabinoside therapy. Blood 27:771–781, 1966.

20. Best JM, Banatvala JE: The effect of a human interferon preparation on vaccine-induced rubella infection. J Biol Stand 3:197–212, 1975.

21. Betts RF, Zaky DA, Douglas RG Jr, et al: Ineffectiveness of subcutaneous cytosine arabinoside in localized herpes zoster. Ann Intern Med 82:778–783, 1975.

22. Bishop DHL: Virion polymerases. In: Fraenkel-Conrat H, Wagner RR (Eds): Comprehensive Virology, 10. New York, Plenum, 1977.

23. Bleidner WE, Harmon JB, Hewes WE, et al: Absorption, distribution and excretion of amantadine hydrochloride. J Pharmacol Exp Ther 150:1–7, 1965.

24. Bodey GP, Gottlieb J, McCredie KB, et al: Adenine arabinoside in cancer chemotherapy. In: Pavan-Langston D (Ed): Adenine Arabinoside: An Antiviral Agent. New York, Raven Press, 1975.

25. Boston Interhospital Virus Study Group and the NIAID-Sponsored Cooperative Antiviral Clinical Study: Failure of high dose 5-iodo-2'-deoxyuridine in the therapy of herpes simplex virus encephalitis. N Engl J Med 292:599–603, 1975.

26. Breeden CJ, Hall TC, Tyler HR: Herpes simplex encephalitis treated with systemic 5-iodo-2' deoxyuridine. Ann Intern Med 65:1050–1056, 1966.

27. Bryson YJ, Connor JD: In vitro susceptibility of varicella zoster virus to adenine arabinoside and hypoxanthine arabinoside. Antimicrob Agents Chemother 9:540–543, 1976.

28. Bryson Y, Connor JD, Sweetman L, et al: Determination of plaque inhibitory activity of adenine arabinoside (9-8-D-arabinofuranosyladenine) for herpesviruses using an adenosine deaminase inhibitor. Antimicrob Agents Chemother 6:98–101, 1974.

29. Bryson YJ, Kronenberg LH: Combined antiviral effects of interferon, adenine arabinoside, hypoxanthine arabinoside, and adenine arabinoside-5'-monophosphate in human fibroblast cultures. Antimicrob Agents Chemother 11:299–306, 1977.

30. Bucher D, Palese P: The biologically active proteins of influenza virus: Neuraminidase. In: Kilbourne ED (Ed): The Influenza Viruses and Influenza. New York, Academic Press, 1975.

31. Burnett JW, Katz SL: A study of the use of 5 iodo-2'-deoxyuridine in cutaneous herpes simplex. J Invest Dermatol 40:7–8, 1963.

32. Burns RP: A double-blind study of IDU in human herpes simplex keratitis. Arch Ophthalmol 70:381–384, 1963.

33. Calabresi P: Clinical studies with systemic administration of antimetabolites of pyrimidine nucleosides in viral infections. Ann NY Acad Sci 130:192–208, 1965.

34. Calabresi P, Cardoso SS, Finch SC, et al: Initial clinical studies with 5-iodo-2'-deoxyuridine. Cancer Res 21:550–559, 1961.

35. Calabresi P, Creasey WA, Prusoff H, et al: Clinical and pharmacological studies with 5-iodo-2'-deoxycytidine. Cancer Res 23:583–592, 1963.

36. Caliguiri LA, Tamm I: Guanidine and 2-(α-hydroxybenzyl)-benzimidazole (HBB): Selective inhibitors of picornavirus multiplication. In: Carter WA (Ed): Selective Inhibitors of Viral Functions. Cleveland. CRC Press, 1973.

37. Carter WA (Ed): Selective Inhibitors of Viral Functions. Cleveland, CRC Press, 1973.

38. Chalmers TC: Effects of ascorbic acid on the common cold. An evaluation of the evidence. Am J Med 58:532–536, 1975.

39. Chang T, Fiumara N: (Abstract) Treatment of recurrent genital herpes with levamisole. 17th Interscience Conference on Antimicrobial Agents and Chemotherapy, NY, 12–14 October 1977, 459.

40. Chang T, Weinstein L: Antiviral activity of isoprinosine in vitro and in vivo. Am J Med Sci 265(2):143–146, 1973.

41. Cheng Y: A rational approach to the development of antiviral chemotherapy: Alternative substrates of herpes simplex virus type 1 (HSV-1) and type 2 (HSV-2) thymidine kinase (TK). Ann NY Acad Sci 284:594–598, 1977.

42. Cheng YC, Goz B, Neenan JP, et al: Selective inhibition of herpes simplex virus by 5'-amino-2', 5'-dideoxy-5-iodouridine. J Virol 15:1284–1285, 1975.

43. Ch'ien LT, Cannon NJ, Whitley RJ, et al: Effect of adenine arabinoside on cytomegalovirus infections. J Infect Dis 130:32–39, 1974.

44. Ch'ien LT, Schabel FM Jr, Alford CA Jr: Arabinosyl nucleosides and nucleotides. In: Carter WA (Ed): Selective Inhibitors of Viral Functions. Cleveland, CRC Press, 227–256, 1973.

45. Cho CT, Liu C, Voth DW, et al: Effects of idoxuridine on *Herpesvirus hominis* encephalitis and disseminated infections in marmosets. J Infect Dis 128:718–723, 1973.

46. Chow AW, Ronald A, Fiala M, et al: Cytosine arabinoside therapy for herpes simplex encephalitis—clinical experience with six patients. Antimicrob Agents Chemother 3:412–417, 1973.

47. Cohen A, Togo Y, Khakoo R, et al: Comparative clinical and laboratory evaluation of the prophylactic capacity of ribavirin, amantadine hydrochloride, and placebo in induced human influenza type A. J Infect Dis 133:A114–A120, 1976.

48. Coker-Vann M, Dolin R: Effect of adenine arabinoside on Epstein-Barr virus in vitro. J Infect Dis 135:447–453, 1977.

49. Coleman VR, Tsu E, Jawetz E: "Treatment-resistance" to idoxuridine in herpetic keratitis (33419). Proc Soc Exp Biol Med 129:761–765, 1965.

50. Connor JD, Sweetman L, Carey S, et al: Effect of adenosine deaminase upon the antiviral activity in vitro of adenine arabinoside for vaccinia virus. Antimicrob Agents Chemother 6:630–636, 1974.

51. Connor JD, Sweetman L, Carey S, et al: Susceptibility *in vitro* of several large DNA viruses to the antiviral activity of adenine arabinoside and its metabolite, hypoxanthine arabinoside: Relation to human pharmacology. *In:* Pavan-Langston D (Ed): Adenine Arabinoside: An Antiviral Agent. New York, Raven Press, 1975.

52. Cooper GM: Phosphorylation of 5-bromodeoxycytidine in cells infected with herpes simplex virus. Proc Natl Acad Sci USA 70:3788–3792, 1973.

53. Cooper PD: Genetics of picornaviruses. *In:* Fraenkel-Conrat H, Wagner RR (Eds): Comprehensive Virology, 9. New York, Plenum, 1977.

54. Cooper PD: The possible role of the equestron as an achilles' heel for chemotheraphy of picornavirus infections. Ann NY Acad Sci 284:650–661, 1977.

55. Corbett MB, Sidell CM, Zimmerman M: Idoxuridine in the treatment of cutaneous herpes simplex. JAMA 196:155–158, 1966.

56. Corey L, Reeves WC, Vontver L, et al: (Abstract) Evaluation of topical ether for treatment of genital herpes simplex virus infection. 17th Inter-science Conference on Antimicrobial Agents and Chemotheraphy, NY, 12–14 October 1977, 292.

57. Coster DJ, McKinnon JR, McGill JI, et al: Clinical evaluation of adenine arabinoside and trifluorothymidine in the treatment of corneal ulcers caused by herpes simplex virus. J Infect Dis 133:A173–A177, 1976.

58. Coulehan JL, Eberhard S, Kapner L, et al: Vitamin C and acute illness in Navajo schoolchildren. N Engl J Med 295:973–977, 1976.

59. Courtney RJ: Herpes simplex virus protein synthesis in the presence of 2-deoxy-D-glucose. Virology 73:286–294, 1976.

60. Creasey WA, Papac RJ, Markiw ME, et al: Biochemical and pharmacological studies with 1-β-D-arabinofuranosylcytosine in man. Biochem Pharmacol 15:1417–1428, 1966.

60a. Davis CM, Van Dersarl JV, Coltman CA Jr: Failure of cytarabine in varicella-zoster infections. JAMA 224:122–123, 1973.

61. Dawber R: Idoxuridine in herpes zoster: Further evaluation of intermittent topical therapy. Br Med J 2:526–527, 1974.

62. DeClercq E: Nonpolynucleotide interferon inducers. *In:* Carter WA (Ed): Selective Inhibitors of Viral Functions, Cleveland, CRC Press, 1973.

63. Dickinson PCT, Chang TW, Weinstein L: Effects of amantadines on influenza b and measles virus infection in children. Antibicrob Agents Chemother 521–526, 1966.

64. Dobersen MJ, Jerkofsky M, Greer S: Enzymatic basis for the selective inhibition of

varicella-zoster virus by 5-halogenated analogues of deoxycytidine. J Virol 20:478–486, 1976.

65. Douglas RG Jr, Betts RF: Effect of induced interferon in experimental rhinovirus infections in volunteers. Infect Immun 9:506–510, 1974.

66. Douglas RG Jr, Betts RF, Simons RL, et al: Evaluation of a topical interferon inducer in experimental influenza infection in volunteers. Antimicrob Agents Chemother 8:684–687, 1975.

67. Dourmashkin RR, Tyrrell DAJ: Electron microscope observations on the entry of influenza virus into susceptible cells. J Gen Virol 24:129–141, 1974.

68. do Valle LA, de Melo PR, Gomes LF, et al: Methisazone in prevention of variola minor among contacts. Lancet 2:976–978, 1965.

69. Drach JC, Shipman C Jr: The selective inhibition of viral DNA synthesis by chemotherapeutic agents: An indicator of clinical usefulness? Ann NY Acad Sci 284:396–409, 1977.

70. Dresner AJ, Seamans ML: Evidence of the safety and efficacy of adenine arabinoside in the treatment of herpes simplex epithelial keratitis. *In:* Pavan-Langston D (Ed): Adenine Arabinoside: An Antiviral Agent. New York, Raven Press, 1975.

71. Dudgeon J, Bhargava SK, Ross CAC: Treatment of adenovirus infection of the eye with 5-iodo-2'-deoxyuridine. A double-blind trial. Br J Ophthal 53:530–533, 1969.

72. Duff R, Rapp F: Oncogenic transformation of hamster embryo cells after exposure to inactivated herpes simplex virus type 1. J Virol 12:209–217, 1973.

73. Durr FE, Lindh HF, Forbes M: Efficacy of 1-β-D-ribofuranosyl-1,2,4-triazole-3-carboxamide against influenza virus infections in mice. Antimicrob Agents Chemother 7:582–586, 1975.

74. Dykes MHM, Meier, P: Ascorbic acid and the common cold. JAMA 231:1073–1079, 1975.

75. Eaglstein WH, Katz R, Brown JA: The effects of early corticosteroid therapy on the skin eruption and pain of herpes zoster. JAMA 211:1681–1683, 1970.

76. Eggers HJ: Successful treatment of enterovirus-infected mice by 2-α-hydroxybenzyl)-benzimidazole and guanidine. J Exp Med 143:1367–1381, 1976.

77. Emodi G, O'Reilly R, Muller A, et al: Effect of human exogenous leukocyte interferon in cytomegalovirus infections. J Infect Dis 133:A199–A204, 1976.

78. Engle CG, Stewart RC: Anti-herpetic activity of 5-iodo-2'-deoxyuridine in presence of its degradation products. (28825). Proc Soc Exp Biol Med 115:43–45, 1964.

79. Eriksson B, Helgstrand E, Johansson NG, et al: Inhibition of influenza virus ribonucleic acid polymerase by ribavirin triphosphate. Antimicrob Agents Chemother 11:946–951, 1977.

80. Fahn S, Craddock G, Kumin G: Acute toxic psychosis from suicidal overdosage of amantadine. Arch Neurol 25:45–48, 1971.

81. Felber TD, Smith EB, Knox JM, et al: Photodynamic inactivation of herpes simplex. Report of a clinical trial. JAMA 223:289–292, 1973.

82. Feldman S, Hughes WT, Darlington RW, et al: Evaluation of topical polyinosinic acid-polycytidylic acid in treatment of localized herpes zoster in children with cancer: A randomized, double-blind controlled study. Antimicrob Agents Chemother 8:289–294, 1975.

83. Fenton RJ, Potter CW: Dose-response activity of ribavirin against influenza virus infection in ferrets. J Antimicrob Chemother 3:263–271, 1977.

84. Field AK: Interferon induction by polynucleotides. *In:* Carter WA (Ed): Selective Inhibitors of Viral Functions. Cleveland, CRC Press, 1973.

85. Field AK, Young CW, Krakoff IH, et al: Induction of interferon in human subjects by poly I:C (35454). Proc Soc Exp Biol Med 136:1180–1186, 1971.

86. Fishaut JM, Connor JD, Lampert PW: Comparative effects of arabinosyl nucleosides upon the postnatal growth and development of the rat. Pediatr Res 8:825–829, 1974.

87. Fox BW: Pharmacology and chemistry of some inhibitors of herpes replication. J Antimicrob Chemother 3:23–32, 1977.

87a. Freeman AI, Al-Bussam N, O'Malley JA, et al: Pharmacologic effects of polyinosinic-polycitidylic acid in man. J Med Virol 1:79–93, 1977.

88. Friedman RM: Antiviral activity of interferons. Bacteriol Rev 41:543–567, 1977.

89. Galbraith AW: Therapeutic trials of amantadine (Symmetrel) in general practice. J Antimicrob Chemother 1:81–86, 1975.

90. Galbraith AW, Schild GS, Oxford JS, et al: Protective effect of aminoadamantane on influenza A2 infections in the family environment. Ann NY Acad Sci 173:29–43, 1970.

91. Galbraith AW, Schild GC, Potter CW, et al: The therapeutic effect of amantadine in influenza occurring during the winter of 1971-2 assessed by double-blind study. J Roy Coll Gen Pract 23:34–37, 1973.

92. Gatmaitan BG, Stanley ED, Jackson GG: The limited effect of nasal interferon induced by rhinovirus and a topical chemical inducer on the course of infection. J Infect Dis 127:401–407, 1973.

93. Gerald PS, Monedjikova V, Enders JF: (Abstract) Genes for susceptibility to viruses. Pediatr Res 8:424, 1974.

94. Gerber P: Activation of Epstein-Barr virus by 5-bromodeoxy-uridine in "virus-free" human cells. Proc Natl Acad Sci USA 69:83–85, 1972.

95. Glasgow LA: Advantages and limitations of animal models in the evaluation of antiviral substances. J Infect Dis 133:A73–A78, 1976.

96. Glasgow LA, Galasso GJ: Isoprinosine: Lack of antiviral activity in experimental model infections. J Infect Dis 126:162–169, 1972.

97. Glazko AJ, Chang T, Drach JC, et al: Species differences in the metabolic disposition of adenine arabinoside. In: Pavan-Langston D (Ed): Adenine Arabinoside: An Antiviral Agent. New York, Raven Press, 1975.

98. Goodman EL, Luby JP, Johnson MT: Prospective double-blind evaluation of topical adenine arabinoside in male herpes progenitalis. Antimicrob Agents Chemother 8:693–697, 1975.

99. Greenberg HB, Pollard RB, Lutwick LI, et al: Effect of human leukocyte interferon on hepatitis B virus infection in patients with chronic active hepatitis. N Engl J Med 295:517–522, 1976.

100. Griffith JF, Fitzwilliam JF, Casagrande S, et al: Experimental herpes simplex virus encephalitis: Comparative effects of treatment with cytosine arabinoside and adenine arabinoside. J Infect Dis 132:506–510, 1975.

101. Grunert RR, Hoffmann CE: Sensitivity of influenza A/New Jersey/8/76 (HswlNl) virus to amantadine-HCl. J Infect Dis 136:297–300, 1977.

102. Grunert RR, McGahen JW, Davies WL: The in vivo antiviral activity of 1-adamantanamine (amantadine). I. Prophylactic and therapeutic activity against influenza viruses. Virology 26:262–269, 1965.

103. Guerra R, Frezzotti R, Bonanni R, et al: A preliminary study on treatment of human herpes simplex keratitis with an interferon inducer. Ann NY Acad Sci 173:823–830, 1970.

104. Guggenheim MA, Baron S: Clinical studies of an interferon inducer, polyriboinosinic-polyribocytidylic acid [poly (I)-ploy (C)], in children. J Infect Dis 136:50–58, 1977.

105. Gurwith MF, Harman CE, Merigan TC: Approach to diagnosis and treatment of herpes simplex encephalitis—A report of two cases. Calif Med 115:63–71, 1971.

106. Hadden JW, Lopez C, O'Reilly RJ, et al: Levamisole and inosiplex: Antiviral agents with immunopotentiating action. Ann NY Acad Sci 284:139–152, 1977.

107. Hall WJ, Douglas RG Jr, Hyde RW, et al: Pulmonary mechanics after uncomplicated influenza A infection. Am Rev Respir Dis 113:141–147, 1976.

108. Hampar B, Derge JG, Martos LM, et al: Synthesis of Epstein-Barr virus after activation of the viral genome in a "virus-negative" human lymphoblastoid cell (Raji) made resistant to 5-bromodeoxyuridine. Proc Natl Acad Sci USA 69:78–82, 1972.

109. Hart DRL, Brightman VJF, Readshaw GG, et al: Treatment of human herpes simplex keratitis with IDU. Arch Ophthalmol 73:623–634, 1965.

110. Hayden FG, Hall WJ, Douglas RG Jr, et al: (Abstract) Aerosolized amantadine HCl: Pharmacokinetics and safety testing in normal volunteers. 17th Interscience Conference on Antimicrobial Agents and Chemotherapy 12–14 October 1977, New York, abstract 279.

111. Hecht SD, Hanna L, Sery TW, et al: Treatment of epidemic keratoconjunctivities with idoxuridine (IUDR). Arch Ophthalmol 73:49–54, 1965.

112. Heiner GG, Fatima N, Russel PK, et al: Field trials of methisazone as a prophylactic agent against smallpox. Am J Epidemiol 94:435–449, 1971.

113. Herrmann EC Jr (Ed): Third Conference on Antiviral Substances. New York, Ann NY Acad Sci 284, 1977.

114. Herrmann EC Jr, Stinebring WR (Eds): Second Conference on Antiviral Substances. Ann NY Acad Sci 173, 1970.

115. Hilfenhaus J, Weinmann E, Majer M, et al: Administration of human interferon to rabies virus-infected monkeys after exposure. J Infect Dis 135:846–849, 1977.

116. Hill DA, Baron S, Perkins JC, et al: Evaluation of an interferon inducer in viral respiratory disease. JAMA 219:1179–1184, 1972.

117. Ho DHW, Frei E: Clinical pharmacology of 1-β-D-arabinofuranosyl cytosine. Clin Pharmacol Ther 12:944–954, 1971.

118. Ho M, Armstrong JA: Interferon. Ann Rev Microbiol 29:131–161, 1975.

119. Hodes DS, Schnitzer TJ, Kalica AR, et al: Inhibition of respiratory syncytial, parainfluenza 3, and measles viruses by 2-deoxy-D-glucose. Virology 63:201–208, 1975.

120. Hoffman CE: Amantadine HCl and related compounds. In: Carter WA (Ed): Selective Inhibitors of Viral Functions. Cleveland, CRC Press, 199–211, 1973.

121. Hoffman CE, Neumayer EM, Haff RF, et al: Mode of action of the antiviral activity of amantadine in tissue culture. J Bacteriol 90:623–628, 1965.

122. Holland JJ, Kiehn ED: Specific cleavage of viral proteins as steps in the synthesis and maturation of enteroviruses. Proc Natl Acad Sci. USA 60:1015–1022, 1968.

123. Holmes B, Quie PG, Windhorst DB, et al: Protection of phagocytized bacteria from the killing action of antibiotics. Nature 210:1131–1132, 1966.

124. Hyndiuk RA, Hull DS, Schultz RO, et al: Adenine arabinoside in idoxuridine unresponsive and intolerant herpetic keratitis. Am J Ophthalmol 79:655–658, 1975.

125. Hyndiuk RA, Okumoto M, Damiano RA, et al: Treatment of vaccinial keratitis with vidarabine. Arch Ophthalmol 94:1363–1364, 1976.

126. Huffman JH, Sidwell RW, Khare GP, et al: In vitro effect of 1-β-D-ribofuranosyl-1,2,4-triazole-3-carboxamide (virazole, ICN 1229) on deoxyribonucleic acid and ribonucleic acid viruses. Antimicrob Agents Chemother 3:235–241, 1973.

127. Illis LS, Merry RTG: Treatment of herpes simplex encephalitis. J Roy Coll Phys Lond 7:34–44, 1972.

128. Ing TS, Rahn AC, Armbruster KFW, et al: Accumulation of amantadine hydrochloride in renal insufficiency. N Engl J Med 291:1257, 1975.
129. Ive FA: A trial of 5 iodo-2′-deoxyuridine in herpes simplex. Br J Dermatol 76:463–464, 1964.
130. Jacobson MF, Baltimore D: Polypeptide cleavages in the formation of poliovirus proteins. Proc Natl Acad Sci USA 61:77–84, 1968.
131. Jamieson AT, Gentry GA, Subak-Sharpe JH: Induction of both thymidine and deoxycytidine kinase activity by herpes viruses. J Gen Virol 24:465–480, 1974.
132. Jamieson AT, Subak-Sharpe JH: Biochemical studies on the herpes simplex virus-specified deoxypyrimidine kinase activity. J Gen Virol 24:481–492, 1974.
133. Jawetz E, Coleman VR, Dawson CR, et al: The dynamics of *IUDR* action in herpetic keratitis and the emergence of *IUDR* resistance *in vivo*. Ann NY Acad Sci 173:282–291, 1970.
134. Jepson CN: Treatment of herpes simplex of the cornea with IDU. Am J Ophthalmol 57:213, 1964.
135. Jerkofsky M, Dobersen MJ, Greer S: Selective inhibition of the replication of varicella-zoster virus by 5-halogenated analogs of deoxycytidine. Ann NY Acad Sci 284:389, 1977.
136. Joklik WK: The mechanism of action of interferon. Ann NY Acad Sci 284:711–716, 1977.
137. Jolley WB, Call TW, Alvord LS, et al: Immunosuppressive activity of ribavirin using the rabbit skin allograft model. Ann NY Acad Sci 284:230, 1977.
138. Jones BR, Coster DJ, Falcon MG, et al: Topical therapy of ulcerative herpetic keratitis with human interferon. Lancet 2:128, 1976.
139. Jones BR, McGill JI, McKinnon JR, et al: Preliminary experience with adenine arabinoside in comparison with idoxuridine and trifluorothymidine in the management of herpetic keratitis. *In:* Pavan-Langston D (Ed): Adenine Arabinoside: An Antiviral Agent. New York, Raven Press, 1975.
140. Jones DB: Adenine arabinoside in herpes simplex keratitis treatment of idoxuridine-failure epithelial disease and combined corticosteroid therapy in stromal keratitis. *In:* Pavan-Langston D (Ed): Adenine Arabinoside: An Antiviral Agent. New York, Raven Press, 1975.
141. Jordan GW, Fried RP, Merigan TC: Administration of human leukocyte interferon in herpes zoster. I. Safety, circulating antiviral activity and host responses to infection. J Infect Dis 130:56–62, 1974.
142. Juel-Jensen BE: Results of the treatment of zoster with idoxuridine in dimethyl-sulphoxide. Ann NY Acad Sci 173:74–82, 1970.
143. Juel-Jensen BE, MacCallum FO: Treatment of herpes simplex lesions of the face with idoxuridine: Results of a double-blind controlled trial. Br Med J 2:987–988, 1964.
144. Juel-Jensen BE, MacCallum FO: Herpes simplex lesions of face treated with idoxuridine applied by spray gun: Results of a double-blind controlled trial. Br Med J 1:901–903, 1965.
145. Juel-Jensen BE, MacCallum FO: Herpes Simplex Varicella and Zoster. Philadelphia, Lippincott, 1972.
146. Kaluza G: Effect of impaired glycosylation on the biosynthesis of Semliki forest virus glycoproteins. J Virol 16:602–612, 1975.
147. Karnofsky DA, Lacon CR: The effects of 1-β-D-arabinofuranosylcytosine on the developing chick embryo. Biochem Pharmacol 15:1435–1442, 1966.
148. Kato N, Eggers HJ: Inhibition of uncoating of fowl plague virus by 1-adamantanamine hydrochloride. Virology 37:632–641, 1969.

149. Kaufman, HE: Ocular antiviral therapy in perspective. J Infect Dis 133:A96–A100, 1976.

150. Kaufman HE, Capella JA, Maloney ED, et al: Corneal toxicity of cytosine arabinoside. Arch Ophthalmol 72:535–540, 1964.

151. Kaufman HE, Centifanto YM, Ellison ED, et al: Tilorone hydrochloride: Human toxicity and interferon stimulation (35576). Proc Soc Exp Biol Med 137:357–360, 1971.

152. Kaufman HE, Meyer RF, Laibson PR, et al: Human leukocyte interferon for the prevention of recurrences of herpetic keratitis. J Infect Dis 133:A165–A168, 1976.

153. Keeney RE: Human tolerance of adenine arabinoside. In: Pavan-Langston D (Ed): Adenine Arabinoside: An Antiviral Agent. New York, Raven Press, 1975.

153a. Kempe CH, Rodgerson D, Sieber OF: Measurement of N-methylisatin β-thiosemicarbazone serum levels. Lancet 1:824–825, 1965.

154. Kern ER, Overall JC Jr, Glasgow LA: *Herpesvirus hominis* infection in newborn mice. I. An experimental model and therapy with iododeoxyuridine. J Infect Dis 128:290–299, 1973.

155. Khakoo R, Watson G, Waldman R, et al: (Abstract) Effect of isoprinosine on induced human influenza A infection. 17th Interscience Conference on Antimicrobial Agents and Chemotherapy, NY, 12–14 October 1977, 146.

156. Kibrick S, Katz AS: Topical idoxuridine in recurrent herpes simplex. Ann NY Acad Sci 173:83–89, 1970.

157. Kilham L, Ferm VH: Congenital anomalies induced in hamster embryos with ribavirin. Science 195:413–414, 1977.

158. Kinkel AW, Buchanan RA: Human pharmacology. In: Pavan-Langston D (Ed): Adenine Arabinoside: An Antiviral Agent. New York, Raven Press, 1975.

159. Kit S, Jorgensen GN, Dubbs DR, et al: Biochemical and serological properties of the thymidine-phosphorylating enzymes induced by herpes simplex virus mutants temperature-dependent for enzyme formation. Virology 69:179–190, 1976.

160. Kitamoto O: Therapeutic effectiveness of amantadine hydrochloride in naturally occurring Hong Kong influenza—double blind studies. Jpn J Tuberc Chest Dis 17:1–7, 1971.

161. Klenk HD, Scholtissek C, Rott R: Inhibition of glycoprotein biosynthesis of influenza virus by D-glucosamine and 2-deoxy-D-glucose. Virology 49:723–734, 1972.

162. Kligman AM: Topical pharmacology and toxicology of dimethyl sulfoxide—Part 1. JAMA 193:796–804, 1965.

163. Kligman AM: Topical pharmacology and toxicology of dimethyl sulfoxide—Part 2. JAMA 193:923–928, 1965.

164. Koplan JP, Monsur KA, Foster SO, et al: Treatment of variola major with adenine arabinoside. J Infect Dis 131:34–39, 1975.

165. Korant BD: Cleavage of viral precursor proteins in vivo and in vitro. J Virol 10:751–759, 1972.

166. Kraybill EN, Sever JL, Avery GB, et al: Experimental use of cytosine arabinoside in congenital cytomegalovirus infection. J Pediatr 80:485–487, 1972.

167. Kurtz SM: Toxicology of adenine arabinoside. In: Pavan-Langston D (Ed): Adenine Arabinoside: An Antiviral Agent. New York, Raven Press, 1975.

168. Laibson PR, Krachmer JH: Controlled comparison of adenine arabinoside and idoxuridine therapy of human superficial dendritic keratitis. In: Pavan-Langston D (Ed): Adenine Arabinoside: An Antiviral Agent. New York, Raven Press, 1975.

169. Laibson PR, Leopold IH: An evaluation of double blind IDU therapy in 100 cases of herpetic keratitis. Trans Am Acad Ophthalmol Otolaryngol 68:22–34, 1964.

170. Lamar JK, Calhoun FJ, Darr AG: Effects of amantadine hydrochloride on cleavage and embryonic development in the rat and rabbit. Toxicol Appl Pharmacol 17:272, 1970.

171. Larson EW, Stephen EL, Walker JS: Therapeutic effects of small-particle aerosols of ribavirin on parainfluenza (Sendai) virus infections of mice. Antimicrob Agents Chemother 10:770–772, 1976.

172. Lauter CB, Bailey EJ, Lerner AM: Microbiologic assays and neurological toxicity during use of adenine arabinoside in humans. J Infect Dis 134:75–79, 1976.

173. Lerner AM, Bailey EJ: Concentrations of idoxuridine in serum, urine, and cerebro-spinal fluid of patients with suspected diagnoses of Herpesvirus hominis encephalitis. J Clin Invest 51:45–49, 1972.

174. Lerner AM, Bailey EJ: Synergy of 9-β-D-arabinofuranosyladenine and human interferon against herpes simplex virus, type 1. J Infect Dis 130:549–552, 1974.

175. Levinson W: Inhibition of viruses, tumors, and pathogenic microorganisms by isatin β-thiosemicarbazone and other thiosemicarbazones. In: Carter WA (Ed): Selective Inhibitors of Viral Functions. Cleveland, CRC Press, 1973.

176. Levy HB, Baer G, Baron S, et al: A modified polyriboinosinic-polycytidylic acid com-plex that induces interferon in primates. J Infect Dis 132:434–439, 1975.

177. Little JW, Hall WJ, Douglas RG Jr, et al: Amantadine effect on peripheral airways abnormalities in influenza. Ann Intern Med 85:177–182, 1976.

178. Longley S, Dunning RL, Waldman RH: Effect of isoprinosine against challenge with A (H₃N₂)/Hong Kong influenza virus in volunteers. Antimicrob Agents Chemother 3:506–509, 1973.

179. Lowy DR, Rowe WP, Teich N, et al: Murine leukemia virus: High-frequency activa-tion in vitro by 5-iododeoxyuridine and 5-bromodeoxyuridine. Science 174:155–156, 1971.

180. Luby JP, Jones SR, Johnson MT, et al: Sensitivities of herpes simplex virus types 1 and 2 and varicella-zoster virus to adenine arabinoside and hypoxanthine arabinoside. In: Pavan-Langston D (Ed): Adenine Arabinoside: An Antiviral Agent. New York, Raven Press, 1975.

181. MacCallum FO, Juel-Jensen BE: Herpes simplex virus skin infection in man treated with idoxuridine in dimethyl sulphoxide. Results of a double-blind controlled trial. Br Med J 2:805–807, 1966.

182. McCracken GH Jr, Luby JP: Cytosine arabinoside in the treatment of congenital cytomegalic inclusion disease. J Pediatr 80:488–495, 1972.

183. McKinnon Jr, McGill JI, Jones BR: A coded clinical evaluation of adenine arabinoside and trifluorothymidine in the treatment of ulcerative herpetic keratitis. In: Pavan-Langston D (Ed): Adenine Arabinoside: An Antiviral Agent. New York, Raven Press, 1975.

184. Magnussen CR, Douglas RG Jr, Betts, RF, et al: Double-blind evaluation of oral ribavirin (virazole) in experimental influenza A virus infection in volunteers. Anti-microb Agents Chemother 12:498–502, 1977.

185. Manders ED, Tilles JG, Huang AS: Interferon-mediated inhibition of virion-directed transcription. Virology 49:573–581, 1972.

186. Mao JCH, Robishow EE, Overby LR: Inhibition of DNA polymerase from herpes simplex virus-infected Wi-38 cells by phosphonoacetic acid. J Virol 15:1281–1283, 1975.

187. Marcus PI, Engelhardt DL, Hunt JM, et al: Interferon action: Inhibition of VSV RNA synthesis induced by virion-bound polymerase. Science 174:593–598, 1971.

188. Marcus PI, Sekellick MJ: Interferon action III. Primary transcription rate of vesicular stomatitis virus is inhibited by interferon action. J Gen Virol (In press).

189. Marks MI: Evaluation of four antiviral agents in the treatment of herpes simplex encephalitis in a rat model. J Infect Dis 131:11–16, 1975.

190. Mate J, Simon M, Juvancz I: Use of viregyt (Amantadine hydrochloride) in the treatment of epidemic influenza. Ther Hung 19:117–121, 1971.

191. Medical Research Council. Herpes Encephalitis Working Party. Lancet (in press).

192. Medrano L, Green H: Picornavirus receptors and picronavirus multiplication in human-mouse hybrid cell lines. Virology 54:515–524, 1973.

193. Mehr KA, Albano L: Failure of levamisole in herpes simplex. Lancet 2:773–774, 1977.

194. Merigan TC, De Clercq E, Finkelstein MS, et al: Clinical studies employing interferon inducers in man and animals. Ann NY Acad Sci 173:746–759, 1970.

195. Merigan TC, Hall TS, Reed SE, et al: Inhibition of respiratory virus infection by locally applied interferon. Lancet 1:563–567, 1973.

196. Merigan TC, Jordon GW, Fried RP: Clinical utilization of exogenous human interferon. Perspect Virol 9:249–265, 1975.

197. Merigan TC, Regelson W: Interferon induction in man by a synthetic polyanion of defined composition. N Engl J Med 277:1283–1287, 1967.

198. Merigan TC (Ed): Antivirals with clinical potential. J Infect Dis 133 (June Supplement): A1–A279, 1976.

199. Metz DH: The mechanism of action of interferon. Cell 6:429–439, 1975.

200. Metz DH, Levin MJ, Oxman MN: Mechanism of interferon action: Further evidence for transcription as the primary site of action in simian virus 40 infection. J Gen Virol 32:227–240, 1976.

201. Miller DA, Miller OJ, Dev VG, et al: Human chromosome 19 carries a poliovirus receptor gene. Cell 1:167–174, 1974.

202. Miller JP, Kigwana LJ, Streeter DG, et al: The relationship between the metabolism of ribavirin and its proposed mechanism of action. Ann NY Acad Sci 284:211–229, 1977.

203. Miller JZ, Nance WE, Norton JA et al: Therapeutic effect of vitamin C. A co-twin control study. JAMA 237:248–251, 1977.

204. Miller RL, Iltis JP, Rapp F: Differential effect of arabinofuranosylthmyine on the replication of human herpesviruses. J Virol 23:679–684, 1977.

205. Monsur KA, Hossain MS, Huq F, et al: Treatment of variola major with cytosine arabinoside. J Infect Dis 131:40–43, 1975.

206. Moshkowitz A, Goldblum N, Heller E: Studies on the antiviral effect of rifampicin in volunteers. Nature 229:422–424, 1971.

207. Moss B: Ansamycins: (A) rifamycin sv derivatives. In: Carter WA (Ed): Selective Inhibitors of Viral Functions. Cleveland, CRC Press, 1973.

208. Moss B, Rosenblum EN, Grimley PM: Assembly of vaccinia virus particles from polypeptides made in the presence of rifampicin. Virology 45:123–134, 1971.

209. Moss B, Rosenblum EN, Grimley PM: Assembly of virus particles during mixed infection with wild-type vaccinia and a rifampicin-resistant mutant. Virology 45:135–148, 1971.

210. Muldoon RL, Stanley ED, Jackson GG: Use and withdrawal of amantadine chemoprophylaxis during epidemic influenza A. Am Rev Resp Dis 113:487–491, 1976.

211. Muller WEG, Zahn RK, Bittlingmaier K, et al: Inhibition of herpesvirus DNA synthesis by 9-β-D-arabinofuranosyladenine in cellular and cell-free systems. Ann NY Acad Sci 284:34–48, 1977.

212. Myers MG, Oxman MN, Clark JE, et al: Failure of neutral-red photodynamic inactivation in recurrent herpes simplex virus infections. N Engl J Med 293:945–949, 1975.

213. Neumayer EM, Haff RF, Hoffmann CE: Antiviral activity of amantadine hydrochloride in tissue culture and *in ovo*. Proc Soc Exp Biol Med 119:393, 1965.

214. Nichols WW: *In vitro* chromosome breakage induced by arabinosyladenine in human leukocytes. Cancer Res 21:1502–1505, 1964.

215. Nolan DC, Lauter CB, Lerner AM: Idoxuridine in herpes simplex virus (type I) encephalitis. Experience with 29 cases in Michigan, 1966–1971. Ann Intern Med 78:243–246, 1973.

216. Nutter RL, Rapp F: The effect of cytosine arabinoside on virus production in various cells infected with herpes simplex virus types 1 and 2. Cancer Res 33:166–170, 1973.

217. O'Day DM, Jones BR, Poirier R, et al: Proflavine photodynamic viral inactivation in herpes simplex keratitis. Am J Ophthalmol 79:941–948, 1975.

218. O'Day DM, Poirier RH, Jones DB, et al: Vidarabine therapy of complicated herpes simplex keratitis. Am J Ophthalmol 81:642–649, 1976.

219. O'Donoghue JM, Ray CG, Terry DW Jr, et al: Prevention of nosocomial influenza infection with amantadine. Am J Epidemiol 97:276–282, 1973.

220. Ogino T, Otsuka T, Takahashi M: Induction of deoxypyrimidine kinase activity in human embryonic cells infected with varicella-zoster virus. J Virol 21:1232–1235, 1977.

221. Okada Y, Kim J: Interaction of concanavalin A with enveloped viruses and host cells. Virology 50:507–515, 1972.

222. Overby LR, Duff RG, Mao JCH: Antiviral potential of phosphonoacetic acid. Ann NY Acad Sci 284:310–320, 1977.

223. Oxford JS: An inhibitor of the particle associated RNA dependent RNA polymerase of influenza A and B viruses. J Gen Virol 18:11–19, 1973.

224. Oxford JS: Inhibition of the replication of influenza A and B viruses by a nucleoside analogue (ribavirin). J Gen Virol 28:409–414, 1975.

225. Oxford JS, Perrin DD: Inhibition of the particle-associated RNA-dependent RNA polymerase activity of influenza viruses by chelating agents. J Gen Virol 23:59–71, 1974.

226. Oxford JS, Perrin DD: Influenza RNA transcriptase inhibitors: Studies *in vitro* and *in vivo*. Ann NY Acad Sci 284:613–623, 1977.

227. Oxman MN, Levin MJ: Interferon and transcription of early virus-specific RNA in cells infected with simian virus 40. Proc Natl Acad Sci USA 68:299–302, 1971.

228. Pachuta DM, Togo Y, Hornick RB, et al: Evaluation of isoprinosine in experimental human rhinovirus infection. Antimicrob Agents Chemother 5:403–408, 1974.

229. Panitch HS, Baringer JR: Experimental herpes simplex encephalitis. Arch Neurol 28:371–375, 1973.

230. Panusarn CH, Stanley ED, Dirda V, et al: Prevention of illness from rhinovirus infection by a topical interferon inducer. N Engl J Med 291:57–61, 1974.

231. Parker JD: A double-blind trial of idoxuridine in recurrent genital herpes. J Antimicrob Chemother 3 (Suppl. A):131–137, 1977.

232. Paterson A, Fox AD, Davies G, et al: Controlled studies of IDU in the treatment of herpetic keratitis. Trans Ophthalmol Soc UK 83:583–591, 1963.

233. Palese P, Compans RW: Inhibition of influenza virus replication in tissue culture by 2-deoxy-2, 3-dehydro-N-trifluoroacetylneuraminic acid (FANA): Mechanism of action. J Gen Virol 33:159–163, 1976.

234. Pauling L: Vitamin C and the Common Cold. San Francisco, WH Freeman & Co, 1970.

235. Pavan-Langston D: Clinical evaluation of adenine arabinoside and idoxuridine in the treatment of ocular herpes simplex. Am J Ophthalmol 80:495–502, 1975.

236. Pavan-Langston D, Buchanan RA, Alford CA Jr (Eds): Adenine Arabinoside: An Antiviral Agent. New York, Raven Press, 1975.

237. Pavan-Langston D, Dohlman CH: A double blind clinical study of adenine arabinoside therapy of viral keratoconjunctivitis. Am J Ophthalmol 74:81–88, 1972.

238. Pavan-Langston D, Dohlman CH, Geary P, et al: Intraocular penetration of adenine arabinoside and idoxuridine. Therapeutic implications in clinical herpetic uveitis. In: Pavan-Langston D (Ed): Adenine Arabinoside: An Antiviral Agent. New York, Raven Press, 1975.

239. Pavan-Langston D, Langston RHS, Geary PA: Prophylaxis and therapy for experimental ocular herpes simplex. Comparison of idoxuridine, adenine arabinoside, and hypoxanthine arabinoside. Arch Ophthalmol 92:417–421, 1974.

240. Pavan-Langston D, North RD Jr, Geary PA, et al: Intraocular penetration of the soluble antiviral, Ara-AMP. Arch Ophthalmol 94:1585–1588, 1976.

241. Peckinpaugh RO, Askin FB, Pierce WE, et al: Field studies with amantadine: Acceptability and protection. Ann NY Acad Sci 173:62–73, 1970.

242. Philippon Am, Plommet MG, Kazmierczak A, et al: Rifampin in the treatment of experimental brucellosis in mice and guinea pigs. J Infect Dis 136:482–488, 1977.

243. Plotkin SA, Stetler H: Treatment of congenital cytomegalic inclusion disease with antiviral agents. Antimicrob Agents Chemother, pp 372–379, 1969.

244. Pollard RB, Smith JL, Neal EA, et al: The effect of adenine arabinoside on chronic hepatitis B virus infection. JAMA (in press, 1978).

245. Poirier RH, Kinkel AW, Ellison AC, et al: Intraocular penetration of topical 3% adenine arabinoside. In: Pavan-Langston D (Ed): Adenine Arabinoside: An Antiviral Agent. New York, Raven Press, 1975.

246. Potter CW, Phair JP, Vodinelich L, et al: Antiviral, immunosuppressive and antitumor effects of ribavirin. Nature 259:496–497, 1976.

247. Prusiner P, Sundaralingam M: A new class of synthetic nucleoside analogues with broad-spectrum antiviral properties. Nature [New Biol.] 244:116–117, 1973.

248. Prusoff WH, Goz B: Potential mechanisms of action of antiviral agents. Fed Proc 32:1679–1687, 1973.

249. Prusoff WH, Ward DC: Nucleoside analogs with antiviral activity. Biochem Pharmacol 25:1233–1239, 1976.

250. Prusoff WH, Ward DC, Lin TS, et al: Recent studies on the antiviral and biochemical properties of 5-halo-5'-amino-deoxyribonucleosides. Ann NY Acad Sci 284:335–341, 1977.

251. Rao AR, Jacobs ES, Kamalakshi S, et al: Chemoprophylaxis and chemotherapy in variola major. Part I. An assessment of CG 662 and marboran in prophylaxis of contacts of variola major. Indian J Med Res 57:477–483, 1969.

252. Rao AR, Jacobs ES, Kamalakshi S, et al: Chemoprophylaxis and chemotherapy in variola major. Part II. Therapeutic assessment of CG 662 and marboran in treatment of variola major in man. Indian J Med Res 57:484–494, 1969.

253. Rao AR, McFadzean JA, Kamalakshi K: An isothiazole thiosemicarbazone in the treatment of variola major in man. Lancet 1:1068–1072, 1966.

254. Ray EK, Halpern BL, Levitan DB, et al: A new approach to viral chemotherapy. Inhibitors of glycoprotein synthesis. Lancet 2:680–683, 1974.

255. Reed SE, Craig JW, Tyrrell DAJ: Four compounds active against rhinovirus: Comparison In vitro and in volunteers. J Infect Dis 133:A128–A135, 1976.

256. Renis HE: Chemotherapy of genital herpes simplex virus type 2 infections of female hamsters. Antimicrob Agents Chemother 11:701–707, 1977.

257. Richman DD, Murphy BR, Baron S, et al: Three strains of influenza A virus (H3N2): Interferon sensitivity *in vitro* and interferon production in volunteers. J Clin Microbiol 3:223–226, 1976.

258. Rizzo M, Biandrate P, Tognoni G, et al: Amantadine in depression: Relationship between behavioural effects and plasma levels. Eur J Clin Pharmacol 5:226–228, 1973.

259. Roome APCH, Tinkler AE, Hilton AL, et al: Neutral red with photoinactivation in the treatment of herpes genitalis. Br J Vener Dis 51:130–133, 1975.

260. Ross AH, Julia A, Balakrishnan C: Toxicity of adenine arabinoside in humans. J Infect Dis 133:A192–A198, 1976.

261. Sabin AB: Amantadine hydrochloride. JAMA 200:135–142, 1967.

262. St Jeor S, Rapp F: Cytomegalovirus replication in cells pretreated with 5-iodo-2'-deoxyuridine. J Virol 11:986–990, 1973.

263. Salido-Rengell F, Nasser-Quinones H, Briseno-Garcia B: The effect of 1-β-D-ribo-furanosyl-1,2,4,triazole-3-carboxamide (ribavirin) in a double-blind study during an outbreak of influenza. Ann NY Acad Sci 284:272–277, 1977.

264. Sammons ML, Stephen EL, Levy HB, et al: Interferon induction in cynomolgus and rhesus monkeys after repeated doses of a modified polyriboinosinic-polyribocytidylic acid complex Antimicrob Agents Chemother 11:80–83, 1977.

265. Scheid A, Choppin PW: Identification of biological activities of paramyxovirus glyco-proteins. Activation of cell fusion, hemolysis, and infectivity by proteolytic cleavage of an inactive precursor protein of Sendai virus. Virology 57: 475–490, 1974.

266. Scheid A, Choppin PW: Protease activation mutants of Sendai virus. Activation of biological properties by specific proteases. Virology 69:265–277, 1976.

267. Schimpff SC, Fortner CL, Greene WH, et al: Cytosine arabinoside for localized herpes zoster in patients with cancer: Failure in a controlled trial. J Infect Dis 130:673–676, 1974.

268. Schofield KP, Potter CE, Edey D, et al: Antiviral activity of ribavirin on influenza invection in ferrets. J Antimicrob Chemother 1:63–69, 1975.

269. Scholtissek C: Inhibition of the multiplication of enveloped viruses by glucose deriva-tives. Curr Top Microbiol Immunol 70:101–119, 1975.

270. Scholtissek C: Inhibition of influenza RNA synthesis by virazole (ribavirin). Arch Virol 50:349–352, 1976.

271. Scholtissek C, Rott R, Hau G, et al: Inhibition of the multiplication of vesicular stomatitis and Newcastle disease virus by 2-deoxy-D-glucose. J Virol 13:1186–1193, 1974.

272. Schwab RS, England AC Jr, Poskanzer DC, et al: Amantadine in the treatment of Parkinson's disease. JAMA 208:1168–1170, 1969.

273. Schwab RS, Poskanzer DC, England AC Jr., et al: Amantadine in Parkinson's disease. JAMA 222:792–795, 1972.

274. Scientific Committee on Interferon: Effect of interferon on vaccination in volunteers. Lancet 1:873–875, 1962.

275. Scientific Committee on Interferon: Experiments with interferon in man. Lancet 1:505–506, 1965.

276. Shaffer JM, Kucera CJ, Spink WW: The protection of intracellular *Brucella* against therapeutic agents and the bactericidal action of serum. J Exp Med 97:77–89, 1953.

277. Shannon WM: Adenine arabinoside: Antiviral activity *in vitro*. *In:* Pavan-Langston D (Ed): Adenine Arabinoside: An Antiviral Agent. New York, Raven Press, 1975.

278. Shealy CN, Weeth JB, Mercier D: Livedo reticularis in patients with parkinsonism receiving amantadine. JAMA 212:1522–1523, 1970.

279. Sidwell RW, Huffman JH, Allen LB, et al: *In vitro* antiviral activity of 6-substituted 9-β-D-ribofuranosylpurine 3′,5′-cyclic phosphates. Antimicrob Agents Chemother 5:652–657, 1974.

280. Sidwell RW, Huffman JH, Khare GP, et al: Broad-spectrum antiviral activity of virazole: 1-β-D-ribofuranosyl-1,2,4-triazole-3-carboxamide. Science 177:705–706, 1972.

281. Sidwell RW, Khare GP, Allen LB, et al: *In vitro* and *in vivo* effect of 1-β-D-ribofuranosyl-1,2,4-triazole-3-carboxamide (ribavirin) on types 1 and 3 parainfluenza virus infections. Chemotherapy 21:205–220, 1975.

282. Sloan BJ: Adenine arabinoside: Chemotherapy studies in animals. *In:* Pavan-Langston D (Ed): Adenine Arabinoside: An Antiviral Agent. New York, Raven Press, 1975.

283. Sloan BJ, Kielty JK, Miller FA: Effect of a novel adenosine deaminase inhibitor (Co-vidarabine, CO-V) upon the antiviral activity *in vitro* and *in vivo* of vidarabine (VIRA-A) for DNA virus replication. Ann NY Acad Sci 284:60–80, 1977.

284. Smorodintsev AA, Zyldnikov DM, Kiseleva AM, et al: Evaluation of amantadine in artifically induced A2 and B influenza. JAMA 213:1448–1454, 1970.

285. Soto AJ, Hall TS, Reed SE: Trial of the antiviral action of isoprinosine against rhinovirus infection of volunteers. Antimicrob Agents Chemother 3:332–334, 1973.

286. Staal SP, Rowe WP: Enhancement of adenovirus infection in Wi-38 and AGMK cells by pretreatment of cells with 5-iododeoxyuridine. Virology 64:513–519, 1975.

286a. Stalder H: Antiviral therapy. Yale J Biol Med 50:507–532, 1977.

287. Stanley ED, Jackson GG, Dirda VA, et al: Effects of a topical interferon inducer on rhinovirus infections in volunteers. J Infect Dis 133:A121–A127, 1976.

288. Stanley ED, Muldoon RE, Akers LW, et al: Evaluation of antiviral drugs: The effect of amantadine on influenza in volunteers. Ann NY Acad Sci 130:44–51, 1965.

289. Steffenhagen KA, Easterday BC, Galasso GJ: Evaluation of 6-azauridine and 5-iododeoxyuridine in the treatment of experimental viral infections. J Infect Dis 133:603–612, 1976.

290. Stephen EL, Dominik JW, Moe JB, et al: Therapeutic effects of ribavirin given by the intraperitoneal or aerosol route against influenza virus infections in mice. Antimicrob Agents Chemother 10:549–554, 1976.

291. Stevens DA, Jordon GW, Waddell TF, et al: Adverse effect of cytosine arabinoside on disseminated zoster in a controlled trial. N Engl J Med 289:873–878, 1973.

292. Streeter DG, Witkowski JT, Khare GP, et al: Mechanism of action of 1-β-D-ribofuranosyl-1,2,4-triazole-3-carboxamide (virazole), a new broad-spectrum antiviral agent. Proc Natl Acad Sci USA 70:1174–1178, 1973.

293. Stringfellow DA, Glasgow LA: Hyporeactivity of infection: potential limitation to therapeutic use of interferon-inducing agents. Infect Immun 6:743–747, 1972.

294. Sugar J, Kaufman HE: Halogenated pyrimidines in antiviral therapy. *In:* Carter WA (Ed): Selective Inhibitors of Viral Functions. Cleveland, CRC Press, 1973, pp 295–311.

295. Summers DF, Maizel JV: Evidence for large precursor proteins in poliovirus synthesis. Proc Natl Acad Sci USA 59:966–971, 1968.

296. Summers DF, Shaw EN, Steward ML, et al: Inhibition of cleavage of large poliovirus-specific precursor proteins in infected HeLa cells by inhibitors of proteolytic enzymes. J Virol 10:880–884, 1972.

297. Sundmacher R, Neumann-Haefelin D, Manthey KF, et al: Interferon in treatment of

dendritic keratitis in humans: A preliminary report. J Infect Dis 133:A160–A164, 1976.

298. Sundmacher R, Neumann-Haefelin D, Cantell K: Successful treatment of dendritic keratitis with human leukocyte interferon. A controlled clinical study. Albrecht von Graefes Arch Klin Ophthalmol 201:39–45, 1976.

299. Sweetman L, Connor JD, Seshamani R, et al: Deamination of adenine arabinoside in cell cultures used for *in vitro* viral inhibition studies. *In:* Pavan-Langston D (Ed): Adenine Arabinoside: An Antiviral Agent. New York, Raven Press, 1975.

300. Swyers JS, Lausch RN, Kaufman HE: Corneal hypersensitivity to herpes simplex. Br J Ophthalmol 51:843–846, 1967.

301. Talley RW, O'Bryan RM, Tucker WG, et al: Clinical pharmacology and human antitumor activity of cytosine arabinoside. Cancer 20:809, 1967.

302. Taylor PK, Doherty NR: Comparison of the treatment of herpes genitalis in men with proflavin photoinactivation, idoxuridine ointment, and normal saline. Br J Vener Dis 51:125–129, 1975.

303. Temin H, Mizutani S: RNA-dependent DNA polymerase in virions of Rous sarcoma virus. Nature 226:1211–1213, 1970.

304. Todaro GJ, Green H: Enhancement by thymidine analogs of susceptibility of cells to transformation by SV40. Virology 24:393–400, 1964.

305. Togo Y, McCracken EA: Chemoprophylaxis and therapy of respiratory viral infections. Double-blind clinical assessment of ribavirin (virazole) in the prevention of induced infection with type B influenza virus. J Infect Dis 133:A109–A113, 1976.

306. Togo Y, Schwartz AR, Hornick RB: Failure of a 3-substituted triazinoindole in the prevention of experimental human rhinovirus infection. Chemotherapy 18:17–26, 1973.

307. Turner W, Bauer DJ, Nimmo-Smith RH: Eczema vaccinatum treated with N-methyl-isatin-β—thiosemicarbazone. Br Med J 1:1317–1319, 1962.

308. Tyrrell DAJ: Interferon and Its Clinical Potential. London, Heinemann, 1976.

309. Vernier VG, Harmon JB, Stump JM, et al: The toxicologic and pharmacologic properties of amantadine hydrochloride. Toxicol Appl Pharmacol 15:642–665, 1969.

310. Waldman RH, Ganguly R: Therapeutic efficacy of inosiplex (isoprinosine) in rhinovirus infection. Ann NY Acad Sci 284:153–160, 1977.

311. Walker JS, Stephen EL, Spertzel RO: Small-particle aerosols of antiviral compounds in treatment of type A influenza pneumonia in mice. J Infect Dis 133:A140–A144, 1976.

312. Wallis C, Melnick JL: Irreversible photosensitization of viruses. Virology 23:520–527, 1964.

313. Wallis, C, Melnick JL: Photodynamic inactivation of animal viruses: A review. Photochem Photobiol 4:159–170, 1965.

314. Walters HE, Paulshock M: Therapeutic efficacy of amantadine HCl. Missouri Med 67:176–179, 1970.

315. Watson GI: Use of amantadine in an epidemic of 'Hong Kong' influenza type A$_2$ in family practice. Practitioner 205:351–357, 1970.

316. Wehrli W, Staehelin M: Actions of the rifamycins. Bacteriol Rev 35:290–309, 1971.

317. Wellings PC, Awdry PN, Bors FH, et al: Clinical evaluation of trifluorothymidine in the treatment of herpes simplex corneal ulcers. Am J Ophthalmol 73:932–942, 1977.

318. Welsh R, Trowbridge RS, Kowalski JB, et al: Amantadine hydrochloride inhibition of early and late stages of lymphocytic choriomeningitis virus-cell interactions. Virology 45:679–686, 1971.

319. Whitley RJ, Chien LT, Buchanan RA, et al: Studies on adenine arabinoside—a model for antiviral chemotherapeutics. Perspect Virol 9:315–333, 1975.

320. Whitley RJ, Chien LT, Nahmias AJ, et al: Adenine arabinoside therapy of neonatal herpetic infections. *In:* Pavan-Langston D, Buchanan RA, Alford CA (Eds): Adenine Arabinoside: An Antiviral Agent. New York, Raven Press, 1975.

321. Whitley RJ, Chien LT, Dolin R, et al: Adenine arabinoside therapy of herpes zoster in the immunosuppressed. NIAID collaborative antiviral study. N Engl J Med 294:1193–1199, 1976.

322. Whitley RJ, Soong SJ, Dolin R, et al: Adenine arabinoside therapy of biopsy-proved herpes simplex encephalitis. N Engl J Med 297:289–294, 1977.

323. Wilkerson S, Finley SC, Finley WH, et al: (abstract) Chromosome breakage in patients receiving ara-A. Clin Res (Abstr) 21:52, 1973.

324. Wingfield WL, Pollack D, Grunert RR: Therapeutic efficacy of amantadine HCl and rimantadine HCl in naturally occurring influenza A2 respiratory illness in man. N Engl J Med 281:579–584, 1969.

325. Woodman DR, Williams JC: Effects of 2-deoxy-D-glucose and 3-deazauridine individually and in combination on the replication of Japanese B encephalitis virus. Antimicrob Agents Chemother 11:475–481, 1977.

326. Woodson B, Joklik WK: The inhibition of vaccinia virus multiplication by isatin-β-thiosemicarbazone. Proc Natl Acad Sci USA 54:946–953, 1965.

327. Wright, PF, Khaw KT, Oxman MN, Shwachman H: Evaluation of the safety of amantadine HCl and the role of respiratory viral infections in children with cystic fibrosis. J Infect Dis 134:144–149, 1976.

328. Yamamoto K, Yamaguchi N, Oda K: Mechanism of interferon-induced inhibition of early simian virus 40 (SV40) functions. Virology 68:58–70, 1975.

329. Zaky, DA, Betts RF, Douglas RG Jr, et al: Varicella-zoster virus and subcutaneous cytarabine: Correlation of *in vitro* sensitivities to blood levels. Antimicrob Agents Chemother 7:229–232, 1975.

330. Zertuche HF, Perches RD: Clinical experiences using the antiviral 1-β-D-ribofuranosyl-1,2,4-triazole-3-carboxamide (ribavirin) in Mexico. Ann NY Acad Sci 284:284–288, 1977.

CHAPTER 9

VIRAL ENTERITIS

Neil R. Blacklow, M.D., David S. Schreiber, M.D. and Jerry S. Trier, M.D.

Introduction

Viral enteritis is a common disease that affects all age groups and occurs in both epidemic and endemic forms. Its frequency as the second most common disease experienced by American civilians was documented by a study of Cleveland families which covered nearly 10 years and encompassed approximately 25,000 illnesses [24]. Although the disease is usually self-limited, it can be lethal in the elderly, debilitated or infant patient. It is of enormous economic importance in terms of employee time lost from work, and it is also likely responsible for many of the common diarrheal syndromes that occur in crowded under-developed areas of the world.

Viral enteritis occurs in at least two epidemiologically distinct clinical forms. One entity is characteristically epidemic in nature, and usually produces a 24–48 hour explosive self-limited illness characterized by varying combinations of diarrhea, vomiting, nausea, abdominal cramps, headache, malaise, myalgia, and low-grade fever. This form of enteritis commonly occurs in family and community-wide outbreaks among school age children, family contacts and adults. It has been given descriptive names, such as viral diarrhea, epidemic diarrhea and vomiting, winter vomiting disease, epidemic collapse, and acute infectious non-bacterial gastroenteritis [11].

The second clinical entity of viral enteritis occurs predominantly in infants and young children, in whom it can produce severe dehydration that requires hospitalization for parenteral fluid therapy [77,85]. Ill

From the Departments of Medicine, University of Massachusetts Medical School, Worcester, Mass. and Harvard Medical School, West Roxbury Veterans Administration Hospital, Peter Bent Brigham Hospital, Boston, Mass.

Supported by Contract DAMD 17-76-C-6052 from United States Army Medical Research and Development Command, Grant R805169-01-1 from the United States Environmental Protection Agency, Grant AMDD17537 from the National Institutes of Health.

infants are usually febrile and experience severe diarrhea that is frequently accompanied by vomiting. This disease form of viral enteritis is usually sporadic, but occasionally can be epidemic. Disease among family contacts of ill infants is uncommon.

Recently, etiologic agents have been uncovered that, for the first time, account for many cases of viral enteritis. Elusive parvovirus-like agents have been shown to be a cause of the epidemic viral enteritis syndrome, and a ubiquitous reovirus-like agent is now known to produce approximately one-half of all infantile enteritis illnesses that require hospitalization. These developments, coupled with recent advances in understanding the pathogenesis of infection, have stimulated this review, which will cover the topic of viral enteritis by a discussion sequentially, of various established and candidate etiologic agents.

Historical Background

Early studies of the etiology of viral enteritis were based on three approaches: epidemiologic surveys, inoculation of animals, and use of human volunteers. In epidemiologic studies, stools from ill and control infants and young children were screened for possible causative agents by standard tissue culture technics. Several surveys of infantile enteritis in the United States resulted in the isolation of a multiplicity of serotypes of known enteric viruses—echovirus, coxsackievirus and adenovirus—in 20 to 50% of ill infants but also in up to 20% of control patients, which made interpretation of the data difficult [8,75,103,104]. Similar problems were encountered in studies from underdeveloped nations in which known enteric viruses were identified in up to 80% of infants with diarrhea but were also recovered from 40–80% of controls [7,68,71]. Most important has been the failure of numerous attempts to recover etiologic agents from epidemiologically distinct, well circumscribed communitywide epidemics of viral enteritis in the United States [11].

The only productive animal inoculation studies of historical interest were reported in 1943 by Light and Hodes, who induced diarrhea in calves with a filterable agent derived from the diarrheal stools of infants [54]. This observation remained ignored and unconfirmed for over 30 years, until a frozen and vacuum-dried specimen of calf stool from the 1943 studies was recently examined by electron microscopy and revealed particles consistent with a reovirus-like agent [38]. Although this ancient specimen appeared to lose its infectiousness for the gnotobiotic calf on recent inoculation, it is likely that the 1943 virus was an isolate of the reovirus-like agent of infantile enteritis.

Early investigators also attempted to induce disease in volunteers,

TABLE 1. Viral Enteritis Agents

Agent	Etiologic Relationship Established	Methods by Which Agent Identified	Characterization of Agent			
			Size	Density	Nucleic Acid	Replication in Cell Culture
A. ESTABLISHED AGENTS						
Parvovirus-like (Norwalk, etc.)	Yes	Immune electron microscopy Volunteer studies	26–27 nm	1.36–1.41 gm/cm³ cesium chloride	Presumed DNA	Negative
Reovirus-like (Rotavirus, Duovirus, etc.)	Yes	Electron microscopy Counterimmunoelectrophoresis Radioimmunoassay Enzyme-linked immunosorbent assay Fluorescent virus precipitin test Animal inoculation Cell culture antigen production Serologic assays	70 nm double-shelled capsid	1.35–1.37 gm/cm³ cesium chloride	Double-stranded segmented RNA	Inefficient, limited
B. CANDIDATE AGENTS						
Adenovirus	No	Electron microscopy	75 nm icosahedral	1.35 gm/cm³ cesium chloride	DNA	Usually negative
Coronavirus-like	No	Electron microscopy	Pleomorphic 120–230 nm, enveloped	?	Presumed RNA	? Inefficient
"Mini-Reovirus"	No	Electron microscopy	30 nm	?	?	?
"Astrovirus"	No	Electron microscopy	28 nm	?	?	?

under controlled conditions, by the oral administration of infectious, bacteria-free fecal filtrates derived from naturally occurring epidemic cases of viral enteritis. Gordon and Jordan uncovered two agents, the Marcy and FS strains, each of which induced short-term homologous immunity on rechallenge studies [36,40]. Cross-challenge studies in volunteers failed to reveal evidence of heterologous immunity and thus suggested that the two agents were not closely related [40]. Similar studies in Japan revealed four disease-producing inocula which, like the Marcy and FS agents, could be passaged serially through multiple generations of volunteers [34,51]. However, none of these agents could be identified or cultivated in the laboratory and, in time, they all were discarded from storage in freezers.

Thus, until the 1970's, little information was available about the etiology of viral enteritis. Recent utilization of new virologic and immunologic technics has finally resulted in the discovery of etiologic agents. These agents will now be discussed.

Current Status of Viral Enteritis Agents

Table 1 summarizes pertinent characteristics of established and candidate viral enteritis agents: It is apparent that there are two groups of agents (parvovirus-like and reovirus-like) which have been shown clearly to produce viral enteritis and have been partially characterized. There are also a number of candidate agents which have been proposed as causes of viral enteritis, but the evidence is inconclusive. Presence of a virus in a diarrheal stool specimen does not by itself establish a causal relationship. A number of additional features are necessary to demonstrate conclusively an etiologic role. These include: finding the virus in the feces of patients during disease, with disappearance of the agent from the stools of most patients during convalescence; demonstration of a viral-specific antibody rise in the serums of convalescent patients when compared with acute phase serums; demonstration of the virus in the stools of a very small percentage of control asymptomatic patients when compared with a very large percentage in stools of ill subjects. It is also highly desirable to achieve transmission of enteritis to experimental animals or human volunteers by administration of the agent and subsequent serial passage of the agent through multiple generations of animals or volunteers. These criteria have yet to be fulfilled for the candidate agents listed in Table 1.

During the past several years, numerous preliminary reports concerning viral enteritis agents have appeared in letters to editors of journals, which at times have been informative and at other times confusing.

Visualization by electron microscopy of virus-like objects in diarrheal stool specimens is difficult to interpret in the absence of additional data. Objects have even been assigned virus names by electron microscopists. Clearly, electron microscopy has proved to be the indispensible tool for the initial identification of the parvovirus-like and reovirus-like agents. However, cataloging of stool objects should be followed by biologic characterization of these objects and by an attempt to fulfill the criteria outlined above. The problem is further compounded by the fact that small round-shaped bacteriophage particles are commonly found in normal human stool specimens. A discussion follows of each of the established and candidate viral enteritis agents that are outlined in Table 1.

PARVOVIRUS-LIKE AGENTS OF EPIDEMIC ENTERITIS

Epidemiology

Five distinct, well circumscribed school, family and community-wide epidemics in the United States and Great Britain have been shown to be caused by infection with parvovirus-like agents [5,11,20,49,90]. The three agents uncovered in the United States, the Norwalk, Hawaii and Montgomery County (MC) agents, named after the sites of the outbreaks, appear distinctive inasmuch as immunity to one of the agents does not appear to confer clinical immunity to the other agents [98]. The Norwalk agent has been the most extensively studied of the parvovirus-like agents and is derived from an outbreak of enteritis in Norwalk, Ohio in 1968 [1]. Rapid spread from an elementary school throughout the community occurred, with an attack rate of approximately 50% and an incubation period of about 48 hours. The two British agents, the W and Ditchling agents, may be immunologically related, based on immune electron microscopic studies; these studies have also shown a lack of relatedness of these two agents with the Norwalk and Hawaii agents [5]. Another possible parvovirus-like agent has also been associated with three English outbreaks of food-poisoning associated with consumption of cockles. [6].

Clinical Features

The clinical and pathogenic features of parvovirus-like agent enteritis have been studied by disease production in healthy volunteers. Bacteria-free and toxin-free fecal filtrates, derived from the outbreaks caused by the Norwalk, Hawaii, MC and W agents, have each induced illness in volunteers when administered orally [20,98]. In addition, the Norwalk agent has undergone extensive serial passage through multiple generations of volunteers without significant alteration in rate of illness or specific symptoms [26]. In contrast to fecal filtrates, throat washings from volunteers with Norwalk illness have failed to produce disease when administered orally to three volunteers [27].

Experimentally induced parvovirus-like agent illness is indistinguishable from the naturally occurring disease. The incubation period is 18–48 hours and symptoms last for 24–48 hours [26]. Symptoms vary among volunteers receiving identical inocula. Approximately two-thirds of inoculated volunteers develop Norwalk agent illness. Some subjects experience mild to severe vomiting without diarrhea, others develop mild to severe diarrhea without vomiting, and still others experience both diarrhea and vomiting [26]. It therefore appears that the descriptive syndromes of "winter vomiting disease" and "viral diarrhea" can be caused by the same agent. Abdominal cramps, headache, malaise, myalgia, low-grade fever, nausea are commonly present. Routine laboratory studies remain normal except for occasional transient mild leukocytosis [26]. No prolonged illness or long-term sequelae have been observed in volunteers who have received parvovirus-like agents [11].

Pathogenesis

A histologic lesion of the proximal small intestine develops during the course of Norwalk and Hawaii agent enteritis which is characterized by altered mucosal architecture, shortening of villi, and hyperplasia of intestinal crypts [2,28,82,83]. Mononuclear cells and polymorphonuclear leukocytes infiltrate the lamina propria, surface cells contain vacuoles and appear cuboidal and mitotic figures in the hyperplastic crypts increase in number [82,83]. Viral particles have not been visualized by electron microscopy in sections of involved mucosa of the small intestine [2,28]. The histologic lesion may shortly precede the onset of symptoms and has developed in a few infected subjects who remained entirely asymptomatic [82,83]. The extent of small intestinal involvement is not known, since only the proximal small intestine has been studied. It is known, however, that a histologic lesion of the gastric antral and fundic mucosa does not develop during enteritis induced by the Norwalk agent [96]. The colonic mucosa has also been reported as normal in a few cases of Norwalk agent-induced enteritis [2,11].

Malabsorption of fat and xylose occurs during Norwalk agent illness, and may persist for at least one week after infection, although clinical symptoms last only 24–48 hours [11,83]. Decreased levels of the brush border enzymes trehalase and alkaline phosphatase occur during disease, with less consistently demonstrable decreases in levels of sucrase and lactase [2]. Proximal jejunal mucosal levels of adenylate cyclase have remained unchanged during clinical Norwalk and Hawaii enteritis [53]. Serial bacteriologic analysis of jejunal contents has shown a modest increase in bacteria during illness which, however, is not correlated with presence or absence of xylose malabsorption [11].

Biophysical Characteristics

Volunteer studies have demonstrated that the parvovirus-like enteritis agents are stable after exposure to 20% ether, acid (pH 2.7) and heat (60°C for 30 minutes) [20,27]. When passed through 60 or 50 nm size filters, these agents are still infectious for volunteers [20,27]. Conclusive proof of their small size has been provided by the technic of negative staining with immune electron microscopy of infectious filtrates. By this method, particles 25–27 nm in diameter have been visualized [5,49,90]. The buoyant density of these particles in cesium chloride is approximately $1.38 gm/cm^3$, with a range of $1.36–1.41 gm/cm^3$ [5,45,70,90]. The Norwalk, Hawaii, MC, W and Ditchling agents have all been shown to possess this density in cesium chloride, and they are also morphologically indistinguishable. These biophysical characteristics are comparable to those of the known DNA-containing parvovirus group, although definitive classification awaits laboratory propagation of these agents.

Laboratory Propagation

Despite intensive efforts by several laboratories, *in vitro* propagation of the parvovirus-like enteritis agents has not been achieved. Experimental animals, such as mice, rabbits, guinea pigs and rhesus monkeys, have been refractory to infection [11]. The parvovirus-like agents have also failed to replicate in a variety of tissue culture and intestinal organ culture systems [27,89]. Thus, the only experimental handles for these agents at present are immune electron microscopy and human infectivity studies.

Diagnostic Tests—Immune Electron Microsopy

The technic of immune electron microscopy (IEM), although cumbersome and time consuming, is the only laboratory diagnostic test currently available for the parvovirus-like agents. IEM involves the incubation of a virus particle-containing fecal filtrate with convalescent serum from a patient known to have had recent infection with the appropriate viral agent. Antibody in the convalescent serum and the viral particles then form aggregates which can be recovered by centrifugation and visualized by electron microscopy after negative staining with phosphotungstic acid [49]. Various technical manipulations, such as the concentration of stool filtrates and alterations of antigen-antibody ratios may be required to achieve optimal conditions for particle visualization by IEM [90]. The Norwalk, Hawaii, MC, W, and Ditchling agents have all been visualized by this technic [5,49,90]. Studies with the Norwalk agent have shown that about half of ill volunteers excrete the 26–27 nm particles in sufficient titer to be detected by IEM of stools during the first 72 hours after onset of symptoms [89]. Particles are not seen prior to onset of symptoms and are detected in less than 20% of stool specimens collected 72 hours or more after disease onset [89].

The IEM technic has been adapted to semiquantitate serum antibody levels to the parvovirus-like agents. This is achieved by determining, with IEM, the degree of coating by antibody of viral particles after a test serum specimen is reacted with a fecal filtrate known to contain the appropriate parvovirus-like particle [28,49,69,90,98]. It should be emphasized, however, that to date the IEM technic has been used only to study experimentally induced infection. It has been too cumbersome to employ either as a diagnostic tool for naturally occurring enteritis or as an assay for routine serologic studies.

Clinical Immunity

At least two forms of clinical immunity have been demonstrated for experimentally induced Norwalk agent enteritis: One group of individuals maintains *long-term immunity*, as evidenced by persistent failure to develop illness both upon an initial challenge and after rechallenge up to 34 months later; a second cohort of individuals develops enteritis on initial exposure and is again susceptible upon long-term homologous rechallenge 27 to 42 months later [69]. *Short-term immunity* following illness, lasting up to 14 weeks, is usually present [27]. Although rises in serum IEM antibody levels occur following Norwalk illness, these responses appear to reflect infection in susceptible persons and not to play a uniformly protective role, since illness can occur in the presence of serum antibody [69]. It is interesting that volunteers who are persistently resistant to illness maintain low or absent serum IEM antibody ratings, and, thus, factors (perhaps genetic) other than serum antibody appear important in immunity to Norwalk enteritis [69].

It is possible that production of local GI tract antibody may be involved in recovery from parvovirus-like enteritis. However, based on the above-noted studies [69], if this is to be the case for Norwalk enteritis, one has to hypothesize the existence of two cohorts of persons: one (persistently immune) capable of producing local antibody on rechallenge, and the other (lacking long-term immunity) incapable of synthesizing sufficient local antibody for long-term protection. Other local mechanisms may be operative in recovery from parvoviral enteritis, such as interferon, in view of the extremely short duration of clinical illness (12–48 hours). However, no interferon has been detected in jejunal secretions, jejunal homogenates, or sera of volunteers with Norwalk agent enteritis [25]. Synthesis of crude IgA by intestinal biopsies *in vitro* obtained from volunteers before and after Norwalk enteritis has been measured [3]. Evidence for increased crude IgA synthesis was found in two-week post-inoculation specimens from both ill and asymptomatic subjects, indicating the need to perform this kind of study in the future with currently unavailable purified viral reagents.

REOVIRUS-LIKE AGENT (HRVLA)
OF INFANTILE ENTERITIS

Epidemiology

A human reovirus-like agent (HRVLA) which has also been referred to as rotavirus, duovirus, orbivirus-like and infantile gastroenteritis virus by various investigators, is now known to be the cause of both sporadic and epidemic outbreaks of enteritis in infants and young children throughout the world [10,21,29,32,47,52,63,66,94]. Several year-long studies have indicated that approximately one-half of all children hospitalized with enteritis are infected with HRVLA [14,22,48,64]. The peak prevalence of HRVLA disease is during the winter months, whereas it is less common during summer [14,31,48,63]. Among hospitalized patients, an unexplained male to female ratio of 3:2 has been observed [48,64,85]. Transmission of infection is presumed to be person-to-person by the fecal-oral route, with an estimated incubation period of 48 hours [22,23]. Nosocomial spread of HRVLA disease among hospitalized pediatric patients has been well documented [33,64,78,94]. HRVLA disease is most common in the 6–24 month old age group but it has also been observed in the neonate [4,14,16,31,48,85,93]. Subclinical infection is known to occur in adult family contacts of ill young patients [35,50]; in one study, 41% of such contacts had evidence of infection, usually by serologic tests and uncommonly by detection of the agent in stool specimens [50]. HRVLA infection in adults can infrequently be associated with mild gastrointestinal symptoms. The subclinical or mild clinical response of adults to HRVLA infection has been ascribed to resistance induced by previous experience with the agent [50].

Clinical Features

The clinical and pathogenetic features of HRVLA enteritis have been studied in hospitalized patients with naturally occurring disease. The indication for hospitalization is usually dehydration, requiring parenteral fluid therapy. Indeed, HRVLA disease is a leading cause for admission to pediatric hospitals. Diarrhea is the hallmark of the disease in infants and, by definition, is present in all patients. The duration of diarrhea varies, but it may last for up to 5 to 8 days and occasionally for longer [35,66,77,85]. Vomiting usually occurs, beginning before diarrhea, although it may develop concomitantly with diarrhea. Fever occurs in three quarters of patients [77]. Associated pharyngeal and tympanic membrane erythema have been described [17,77]. Death due to HRVLA disease, although rare, has been reported [63].

Pathogenesis

Less information is known about the pathogenesis of HRVLA enteritis than that produced by the Norwalk agent because studies have been limited to the uncontrolled evaluation of sick infants. Duodenal biopsies have been obtained one to five days after disease onset and have revealed mild to severe histologic abnormalities similar to those described with parvovirus-like agent enteritis [9]. In contrast to studies with the parvovirus-like agents, HRVLA particles have been visualized by electron microscopy in intestinal epithelial cells of duodenal biopsy specimens; indeed, the HRVLA was first discovered by its presence in such biopsy specimens [9]. Histology has reverted to normal, with absence of HRVLA particles, four to eight weeks after disease onset [9]. The gastric and colonic mucosa have been reported as normal in the few HRVLA-infected infants in whom they have been examined [63].

There is evidence that the HRVLA can cause small intestinal dysfunction. D-xylose has been administered intraduodenally to 6 infants who harbored the agent in secretions aspirated from the small intestine. One-hour blood xylose levels were low in all six patients [58].

Biophysical Characteristics

The HRVLA was first identified by electron microscopy of biopsies of duodenal mucosa taken from young children with enteritis [9] and was subsequently recognized in negatively stained electron microscopic preparations of stool suspensions from ill children [10,31]. The virus particle is approximately 70 nm in diameter [39,47,56] and has been described as having a double-shelled capsid [31,32]. It appears to contain a 37 nm diameter core, surrounded by an electron-lucent layer from which capsomeres radiate. The surface of the virus is composed of 32 large morphologic units or capsomeres [56]. Some virus particles lack the outer shell and measure 60 nm in diameter; in addition, empty shells that lack the central core are commonly seen. At present, the role of the various viral structural components in infectivity and antigenic recognition is not fully understood. The density of the complete virus in cesium chloride is 1.36–1.37gm/cm^3, and it is 1.29–1.30gm/cm^3 for empty-shelled particles [46,73,76,88]. The viral genome consists of eleven segments of double-stranded RNA [41,74,79]. The virus is structurally quite stable, since it has been recognized by electron microscopy after storage at −20°C for 9 years [4]. It is not known if infectivity remains after such prolonged storage.

Laboratory Propagation

To date, the HRVLA has not been grown efficiently to high titer in tissue or organ culture systems. As a result, it has not been possible to obtain large quantities of HRVLA that can be used for routine diagnostic serologic tests or for detailed biophysical characterization beyond that described above. One laboratory has reported that HRVLA fluorescent-stainable antigen is produced in mucosal cells of human fetal intestinal organ cultures infected with the agent [99]. However, antigen is formed slowly and inefficiently in this system and only with certain inocula. In addition, limited availability of this kind of tissue has precluded practical use of this technic for diagnostic purposes or for laboratory studies with the agent. Of more practical use is the recognition by two laboratories that the HRVLA will form fluorescent-stainable antigen in the cytoplasm of monolayer cell cultures of human, monkey, calf and pig origin [15,91,93]. HRVLA-containing fecal supernates or filtrates from ill infants are centrifuged onto these cells which produce easily detectable viral-specific antigens in less than 24 hours. However, the HRVLA cannot be serially passaged into fresh cell cultures, indicating that incomplete viral replication is taking place [91].

Under experimental conditions, the HRVLA will infect gnotobiotic piglets, calves and lambs as well as newborn colostrum-deprived rhesus monkeys [13,59,62,65,86,92,100]. These animals experience diarrhea after oral inoculation of HRVLA, and virus particles are detectable in the stool.

Diagnostic Tests

In spite of the fact that the HRVLA fails to replicate efficiently in cell culture, a number of technics are now available for diagnosis of this infection. These include detection of the virus in stool specimens by electron microscopy, counterimmunoelectrophoresis, radioimmunoassay, enzyme-linked immunosorbent assay, fluorescent virus precipitin test, and production of HRVLA antigen in cell culture. In addition, several serologic assays for the virus have been developed, most of which are based on the close immunologic relatedness between the HRVLA and similar reovirus-like agents of other animal species that produce enteritis in these neonatal animals [32,43,81,84,91,97]. A discussion follows of each of the technics currently used to diagnose HRVLA infection.

The first and most widely used technic has been electron microscopy, by which the 70 nm HRVLA particles are easily demonstrated in stool specimens passed during acute illness [10,31,47,63]. There are few technical problems with this method, and relatively little processing of stool samples is necessary for specimens to be negatively stained with phosphotungstic acid and rendered suitable for electron microscopy. This is in striking contrast to the vagaries encountered in detection of the parvovirus-like agents in stool specimens, which requires prior adjustment of antigen-antibody ratios and concentration of stool filtrates in order to visualize the extremely small parvovirus-like particles. HRVLA particles are detectable during acute illness and are commonly shed for up to 8 days after disease onset, and rarely longer [52]. The particles are infrequently seen in stools of healthy infants and children: One cumulative report indicated that the HRVLA has been visualized in 396 out of 827 (48%) of children with acute enteritis and in only 2 of 357 asymptomatic children [22].

Although electron microscopy is a simple and reliable technic, it is time-consuming and also requires trained personnel and expensive specialized equipment. As a result, other technics have been developed to detect HRVLA antigen in stools of children with HRVLA enteritis. Counterimmunoelectrophoresis can be used to screen large numbers of specimens rapidly, unlike electron microscopy. Reports from different laboratories have indicated that it is equivalent to or less than electron microscopy in sensitivity of detection of the HRVLA in stool specimens [61,87,95]. Solid-phase radioimmunoassay has been used to diagnose HRVLA in diarrheal stools and is equivalent to or even greater than electron microscopy in sensitivity [42,60]. Radioimmunoassay also offers the advantage of being suitable for the rapid study of large numbers of specimens; however, it does require radioactive reagents and expensive radiation-counting equipment. A variation on the radioimmunoassay technic, the enzyme-linked immunosorbent assay (ELISA), uses similar methodology but replaces radiolabeled iodine with the enzyme alkaline phosphatase in linkage to the specific antibody employed in the test system [101]. ELISA is as sensitive as radioimmunoassay but does not require use of sophisticated technical equipment. A fluorescent virus precipitin test uses indirect immunofluorescence to detect the HRVLA in stools after HRVLA antigen in stool is complexed with specific antibody [72,102]. This test is as sensitive as electron microscopy, but it cannot screen large numbers of specimens at one time and it also requires specialized fluorescence equipment and a trained staff. Finally, the HRVLA can be detected by centrifugation of stool extracts onto cell culture monolayers [15,91,93], as we have discussed above under "Laboratory Propagation." This technic appears to be slightly less sensitive than electron microscopy but it does not require expensive equipment; it is, however, not practical for large-scale studies or rapid diagnosis.

Serum serologic tests have been developed for the HRVLA, and seroconversion has been compared with the efficacy of stool examination by electron microscopy. Significant rises in antibody titer have been shown to HRVLA stool antigen by means of a complement fixation (CF) test using acute and convalescent sera of infants who excreted the agent in their stools [47]. A close concordance has been demonstrated between seroconversion by CF and detection by electron microscopy of HRVLA in diarrheal stool specimens [48].

Because of the limited quantity of HRVLA antigen available, serologically related animal reovirus-like agents have frequently been employed as substitute antigens in serologic tests in place of the HRVLA [29,32,43,44,66,81,91]. Morphologically identical animal reovirus-like agents have been found associated with acute enteritis in feces from calves, mice, piglets, foals, lambs, and rabbits, and other reovirus-like agents have also been recovered from a rectal swab from a monkey (SA11 agent) and from the intestinal washings of sheep and cattle (O agent) [32,43,81,84,91,97]. Several of these agents have been widely used in serologic tests (CF, immunofluorescence and neutralization) since they are capable of replicating to high titer in cell culture, thereby producing large quantities of antigen, which are unavailable for the HRVLA. In comparative CF tests, the use of crude stools containing HRVLA antigen is somewhat more efficient in detecting human antibody responses than is use of the animal agents [12,48], but the animal agents have, nonetheless, proved to be quite practical and useful. Convenient immunofluorescence tests, using cell culture-grown reovirus-like agents from calves and monkey sources, have detected seroconversions in HRVLA-infected infants with a high degree of concordance between electron microscopic detection of the HRVLA and seroconversion by immunofluorescence [30,66,81].

Clinical Immunity

Prevalence studies indicate the rapid acquisition of serum antibodies to the HRVLA during the ages of 6 to 24 months [12,35,37,44,48,66]. A majority of adults and children over 2 years of age possess serum CF and immunofluorescent-stainable antibodies, presumably of the IgG class, indicating the ubiquitous nature of the HRVLA. Antibody, likely maternal in origin, is commonly present in neonates.

In infants and young children with presumed primary infection, serum antibodies that are probably of the IgM class are produced during acute illness and early convalescence and disappear during late convalescence [23,52,67]. Complement-fixing antibody that appears at this time is sensitive to 2-mercaptoethanol, and IgM antibody, detectable by immunofluorescence tests with the reovirus-like agent of calves, also develops.

Many patients who demonstrate a rise in serum antibody titer by either CF or immunofluorescence after HRVLA enteritis have significant antibody levels prior to infection [48]. Thus, it is clear that presence of these serum anti-HRVLA antibodies alone is not sufficient for immunity. What is clear is that children aged 6 to 24 months are more susceptible to infection and disease, regardless of the presence or absence of serum antibody. At present, reinfection of patients with the same strain of enteritis-inducing HRVLA has not been documented, nor has it been shown that there is more than one antigenic variety of HRVLA.

CANDIDATE VIRAL AGENTS

Adenoviruses

Evidence that adenoviruses are a cause of enteritis must still be regarded as equivocal. These agents can be shed chronically in the stools of asymptomatic children for several months. Controlled epidemiologic studies have revealed adenoviruses in many control as well as ill patients [8,75,103,104]. Recent careful longitudinal surveys of hospitalized children with enteritis have revealed adenoviruses in some patients [14,22,33,48,64]; however, serologic responses to adenovirus infection have been found in similar percentages of hospitalized diarrheal and control patients [48], implying that it is unlikely that adenoviruses have an important role in infantile diarrhea requiring hospitalization.

Nonetheless, evidence exists that adenoviruses may produce nosocomial enteritis among hospitalized long-stay infants and young children [33,64]. These agents have been found by electronmicroscopy in this setting during acute illness, with disappearance of adenovirus during convalescence. Many of these adenoviruses can be visualized by electron microscopy of diarrheal feces but are unable to be cultivated in cell culture (unlike conventional adenoviruses that produce acute respiratory tract disease).

By means of intestinal intubation studies, three infants with acute enteritis have been shown to harbor adenovirus in small intestinal secretions and at the same time to show abnormally low absorption of xylose [58].

Coronavirus-like Agent

Coronavirus-like particles have been visualized by electron microscopy of stool specimens collected from three outbreaks of nonbacterial gastroenteritis that have been alluded to by one research laboratory [18,19]. These virus-like particles are pleomorphic, 120–230 nm in size, and closely resemble known nonenteric coronaviruses. Particle-containing stool specimens produce cytopathic effects in organ cultures of human fetal small intestine [18]. Ultrastructural changes have been described in these inoculated cultures that are very suggestive of the replication of coronaviruses [19]. Intracytoplasmic fluorescence, presumed to be coronaviral, has been demonstrated in inoculated organ cultures and human embryonic kidney cell monolayers by reaction with convalescent serum from an ill patient [18].

Similar coronavirus-like particles have been seen in stool specimens from normal patients and chronic tropical sprue patients in southern India [57]. In addition, they have been seen in 18 hospitalized Australian aboriginal infants during an outbreak of enteritis in which 92 infants were studied [80]; however, most cases of enteritis in this outbreak were ascribed to the reovirus-like agent.

It is clear that a relationship of coronavirus-like stool particles to viral enteritis has not been established. The criteria described earlier under "Current Status of Viral Enteritis Agents" have not been met. It is also interesting that several extensive longitudinal studies of viral enteritis have failed to reveal coronavirus-like particles [14,22,31,48,55,64]. Nonetheless, it is known that coronaviruses produce enteritis in other animal species [84], and this lends credence to the hypothesis that the same may be true for man, particularly if one remembers the close relationship between reovirus-like enteritis agents of man and animals.

"Mini-Reovirus"

In one study, a 30 nm "mini-reovirus" particle has been seen by electron microscopy in diarrheal stools of 104 hospitalized infants with enteritis [64]. The particle is described as possessing a double-shelled capsid and looks similar to the HRVLA, but is much smaller. The particle was found during illness and disappeared in convalescence and it bred true in frequent nosocomial cases of single room outbreaks in that patients with secondary and tertiary cases of diarrhea excreted the particle. A limited number of immune electron microscopy studies suggested that serum antibody was absent during illness but developed in convalescence. Parallel electron microscopic studies of stools from normal children were not reported. Strongly suggestive, but not conclusive, evidence for the "mini-reovirus" particle as a cause of viral enteritis now exists from this one study, and confirmatory reports are awaited.

"Astrovirus"

A 28 nm virus-like particle that appears different from parvovirus to experienced electron microscopists has been described in several infants and young children hospitalized with enteritis [55,64,80]. The small round-shaped particle is described as possessing stain-filled surface hollows and a 5- or 6-pointed star-shaped periphery. However, no biologic characterization of these particles has been performed, no studies of matched control populations have been described, no serologic studies have been reported, and no extensive studies of convalescent stools have been performed. These particles have also failed to be described in extensive longitudinal studies of viral enteritis [14,22,31,48]. At this stage, they should be regarded as objects visualized under the electron microscope and as yet they clearly are not proven as viruses.

FUTURE RESEARCH

Remarkable progress has been achieved during the 1970's in our understanding of new etiologic agents that now explain the cause of many cases of viral enteritis. In addition, we are beginning to understand pathophysiologic and immunologic events that occur in association with viral enteritis. However, these advances merely provide the framework for much more that needs to be learned.

We still need to understand the mechanism(s) by which viral enteritis agents enter intestinal mucosal cells—are there specific viral receptors on these cells, or are nonspecific transport mechanisms operative? We already know that for the HRVLA the age of the host is a critical determinant of susceptibility to infection and this finding certainly implies that maturation of the intestine may be important in resistance to infection.

Etiologic agents need to be cultivated *in vitro* so that we can better understand the biology of these agents and have them characterized further. *In vitro* cultivation will also greatly aid the study of mechanisms by which these agents infect.

We also need to understand more completely the immunologic mechanisms that are involved in protection against infection. The finding that there are two forms of clinical immunity to the parvovirus-like Norwalk agent is provocative and carries with it the implication that there may be a genetically determined host susceptibility to infection with this agent. More also needs to be known about other potential factors involved in susceptibility and resistance: the comparative roles of serum and local gastrointestinal tract-secreted antibodies, interferon, presence of specific viral receptors on intestinal epithelial cells, and possible roles of structural or functional changes associated with maturation of the human intestine.

Some of these features will need to be understood more completely to provide the basis for development of methods for immunoprophylaxis and/or chemotherapy of viral enteritis. One possible approach may be to take advantage of the close immunologic relationships among reovirus-like agents of animal species by administering these agents to man in an attempt to induce immunity to HRVLA disease without production of significant illness.

REFERENCES

1. Adler JL, Zickl R: Winter vomiting disease. J Infect Dis 119:668–673, 1969.
2. Agus SG, Dolin R, Wyatt RG et al: Acute infectious nonbacterial gastroenteritis: Intestinal histopathology. Ann Intern Med 79:18–25, 1973.
3. Agus SG, Falchuk ZM, Sessoms CS et al: Increased jejunal IgA synthesis in vitro during acute infectious nonbacterial gastroenteritis. Am J Dig Dis 19:127–131, 1974.
4. Albrey MB, Murphy AM: Rotaviruses and acute gastroenteritis of infants and children. Med J Aust 1:82–85, 1976.
5. Appleton H, Buckley M, Thom BT et al: Virus-like particles in winter vomiting disease. Lancet 1:409–411, 1977.
6. Appleton H, Pereira MS: A possible virus etiology in outbreaks of food-poisoning from cockles. Lancet 1:780–781, 1977.
7. Behbehani AN, Shafa F, Mirakitani FK et al: Viral enteric infections among diar-rheal and non-diarrheal infants in Tehran, Iran. J Trop Med Hyg 72:149–152, 1969.
8. Behbehani AN, Wenner HA: Infantile diarrhea. A study of the etiologic role of viruses. Am J. Dis Child 111:623–629, 1966.
9. Bishop RF, Davidson GP, Holmes IH et al: Virus particles in epithelial cells of duodenal mucosa from children with acute nonbacterial gastroenteritis. Lancet 2:1281–1283, 1973.
10. Bishop RF, Davidson GP, Holmes IH et al: Detection of a new virus by electron microscopy of fecal extracts from children with acute gastroenteritis. Lancet 1:149–151, 1974.
11. Blacklow NR, Dolin R, Fedson DS et al: Acute infectious nonbacterial gastroen-teritis: Etiology and pathogenesis. Ann Intern Med 76:993–1008, 1972.
12. Blacklow NR, Echeverria P, Smith DH: Serologic studies with reovirus-like enteritis agent. Infect Immun 13:1563–1566, 1976.
13. Bridger JC, Woode GN, Jones JM et al: Transmission of human rotavirus to gnotobiotic piglets. J Med Microbiol 8:565–567, 1975.

14. Bryden AS, Davies HA, Hadley RE et al: Rotavirus enteritis in the West Midlands during 1974. Lancet 2:241–243, 1975.

15. Bryden AS, Davies HA, Thouless ME, Flewett TH: Diagnosis of rotavirus infection by cell culture. J Med Microbiol 10:121–125, 1977.

16. Cameron DJS, Bishop RF, Davidson GP et al: New virus associated with diarrhea in neonates. Med J Aust 1:85–86, 1976.

17. Carr ME, McKendrick GDW, Spyridakis T: The clinical features of infantile gastroenteritis due to rotavirus. Scand J Infect Dis 8:241–243, 1976.

18. Caul EO, Clarke SKR: Coronavirus propagated from patient with nonbacterial gastroenteritis. Lancet 2:953–954, 1975.

19. Caul EO, Egglestone SI: Further studies on human enteric coronaviruses. Arch Virol 54:107–117, 1977.

20. Clarke SKR, Cook GT, Egglestone SI et al: A virus from epidemic vomiting disease. Br Med J 3:86–89, 1972.

21. Cruickshank JG, Zilberg B, Axton JHM: Virus particles and gastroenteritis in black and white children in Rhodesia. S Afr Med J 49:859–862, 1975.

22. Davidson GP, Bishop RF, Townley RRW et al: Importance of a new virus in acute sporadic enteritis in children. Lancet 1:242–246, 1975.

23. Davidson GP, Goller I, Bishop RF et al: Immunofluorescence in duodenal mucosa of children with acute enteritis due to a new virus. J Clin Pathol 28:263–266, 1975.

24. Dingle JH, Badger GF, Feller AE, et al: A study of illness in a group of Cleveland families. I. Plan of study and certain general observations. Am J Hyg 58:16–30, 1953.

25. Dolin R, Baron S: Absence of detectable interferon in jejunal biopsies, jejunal aspirates and sera in experimentally induced viral gastroenteritis in man. Proc Soc Exp Biol Med 150:337–339, 1975.

26. Dolin R, Blacklow NR, Dupont H et al: Transmission of acute infectious nonbacterial gastroenteritis to volunteers by oral administration of stool filtrates. J Infect Dis 123:307–312, 1971.

27. Dolin R, Blacklow NR, Dupont H et al: Biological properties of Norwalk agent of acute infectious nonbacterial gastroenteritis. Proc Soc Exp Biol Med 140:578–583, 1972.

28. Dolin R, Levy AG, Wyatt RG et al: Viral gastroenteritis induced by the Hawaii agent. Am J Med 59:761–768, 1975.

29. Echeverria P, Blacklow NR, Smith DH: Role of heat-labile toxigenic Escherichia coli and reovirus-like agent in diarrhea in Boston children. Lancet 2:1113–1116, 1975.

30. Echeverria P, Ho MT, Blacklow NR et al: Relative importance of viruses and bacteria in the etiology of pediatric diarrhea in Taiwan. J Infect Dis 136:383–390, 1977.

31. Flewett TH, Bryden AS, Davies H: Diagnostic electron microscopy of faeces. J Clin Pathol 27:603–614, 1974.

32. Flewett TH, Bryden AS, Davies H: Relation between viruses from acute gastroenteritis of children and newborn calves. Lancet 2:61–63, 1974.

33. Flewett TH, Bryden AS, Davies H: Epidemic viral enteritis in a long-stay children's ward. Lancet 1:4–5, 1975.

34. Fukumi H, Hakaya R, Hatta S et al: An indication as to identify between the infectious diarrhea in Japan and the afebrile infectious non-bacterial gastroenteritis by human volunteer experiments. Jpn J Med Sci Biol 10:1–17, 1957.

35. Gomez-Baretto J, Palmer E, Nahmias AJ et al: Acute enteritis associated with reovirus-like agents. JAMA 235:1857–1860, 1976.

36. Gordon I, Ingraham HS, Korns RF: Transmission of epidemic gastroenteritis to human volunteers by oral administration of fecal filtrates. J Exp Med 80:409–422, 1947.

37. Gust ID, Pringle RC, Barnes GL et al: Complement-fixing antibody response to rotavirus infection. J Clin Microbiol 5:125–130, 1977.
38. Hodes HL: Viral gastroenteritis. Am J Dis Child 131:729–731, 1977.
39. Holmes IH, Ruck BJ, Bishop RF et al: Infantile enteritis viruses: Morphogenesis and morphology. J Virol 16:937 943, 1975.
40. Jordan WS, Gordon I, Dorrance WR: A study of illness in a group of Cleveland families. VII. Transmission of acute non-bacterial gastroenteritis to volunteers: evidence for two different etiologic agents. J Exp Med 98:461–475, 1953.
41. Kalica AR, Garon CF, Wyatt RG et al: Differentiation of human and calf reovirus-like agents associated with diarrhea using polyacrylamide gel electrophoresis of RNA. Virology 74:86–92, 1976.
42. Kalica AR, Purcell RH, Sereno MM et al: A microtiter solid phase radioimmunoassay for detection of the human reovirus-like agent in stools. J Immunol 118:1275–1279, 1977.
43. Kapikian AZ, Cline WL, Kim HW et al: Antigenic relationships among five reovirus-like (RVL) agents by complement fixation (CF) and development of new substitute CF antigens for the human RVL agent of infantile gastroenteritis. Proc Soc Exp Biol Med 152:535–539, 1976.
44. Kapikian AZ, Cline WL, Mebus CA et al: New complement-fixation test for the human reovirus-like agent of infantile gastroenteritis. Lancet 1:1056–1061, 1975.
45. Kapikian AZ, Gerin JL, Wyatt RG et al: Density in cesium chloride of the 27 nm "8FIIa" particle associated with acute infectious nonbacterial gastroenteritis: Determination by ultracentrifugation and immune electron microscopy. Proc Soc Exp Biol Med 142:874–877, 1973.
46. Kapikian AZ, Kalica AR, Shih JW et al: Buoyant density in cesium chloride of the human reovirus-like agent of infantile gastroenteritis by ultracentrifugation, electron microscopy and complement fixation. Virology 70:564–569, 1976.
47. Kapikian AZ, Kim HW, Wyatt RG et al: Reovirus-like agent in stools: Association with infantile diarrhea and development of serologic tests. Science 185:1049–1053, 1974.
48. Kapikian AZ, Kim HW, Wyatt RG et al: Human reovirus-like agent as the major pathogen associated with "winter" gastroenteritis in hospitalized infants and young children. N Engl J Med 294:965–972, 1976.
49. Kapikian AZ, Wyatt RG, Dolin R et al: Visualization by immune electron microscopy of a 27-nm particle associated with acute infectious nonbacterial gastroenteritis. J Virol 10:1075–1081, 1972.
50. Kim HW, Brandt CD, Kapikian AZ et al: Human reovirus-like agent infection: Occurrence in adult contacts of pediatric patients with gastroenteritis. JAMA 238:404–407, 1977.
51. Kojima S, Fukumi H, Kusama H et al: Studies on the causative agent of infectious diarrhea; records of the experiments on human volunteers. Jpn Med J 1:467–476, 1948.
52. Konno T, Suzuki H, Imai A, Ishida N: Reovirus-like agent in acute epidemic gastroenteritis in Japanese infants: Fecal shedding and serologic response. J Infect Dis 135:259–266, 1977.
53. Levy AG, Widerlite L, Schwartz CJ et al: Jejunal adenylate cyclase activity in human subjects during viral gastroenteritis. Gastroenterology 70:321–325, 1976.
54. Light JS, Hodes HL: Studies on epidemic diarrhea of the newborn: Isolation of a filtrable agent causing diarrhea in calves. Am J Public Health 33:1451–1454, 1943.
55. Madeley CR, Cosgrove BP, Bell EJ, Fallon RJ: Stool viruses in babies in Glasgow 1. Hospital admissions with diarrhea. J Hyg 78:261–273, 1977.

56. Martin ML, Palmer EL, Middleton PJ: Ultrastructure of infantile gastroenteritis virus. Virology 68:146–153, 1975.

57. Mathan M, Mathan VI, Swaminathan SP et al: Pleomorphic virus-like particles in human faeces. Lancet 1:1068–1069, 1975.

58. Mavromichalis J, Evans N, McNeish AS et al: Intestinal damage in rotavirus and adenovirus gastroenteritis assessed by D-xylose malabsorption. Arch Dis Child 52:589–591, 1977.

59. Mebus CA, Wyatt RG, Sharpee RL et al: Diarrhea in gnotobiotic calves caused by the reovirus-like agent of human infantile gastroenteritis. Infect Immun 14:471–474, 1976.

60. Middleton PJ, Holdaway MD, Petric M et al: Solid-phase radioimmunoassay for the detection of rotavirus. Infect Immun 16:439–444, 1977.

61. Middleton PJ, Petric M, Hewitt CM et al: Counterimmunoelectro-osmophoresis for the detection of infantile gastroenteritis virus (orbi-group) antigen and antibody. J Clin Pathol 29:191–197, 1976.

62. Middleton PJ, Petric M, Szymanski MT: Propagation of infantile gastroenteritis virus (Orbi-Group) in conventional and germfree piglets. Infect Immun 12:1276–1280, 1975.

63. Middleton PJ, Szymanski MT, Abbott GD et al: Orbivirus acute gastroenteritis of infancy. Lancet 1:1241–1244, 1974.

64. Middleton PJ, Szymanski MT, Petric M: Viruses associated with acute gastroenteritis in young children. Am J Dis Child 131:733–737, 1977.

65. Mitchell JD, Lambeth LA, Sosula L et al: Transmission of rotavirus gastroenteritis from children to a monkey. Gut 18:156–160, 1977.

66. Orstavik I, Figenschau KJ, Haug KW, Ulstrup JC: A reovirus-like agent (rotavirus) in gastroenteritis of children. Scand J Infect Dis 8:1–5, 1976.

67. Orstavik I, Haug KW: Virus-specific IgM antibodies in acute gastroenteritis due to a reovirus-like agent (rotavirus). Scand J Infect Dis 8:237–240, 1976.

68. Parks WD, Queiroga LT, Melnick JL: Studies of infantile diarrhea in Karachi, Pakistan, II. Multiple virus isolations from rectal swabs. Am J Epidemiol 85:469–478, 1967.

69. Parrino TA, Schreiber DS, Trier JS et al: Clinical immunity in acute gastroenteritis caused by Norwalk agent. N Engl J Med 297:86–89, 1977.

70. Paver WK, Caul EO, Clarke SKR: Comparison of a 22 nm virus from human faeces with animal parvoviruses. J Gen Virol 22:447–450, 1974.

71. Pelon W: Viral flora of the human alimentary tract. Am J Dig Dis 10:853–863, 1965.

72. Peterson MW, Spendlove RS, Smart RA: Detection of neonatal calf diarrhea virus, infant reovirus-like diarrhea virus, and a coronavirus using the fluorescent virus precipitin test. J Clin Microbiol 3:376–377, 1976.

73. Petric M, Szymanski MT, Middleton PJ: Purification and preliminary characterization of infantile gastroenteritis virus (Orbivirus group). Intervirology 5:233–238, 1975.

74. Petric M, Tam JS, Middleton PJ: Preliminary characterization of the nucleic acid of infantile gastroenteritis virus (orbivirus group). Intervirology 7:176–180, 1976.

75. Ramos-Alvarez M, Sabin AB: Enteropathogenic viruses and bacteria role in summer diarrheal diseases of infancy and early childhood. JAMA 167:147–156, 1958.

76. Rodger SM, Schnagl RD, Holmes IH: Biochemical and biophysical characteristics of diarrhea viruses of human and calf origin. J Virol 16:1229–1235, 1975.

77. Rodriguez WJ, Kim HW, Arrobio JO et al: Clinical features of acute gastroenteritis associated with human reovirus-like agent in infants and young children. J Pediatr 91:188–193, 1977.

78. Ryder RW, McGowan JE, Hatch MH, Palmer EL: Reovirus-like agent as a cause of nosocomial diarrhea in infants. J Pediatr 90:698–702, 1977.

79. Schnagl RD, Holmes IH: Characteristics of the genome of human infantile enteritis virus (rotavirus). J Virol 19:267–270, 1976.

80. Schnagl RD, Holmes IH, Moore B et al: An extensive rotavirus outbreak in Aboriginal infants in central Australia. Med J Aust 1:259–260, 1977.

81. Schoub BD, Lecatsas G, Prozesky OW: Antigenic relationship between human and simian rotaviruses. J Med Microbiol 10:1–6, 1977.

82. Schreiber DS, Blacklow NR, Trier JS: Small intestinal lesion induced by Hawaii agent acute infectious nonbacterial gastroenteritis. J Infect Dis 129:705–708, 1974.

83. Schreiber DS, Blacklow NR, Trier JS: The mucosal lesion of the proximal small intestine in acute infectious nonbacterial gastroenteritis. N Engl J Med 288:1318–1323, 1973.

84. Schreiber DS, Trier JS, Blacklow NR: Recent advances in viral gastroenteritis. Gastroenterology 73:174–183, 1977.

85. Shepherd RW, Truslow S, Walker-Smith JA et al: Infantile gastroenteritis: A clinical study of reovirus-like agent infection. Lancet 2:1082–1084, 1975.

86. Snodgrass DR, Madeley CR, Wells PW, Angus KW: Human rotavirus in lambs: infection and passive protection. Infect Immun 16:268–270, 1977.

87. Spence L, Fauvel M, Petro R, Bloch S: Comparison of counterimmunoelectrophoresis and electron microscopy for laboratory diagnosis of human reovirus-like agent-associated infantile gastroenteritis. J Clin Microbiol 5:248–249, 1977.

88. Tam JS, Szymanski MT, Middleton PJ, Petric M: Studies on the particles of infantile gastroenteritis virus (orbivirus group). Intervirology 7:181–191, 1976.

89. Thornhill TS, Kalica AR, Wyatt RG et al: Pattern of shedding of the Norwalk particle in stools during experimentally induced gastroenteritis in volunteers as determined by immune electron microscopy. J Infect Dis 132:28–34, 1975.

90. Thornhill TS, Wyatt RG, Kalica AR et al: Detection by immune electron microscopy of 26–27 nm virus-like particles associated with two family outbreaks of gastroenteritis. J Infect Dis 135:20–27, 1977.

91. Thouless ME, Bryden AS, Flewett TH et al: Serological relationships between rotaviruses from different species as studied by complement fixation and neutralization. Arch Virol 53:287–294, 1977.

92. Torres-Medina A, Wyatt RG, Mebus CA et al: Diarrhea caused in gnotobiotic piglets by the reovirus-like agent of human infantile gastroenteritis. J Infect Dis 133:22–27, 1976.

93. Totterdell BM, Chrystie IL, Banatvala JE: Rotavirus infections in a maternity unit. Arch Dis Child 51:924–928, 1976.

94. Tufvesson B, Johnsson T: Occurrence of reo-like viruses in young children with acute gastroenteritis. Acta Pathol Microbiol Scand (B) 84:22–28, 1976.

95. Tufvesson B, Johnsson T: Immunoelectroosmophoresis for detection of reo-like virus: methodology and comparison with electron microscopy. Acta Pathol Microbiol Scand B 84:225–228, 1976.

96. Widerlite L, Trier JS, Blacklow NR et al: Structure of the gastric mucosa in acute infectious nonbacterial gastroenteritis. Gastroenterology 68:425–430, 1975.

97. Woode GN, Bridger JC, Jones JM et al: Morphological and antigenic relationships between viruses (rotaviruses) from acute gastroenteritis of children, calves, piglets, mice and foals. Infect Immun 14:804–810, 1976.

98. Wyatt RG, Dolin R, Blacklow NR et al: Comparison of three agents of acute infectious nonbacterial gastroenteritis by cross-challenge in volunteers. J Infect Dis 129:709–714, 1974.

99. Wyatt RG, Kapikian AZ, Thornhill TS et al: In vitro cultivation in human fetal intestinal organ culture of a reovirus-like agent associated with nonbacterial gastroenteritis in infants and children. J Infect Dis 130:523–528, 1974.

100. Wyatt RG, Sly DL, London WT et al: Induction of diarrhea in colostrum deprived newborn rhesus monkeys with human reovirus-like agent of infantile gastroenteritis. Arch Virol 50:17–27, 1976.

101. Yolken RH, Kim HW, Clem T et al: Enzyme-linked immunosorbent assay (ELISA) for detection of human reovirus-like agent of infantile gastroenteritis. Lancet 2:263–267, 1977.

102. Yolken RH, Wyatt RG, Kalica AR et al: Use of free viral immunofluorescence assay to detect human reovirus-like agent in human stools. Infect Immun 16:467–470, 1977.

103. Yow MD, Melnick JL, Blattner RJ et al: The association of viruses and bacteria with infantile diarrhea. Am J Epidemiol 92:33–39, 1970.

104. Yow MD, Melnick JL, Phillips CA et al: An etiologic investigation of infantile diarrhea in Houston during 1962–63. Am J Epidemiol 83:255–261, 1966.

CHAPTER 10

CHANGING CONCEPTS OF INFECTIOUS DISEASES

Dorothy M. Horstmann, M.D.

The title, "Changing Concepts of Infectious Diseases," provides a wide range of possible approaches. I have chosen to consider the subject in a biologic and historical framework, which allows me to select for discussion both old and new developments that have profoundly influenced thinking about infections over the years. But first, to set the stage, a brief digression to emphasize the importance of understanding and controlling infectious diseases because of their enormous potential in shaping the destinies of peoples and nations.

In his lively book, *Plagues and People,* William McNeill provides a fascinating account of the interaction of humans, parasites, and history, beginning with early man [1]. The influence of various catastrophes due to infection on the evolution of urban cultures and of civilization itself has been profound. The decline of Athens began with an epidemic of a new disease in 430–429 B.C. Its nature is obscure, but Athens never quite recovered from its ravages. Other formidable examples are the devastating effect of plague—The Black Death—on European civilization in the 14th century, and of cholera in the 19th.

Wars and plagues go together, and there is no dearth of documentation of this. In relatively recent times, there was the 1918–1919 pandemic of influenza, the greatest medical disaster of this century. In those two years, influenza is conservatively estimated to have killed 20 million persons; the true number is undoubtedly far greater. Alfred Crosby, in his recent book *Epidemic and Peace, 1918* [2] has reviewed the effects of the disease not only on the course of World War I, in which the armies of both sides were severely compromised as a result of it, but on the peace negotiations, since one after another of the main players in that drama became desperately ill with influenza. Yet almost nowhere in his-

From Yale University School of Medicine, New Haven, Conn.

Presented at the first Fae Golden Kass Lecture, Radcliffe Institute, Cambridge, Mass., February 2, 1977.

tory books, novels, or other writings of the period is the impact of this plague recognized—or even mentioned. An exception is the classic short story by Katherine Ann Porter, *Pale Horse, Pale Rider* [3], which is a moving fictional account of the tragedy that the epidemic brought to ordinary people.

There are many other examples. The American Indians were subdued as much by measles and smallpox as by the early settlers. The extraordinary story of the conquest of Mexico by Cortez and his small band of Spaniards who faced a huge army of Aztecs, has long puzzled historians. Superior arms and skills were not enough to account for the result. McNeil has uncovered a plausible answer: an epidemic of smallpox was raging in Mexico City at the time of the major battle which drove Cortez out of the city; as a result, the Aztecs were unable to follow up their original victory over the defeated and demoralized Spaniards, and although the odds were in their favor, they ended up the losers in the contest [1].

Such episodes illustrate important concepts relating to infectious disease which were not grasped until several centuries later. Why for instance did the Indians and the Aztecs go down at such an alarming rate, while the European invaders suffered relatively little from the same disease? All the evidence indicates that the Spaniards brought smallpox with them and introduced it into a population of susceptibles who had never been exposed to it before. Under such circumstances, a "new" disease is highly virulent, and the Aztecs succumbed in droves. The Spaniards, to whom the infection was no stranger, had acquired a degree of immunity, partly through evolutionary selection of those with genetic resistance, but also as a result of previous experience with the agent; for the most part, they were therefore protected.

An understanding of such host-parasite relationships has been slow in evolving and they are still poorly understood in the case of a number of infections. In general, the view held by most persons is that infectious agents—bacteria, viruses, and other parasites—are all bad characters that cause minor illnesses, severe disease, and sometimes death. The feeling is that they should be avoided at all costs, and eliminated if possible. But as research in microbiology and epidemiology has progressed over the past hundred years, we have come to see the situation in a different light, and recognize that at least some microorganisms have a good side to them. In fact, it turns out that in many instances an infectious agent performs a beneficial function for the humans it attacks. Thus, a number of potentially disease-producing viruses frequently invade and multiply in complete silence; they set up acute infections without disturbing the host in anyway, yet at the same time they induce protective immunity that lasts for life. Other viruses are capable of establishing a more permanent type of symbiotic relationship in which they may live happily with their hosts for years. Here, as in all host-parasite interactions, an equilibrium is established and only when something upsets the balance does disease result. The equilibrium that determines whether an invading organism proliferates to the detriment of its host is an exceedingly complex affair at all levels—molecular, cellular, the total organism, and the social environment. The actual mechanisms involved at each stage are poorly understood despite the remarkable advances in biomedical research in recent decades.

From this sketchy background I should like to turn now to a consideration of certain specific infections—old ones and "new" ones— as illustrations of the ways in which concepts of infectious diseases have altered over the years as new discoveries, some of them quite accidental, have been made. Since I am most familiar with virus infections, I shall deal only with them.

First, poliomyelitis. Its history is a dramatic one and tells a great deal about the slow, painstaking manner in which scientific advances are made [4]. Poliomyelitis is no longer a problem in the United States but it is still a frequent visitor in many of the developing countries of the world. It is a very old disease, at least as old as written history. Archeologic confirmation of its antiquity is based on a beautiful Egyptian stele of the Eighteenth Dynasty, 1580–1350 B.C., which shows a young man, apparently a priest, with a withered and shortened left leg, his left foot held in the characteristic equinus position. This picture is typical of the flaccid paralysis induced by poliomyelitis—and by almost nothing else.

It is astonishing that so old and dramatic a disease should have been so slow in coming to clinical recognition. It was not until the late 18th century A.D. that the first recognizable description appeared in the medical literature. In the following years, beginning in 1830, sporadic cases and some small clusters of cases of "infantile paralysis" in young children were reported by physicians both in Europe and America. At this time there was no idea that the disease was due to an infectious agent. Contact between cases was not a feature, and there was thus no consideration of the possibility of contagion. However, when in the latter part of the 19th century larger and larger epidemics began to occur, first in Scandinavia and then in the United States, it struck some physicians that the disease must be contagious. This was denied by others, who noted only rare instances of two cases in the same family, and no connection between the other children who developed paralysis. The controversy raged until the early 20th century when Ivar Wickman, a Swedish pediatrician, became interested in the disease. There was a huge epidemic in

Sweden in 1905, with more than 1000 cases reported. It was by far the largest outbreak so far anywhere in the world. Cases occurred all over Sweden, but it was the small villages rather than the cities that were the hardest hit. This was an advantage to Wickman, who set out to examine in detail the patterns of disease in families, schools, and small communities. He soon came to the realization that while paralysis is the most spectacular aspect of poliomyelitis, it is not the whole story: many patients had only minor symptoms and signs and no paralysis at all. There had been previous suggestions that this might be the case, but Wickman was the first to grasp the implication in terms of the epidemiology of the disease. He documented all possible cases and came to the firm conclusion that poliomyelitis was an infectious disease, that it was spread through contagion, and that those with minor illnesses were as dangerous to the community as the frank paralytic cases. In one village, he estimated that more than 50 per cent of cases were of the non-paralytic type. The findings strongly suggested that the infection must be spread in large part through the intermediary of such cases—a concept that required reevaluation of the whole clinical and epidemiologic picture of poliomyelitis.

Wickman's discovery was of tremendous importance in several ways: First, it provided an explanation for the peculiar erratic occurrence of cases of paralysis, with no apparent connection between them; secondly, the fact that paralysis was not an essential part of the disease opened up a whole new range of possibilities concerning the nature of the infection, the primary sites of multiplication of the agent, and the mode of spread from person to person. Other Swedish investigators, led by Carl Kling, pursued these questions in the laboratory as soon as the causative agent—poliomyelitis virus—was isolated in Vienna in 1908 by Landsteiner and Popper. By 1912 the Swedish team had many of the answers to the puzzle in hand: they knew that not only was the virus present in the CNS, but it was also shed from the throat and excreted from the intestinal tract of infected persons. Their work contained the key to the pathogeneis and epidemiology of the infection which ultimately formed the basis of control of the disease. But such control, in the form of effective preventive measures, was not achieved until some forty years later.

Why did it take so long for successful vaccines to be developed? The reasons are several. Certain authorities questioned the validity of the 1912 Swedish observations, which, it is true, were based on experiments using rather crude technics. But of greater importance was the resistance of investigators of the time—particularly the Americans—to accept the new concepts concerning the infection, to give up the idea that the virus could propagate only in nervous tissue. By using in their investigation a strain that had been passaged many times in monkeys by brain to brain transfer, they worked with virus that *had* indeed become adapted to grow only in the nervous system, and their experiments therefore gave the results they were looking for. The problem was that these results had nothing to do with the infection in humans, and translation of the findings to the naturally occurring disease led to erroneous interpretations which had some unfortunate—even disastrous—effects when practices based upon them were put into effect. It required another 30 years before the record was finally set straight. Not until the 1940s was it fully documented and generally accepted that poliovirus induces mainly an intestinal infection, and the paralytic disease is a relatively rare complication. And it was only when the true nature of the infection and of the disease were understood that progress could be made toward developing a vaccine for prevention of paralytic poliomyelitis [4].

The story of polio is a good example of how new concepts of infectious disease evolve and change, and how they sometimes have a hard time becoming established. Progress is often slow—a few steps forward and not infrequently a step or two backward, as we inch along toward our goals. The story also illustrates the immense power of strong personalities in shaping the history of science as well as of other fields. This should not be surprising since, of course, scientists are people first, and subject to the same pressures and drives that influence the rest of mankind.

Turning now to rubella (German measles), a disease that has had a briefer history than poliomyelitis, but like it has led to new perceptions of the biologic behavior of certain viruses. Rubella was not accepted as a separate and distinct clinical entity until the 1880s, although it had been recognized as such by certain clinicians as early as the 1750s. Between 1880 and 1941, it was regarded as a mild, inconsequential rash disease of childhood, with rare complictions. It was of no particular interest to physicians or public health workers. Then suddenly in 1941 all this changed: rubella was hurled into the limelight through the perspicacity of one man, Dr. Norman Gregg, an Australian ophthalmologist, who published a paper in the Transactions of the Ophthalmological Society of Australia entitled "Congenital Cataract following German Measles in the Mother" [5]. Gregg's remarkable observations followed in the wake of an extremely large and severe outbreak of rubella in Australia after a 17 year period of minimal incidence. As a result, many young adults were susceptible, and many pregnant women became infected. In searching for an environmental cause for the subsequent epidemic of congenital cataracts, Gregg discovered that the mothers of virtually all the affected infants had experienced rubella early in gestation—often even before they realized that they were pregnant.

And so with Gregg, in 1941, begins the modern history of rubella. One cannot help but wonder how and why it took so long for the teratogenic potential of the virus to be recognized. There was a huge epidemic in the United States in 1935, comparable to the one in 1964. Hundreds of thousands of cases occurred and many must have been in pregnant women, yet nowhere is there any mention of a resulting epidemic of congenital disease in the period following some 7 to 9 months or more later. It is a good illustration of how we tend to see only what we are looking for, as the history of medicine continually reminds us.

Gregg's discovery had a profound impact not only on the subsequent history of rubella but on the whole field of congenital abnormalities, for it focused attention on the possibility that many malformations previously thought to be of genetic or developmental origin might in fact result from environmental agents, including infectious ones. The harvest of discovery has been rich: Cytomegaloviruses, herpes, toxoplasma, and other agents have subsequently been found to induce persistent infections in the fetus which continue into postnatal life. In the case of rebella, isolation of the virus proved a difficult problem; it was not solved until 1962, when Weller and Neva at Harvard, and Parkman, Buescher, and Artenstein at Walter Reed, simultaneously reported success in growing it in tissue culture [6,7]. It was fortunate that this breakthrough occurred before the great 1964 outbreak of the disease in the United States, for with virologic and serologic tools in hand it was possible to learn an enormous amount about the fetal infection [8]. The most important observations were that (1) the virus sets up a chronic infection in target organs, and abortus specimens obtained many weeks after the maternal disease still yielded the virus; (2) at birth infected infants shed large amounts of virus from the throat, and excretion from this site continued over a period of months, the percentage of virus-positive infants gradually diminishing over the first year of life but continuing into the second year in a few cases. Virus was demonstrated to persist in the lens of the eye for three years in a child with congenital cataract; (3) the small size of affected infants and the eventual clearing of the virus from infected tissues, seems to be best explained on the basis that rubella is not a lytic virus, that it infects cells and persists in them without inducing cytopathology, and without interfering with cell division—up to a point. There is a limitation imposed upon a clone of infected cells, however, and that consists of a shortened life span. Thus, infected clones begin to drop out in fetal life, with the result that the infant is small at birth even though of normal gestational age, and his organs and tissues have a greatly reduced number of cells. The fallout continues into postnatal life, and only when all infected clones have disappeared is there clearance of the virus from the organism [9,10]. The peculiar behavior of rubella virus in fetal life, which is quite different from its pathogenic potential in infections acquired postnatally, has parallels in cytomegalovirus and other intrauterine virus-host interactions. The mechanisms involved at the celluar and molecular levels are not at all understood. They pose challenging problems for investigation.

The next disease for discussion is caused by a "new" virus, and provides us with new concepts of the versatility of viruses in inducing infections and possibly, tumors [11,12]. I refer to infectious mononucleosis, a disease that occurs mainly in young adults, frequently university students; only since 1968 has the etiologic agent, Epstein-Barr virus, been known [13]. The story of how this was discovered is a remarkable one, full of surprises, and heavily indebted to serendipity.

Infectious mononucleosis has been recognized as a clinical syndrome since 1889, when Pfeiffer reported cases which he labeled "glandular fever." The classic description, however, which included not only the typical symptoms and signs but also the unusual hematologic findings, was published by Sprunt and Evans in 1920. At the time, the disease was recognized as an infectious one, probably due to a virus. But there were many puzzling features, such as the remarkable age distribution, with a peak incidence in the 15–24 year olds. Why were young children, the common target of most infections, spared? Epidemiologically, the pattern has similarities to that of poliomyelitis and, as hypothesized by Evans, the presumption was that mild or inapparent infections must occur in childhood, but only in the susceptible young adult does the full blown clinical picture emerge [11]. With the introduction of practical tissue culture methods in the 1950s, a number of investigators renewed efforts to isolate an agent, using all of the known tricks of the virologist. All such efforts ended in failure and frustration.

The denouement finally came about accidently. The story begins far away in East Africa, where Dr. Dennis Burkitt, an English surgeon assigned there, was struck by the high incidence of an unusual tumor of the jaw in children living in a particular geographic area, namely a band across the middle of Africa which was a high malaria belt. Burkitt reported his observations in 1958. The fact that the cases occurred primarily where there were many mosquito-borne infections gave rise to the idea that the tumor might be virus-induced—possibly by some new arbovirus. The next chapter takes us to London, where several years later, in 1964, Epstein and Barr received specimens of Burkitt lymphoma tumors of African children, and proceeded to grow them in tissue culture. Thinking in terms of a possible virus etiology, they examined the tissue outgrowths by electron microscopy. Amazingly, they saw typical herpes-like virus particles in the cells [14]. The agent turned out to be a previously unrecognized member of the herpes group with no antigenic relationship to any of the others. Epstein-Barr virus, or EBV as it came to be called, was probably the first virus to be discovered by electron microscopy.

The problem of the relationship of EBV to the etiology of the tumor, Burkitt lymphoma, drew many investigators into the field, including Werner and Gertrude Henle, of the University of Pennsylvania. They succeeded in developing a serologic test to detect antibodies to the agent, and were able to show that all patients wit Burkitt lymphoma had high titers to EBV. As sera from more patients were tested, it was found that among those with leukemia and various malignancies a certain percentage were also antibody-positive, indicating that they had been infected at some time in the past. Furthermore, normal persons with no history of disease also possessed antibodies, the percentage reacting increasing with age.

All this was very puzzling, and the role of EBV in Burkitt lymphoma was not at all clear. The next development occurred in the Henle's laboratory: One of their technicians who had been working with EBV fell ill with infectious mononucleosis. Her sera, collected before the illness, consistently lacked EBV antibody, but after recovery, she had a high antibody titer to the virus [13]. This observation raised the possibility of an association between IM and the new virus; perhaps the long sought etiologic agent had been discovered at last. The Henles were quick to capitalize on this possibility, and turned to colleagues at Yale, where infectious mononucleosis had long been a particular interest ever since Dr. John Paul, in the early 1930s, again quite serendipitously, had discovered the heterophile antibody test which remains today the definitive diagnostic procedure [15]. Because IM is a disease that has a high incidence in university students, in the late 1950s, Dr. Paul and Dr. James Niederman had started a collection of serum from incoming Yale College freshmen, and from cases of infectious mononucleosis as they occurred throughout the ensuing 4 years. The results of tests for antibodies to EB virus on these sera were crucial in providing presumptive evidence that EBV is the causative agent of IM: The results showed that the disease never occurred in those who possessed antibody at the time they entered Yale college; only students who lacked antibody became ill, and all who developed the disease acquired antibody during the course of the illness [11]. These findings were subsequently confirmed and extended by Niederman and Evans of Yale, and in other laboratories in the U.S. and England.

It was not until several years later, however, that isolation and definite identification of the virus from throat washings of patients with infectious mononucleosis was achieved. Part of the difficulty in accomplishing this lay in the cumbersome methods available for growing the virus and detecting its presence. The agent cannot be propagated in tissue cultures in the manner of other herpes viruses. The technic currently in use for isolating it from throat washings depends on the ability of EBV to transform uninfected human blood leukocytes into continuous cell lines. This assay usually requires 30 to 90 days for completion; it is therefore not a practical diagnostic method but rather a research tool. The investigations of Miller and Niederman [16] showed that not only is the virus present in throat washings in acute cases, but excretion in oropharyngeal fluids continues intermittently for months, sometimes for more than a year.

Another remarkable finding was that once infection occurs, the agent can be detected in circulating lymphocytes on cultivation. In tissue cultures, such cells form continuous lines spontaneously, whereas with few exceptions, uninfected lymphocytes do not. Furthermore, the virus persists in some form in the circulating lymphocytes, apparently for life; it has been shown to be present in cells grown out more than 25 years after the host experienced infectious mononucleosis. EBV, like other herpes viruses, thus has a remarkable capacity to persist indefinitely in latent form in the infected host without causing any deleterious effects.

As more information has been gathered about the behavior of EBV in human populations, new concepts concerning the epidemiology of the infection and its mode of spread have also emerged, and older ideas have been confirmed. Serologic studies, for instance, have documented that the infection is a common one in childhood, that it is most often completely inapparent or associated with mild nonspecific symptoms. Only when infection is delayed until young adult life is it expressed as a clinically recognizable syndrome, namely infectious mononucleosis. Furthermore, infection rates have been shown to vary in different parts of the world according to socioeconomic levels. Thus, in areas where poverty and crowding are common—as in Barbados, Uganda, Indonesia—90–95% of children have already been infected and acquired antibody by 4 to 6 years of age [11]. In such populations there are almost no susceptible young adults and infectious mononucleosis is virtually unknown. In more affluent societies, however, in Europe and in the United States, only 30–40% of children are infected by the time they reach 4 to 6 years of age, and a substantial number are still susceptible as teenagers and young adults; among these are the individuals who develop classic IM on exposure.

Answers to another question, namely, what form does exposure to EBV take, have also been provided by recent investigations. One of the puzzling features of the infection has been that it spreads readily in two groups—young preschool children and young adults—but very little dissemination of the virus occurs in those 5 to 14 years old. The explanation for this peculiar age distribution is provided by recent observations of Niederman and Miller and their colleagues indicating that the virus is excreted primarily into the saliva, thus suggesting that cells in the parotid gland might be the primary sites of virus multiplication [17]. This discovery makes it clear why infection occurs in young children who are prone to exchange saliva in one way or another, and in young adults whose affectionate habits have given infectious mononucleosis the name of "kissing disease."

With so much new information about EB virus and infectious mononucleosis, have there been comparable developments in information about the role of the agent in Burkitt lymphoma, and nasopharyngeal carcinoma, another malignancy which also appears to be associated in some way with EBV? At this stage, herpes viruses are prime candidates as causative agents in certain cancers in humans. There are a number of examples of malignant tumors in lower animals in which herpes viruses have been shown to play an etiologic role. These include Marek's disease in chickens, the Lucké frog kidney carcinoma, and leukemia and lymphosarcomas in New World monkeys induced by several simian herpes viruses. It would seem reasonable in biologic terms that herpes viruses of humans—incluing EBV—might behave similarly under certain circumstances. The evidence linking Epstein-Barr virus with Burkitt lymphoma is impressive [12]. Thus, the cells of the tumor contain the EBV genome and several EBV antigens, and EBV-producing cell lines can be derived from the tumors. Patients with Burkitt lymphoma have elevated antibody titers to EBV; they also possess certain unique EBV-related antibodies. The etiologic relationship of EBV with Burkitt lymphoma is strengthened by the ability of the virus to readily transform normal lymphocytes *in vitro*; such cells are "immortalized," and grow as continuous lymphoblastoid cell lines indefinitely. In addition, Shope and Miller have shown that inoculation of the virus into marmosets, a species of New World monkeys, induces lymphomas with pathologic features similar to Burkitt lymphoma [12].

At the present state of knowledge, however, there are many puzzling questions still unanswered concerning the biology of EB virus. This agent causes a high rate of infection the world over, resulting in the disease, infectious mononucleosis, in a small proportion, depending on age and socioeconomic factors; in addition, in a particular geographic area in Africa it is associated with a characteristic malignant tumor of childhood. This striking geographical concentration of Burkitt lymphoma is not completely understood, but immunosuppression resulting from chronic malaria, which has a very high incidence in the area, may be a significant contributing factor. The explanation of the diverse behavior of EBV requires more information than we now possess concerning cell-virus relationships, molecular events in virus replication, inhibitory factors in cells which prevent cell transformation *in vivo*, and the complex nature of host and viral factors which modulate the outcome of infection over a wide range of patterns from inapparent to, possibly, malignant tumor. The further elucidation of these problems will provide not only new insights into the working of EB virus, but should also contribute substantially to a better understanding of viral oncogenesis generally.

Finally, I should like to turn to another relatively new field which has expanded the boundaries of infectious disease into quite unexpected territory. I refer to the so-called slow virus infections. Slow in this terminology refers not to the viuses, but to the delay between the time when infection is established, and the appearance of clinical manifestations of disease. There are a number of infections of man and animals which have extremely prolonged incubation periods—months to years. In all, there is a long period of persistence in the host without cell or tissue damage until something upsets the balance and progressive disease ensues. Most of the infections that fall into this category attack the central nervous system [18]. Two types of agents are involved, the first being the so-called *conventional* ones which are members of known virus families. These agents have standard virus structure, can be seen by electron microscopy both inside and outside of cells, have nucleic acid genomes, are antigenic and induce immune responses, cause inflammatory and degenerative lesions in the host tissues, and are capable of inducing disease affecting the CNS and sometimes other organs and tissues. Five diseases belonging to this group—2 in animals, 3 in man—are of special interest. In each, a member of a different virus family is involved. The two diseases of lower animals are Visna of sheep, and lymphocytic choriomeningitis of mice. In man, rabies has been the one known the longest; its incubation period may last months to several years. Measles virus (and more rarely rubella) has been associated with a late manifestation known as subacute sclerosing panencephalitis, or SSPE, first recognized in the mid 1960s. This is a uniformly fatal encephalitis in children, occurring usually 5 to 10 years after the original disease. Measles virus nucleocapsids can be seen in brain tissue by electron microscopy, accompanied by a marked chronic inflammatory response with little necrosis. It is not clear whether in the pathogenesis of the disorder, the agent, or the host, or both are responsible for the CNS damage. The third human disease is progressive multifocal leukoencephalopathy (PML), long thought to be a degenerative process of the CNS, until in 1965 virus-like particles were observed in brain sections by electron microscopy [19]. It is a rare condition, occurs almost exclusively in immunosuppressed individuals, and causes demyelinating lesions in the white matter of the brain. Several members of the papovavirus family of tumor viruses have been recovered from infected tissues.

The other group of agents causing slow virus infections are classified as *unconventional* and they are indeed bizarre: No virus partices are recognizable in involved cells and the only cytopathology demonstrable by electron microscopy consists of intracellular vacuoles loaded with coiled up sheets of unit membrane, the same membrane forming the walls of the vacuoles. There is no evidence that the viruses possess nucleic acid genomes; they are not antigenic and no immune responses have thus far been demonstrated. The agents have remarkable stability and are not inactivated by heat, even by boiling, or by ultraviolet irradiation, or chemicals such as formalin. No inflammatory reaction occurs in infected tissue, only degenerative lesions, and these are confined to the CNS. Currently four diseases due to unconventional agents are recognized. Two are animal diseases, scrapie in sheep, and tranmissible mink encephalopathy; two are diseases of humans, namely, kuru, and Creuzfeldt-Jacob disease. Scrapie was the first to be recognized as an infection, in France in 1936, and in Scotland a year later [20]. The most dramatic is kuru, a progressive degenerative brain disease confined to a tribe of New Guinean natives, and occurring largely in women and children [21]. It was for his investigations of kuru and the elucidation of its nature that Carleton Gajdusek received the Nobel prize in medicine in 1976. His extensive epidemiologic studies resulted in the conclusion that the disease was infectious, and that transmission occurred through contamination with brain tissue during the rite of ritual cannibalism. The women were the ones who officiated at this ceremony; they handled the brain tissue—bare handed—made it into a puree and scooped it into bamboo tubes for cooking. With infants in their arms, and toddlers playing about, there were many opportunities for contamination of children. The incubation period of kuru can be as long as 15 to 20 years or even longer. But once the disease begins, with tremors and ataxia, it gradually progresses within months to dysarthria, emotional lability, mental deterioration, immobility, cachexia, and death, usually within 6 to 9 months.

While there were many epidemiologic features of kuru that suggested infection, early efforts to recover an agent by various technics were all unsuccessful. Finally, however, when brain tissue from fatal cases was inoculated intracerebrally into chimpanzees, a disease resembling kuru both clinically and pathologically developed. The incubation period in the animals ranged between 16 and 38 months. Subsequently, serial passage from chimpanzee to chimpanzee was accomplished, and more recently the disease has also been transmitted in New World monkeys. As the nature of kuru and its mode of transmission were documented, the practice of ritual cannibalism ceased, and kuru, which formerly accounted for 50% of the deaths in the tribe, has greatly declined. It will have disappeared within 20 years.

The work of Gajdusek, Gibbs, and their colleagues in unravelling the mysteries of kuru, the emergence of SSPE as a measles virus-associated condition, and the identification of other new slow virus infections have had far reaching implications. As a result, consideration has been given to the possibility that various dymelinating diseases of the CNS long classified as degenerative, might also be virus induced [20]. This has already been shown to be the case with Creutzfeldt-Jacob disease, a presenile dementia; as in kuru, the infectious etiology has been demonstrated by reproducing the clinical and pathologic findings on intra-cerebral inoculation of chimpanzees [21]. The discovery of these new kinds of infection which induce none of the usual signs of infection—no fever, no cells in the spinal fluid, no inflammatory lesions in brain tissue—opens up the possibility that other more common CNS diseases might also be caused by infectious agents. Multiple sclerosis is a prime suspect in this connection. There are others, and the question has been raised as to whether the progressive degenerative changes usually associated with senescence might be viral induced. It is well known that a profusion of latent viruses inhabit apparently normal tissues of normal animals. Monkeys, mice, sheep, have all been found to harbor agents in tissues that are sterile by conventional tissue culture and other tests. Human tissues are no exception. Adenoids regularly contain latent viruses that can be revealed by special technics; primary infection with herpes virus is followed by a state of permanent latency in which the virus remains in sensory ganglia cells; some persons infected with hepatitis virus type B remain carriers for many years; herpes zoster—or shingles—in older adults is due to reactivation of the virus that established itself during the course of chickenpox in childhood. Cytomegaloviruses, rubella, and papovaviruses are a few of the other examples of agents capable of long persistence in the human host.

From all this it is clear that the cells of the normal human body harbor a number of viral agents as incompletely replicated provirus. Such host-virus relationships may well lead to gradual decline in cell function over the years, eventually resulting in some type of pathology manifested as a specific disease, or simply as aging [22]. In addition, alteration in cell-immune properties may also be induced by persistent virus infection, eventually leading to cell transformation and possibly to autoimmune disorders. We are clearly just at the beginning of an era of exploration of a whole new range of pathogenetic mechanisms involved in infectious diseases. The harvest in the next decades is bound to be a rich and exciting one, with many potential benefits for human health.

This has been but a superficial and largely personal survey of a few of the many changing concepts of infectious disease, old and new. The present is a time of unparalleled intellectual activity in the fields of microbiology and immunology. Many investigators are probing the molecular events associated with infection, while others who are more biologically oriented are taking a broader tack, looking at interactions between host cells and microbial agents, and attempting to relate these both to molecular events and to disease in the whole organism. Changes in concepts, as medical history illustrates so well, emerge gradually, but there seems little doubt that during the next few decades this will be continuing at an accelerated pace. I predict an exciting life for future investigators in the infectious disease field—exciting and immensely rewarding.

REFERENCES

1. McNeill H: Plagues and People. Garden City, N.Y., Anchor Press/Doubleday, 1976.
2. Crosby W: Epidemic and Peace, 1918. Greenwich, Conn., Greenwood Press, 1976.
3. Porter KA: Pale Horse, Pale Rider. *In:* Phillips W (Ed): Great American Short Novels. New York, Dial Press, 1946.
4. Paul, JR: A History of Poliomyelitis. New Haven, Conn., Yale University Press, 1971.
5. Gregg NMcA: Congenital cataract following German measles in the mother. Trans Ophthalmol Soc Australia 3:35–46, 1941.
6. Weller TH, Neva FA: Propagation in tissue culture of cytopathic agents from patients with rubella-like illness. Proc Soc Exp Biol Med 111:215–225, 1962.
7. Parkman PO, Buescher EL, Artenstein MS: Recovery of rubella virus from army recruits. Proc Soc Exp Biol Med 111:225–230, 1962.
8. Krugman S (Ed): Rubella Symposium. Am J Dis Child 110:1965.
9. Naeye RL, Blanc W: Pathogenesis of congenital rubella. JAMA 194:1277–1283, 1965.
10. Simons MJ: Congenital rubella. An immunological paradox? Lancet 2:1275–1278, 1968.

11. Evans AS, Niederman JC: Epstein-Barr virus. *In:* Evans AS (Ed): Viral Infections of Humans, Epidemiology and Control. New York, Plenum, 1976, pp 209–233.

12. Miller G: Epidemiology of Burkitt lymphoma. *ibid*, pp 481–499.

13. Henle G, Henle W, Diehl V: Relation of Burkitt's tumor-associated herpes type virus to infectious mononucleosis. Proc Natl Acad Sci USA 59:94–101, 1968.

14. Epstein MA, Achong BG, Barr YM: Virus particles in cultured lymphoblasts from Burkitt lymphoma cells. Lancet 1:702–703, 1964.

15. Paul JR, Bunnell WW: The presence of heterophile antibodies in infectious mononucleosis. Am J Med Sci 183:91–104, 1932.

16. Miller G, Niederman JC, Andrews LL: Prolonged oropharyngeal excretion of Epstein-Barr virus after infectious mononucleosis. N Engl J Med 288:229–232, 1973.

17. Niederman JC, Miller G, Pearson HA et al: Infectious mononucleosis. Epstein-Barr virus shedding in saliva and the oropharynx. N Engl J Med 294:1355–1359, 1976.

18. Brody JA, Gibbs CJ: Chronic neurological diseases: subacute sclerosing panencephalitis, progressive multifocal leukoencephalopathy, kuru, Creutzfeldt-Jacob disease. *In:* Evans AS (Ed): Viral Infections of Humans: Epidemiololgy and Control. New York, Plenum, 1976, pp 519–537.

19. Zu Rhein GM: Particles resembling papova viruses in human cerebral demyelinating disease. Science 148:1477–1479, 1965.

20. Hadlow WJ, Ecklund CM: A virus induced encephalopathy of sheep. *In:* Zimmerman HM (Ed): Infections of the Nervous System. Proc. Assoc. Research in Nervous and Mental Diseases. Baltimore, Williams & Wilkins, 1968, 44, pp 281–306.

21. Gajdusek DC, Gibbs CJ: Subacute and chronic diseases caused by atypical infections with unconventional viruses in aberrant hosts. *In:* Persistent Virus Infections. Perspectives in Virology, New York, Academic Press, 1973, pp 279–311.

22. Gajdusek DC: Slow virus infection and activation of latent infections in aging. Adv Gerontol Res 4:201–218, 1972.

INDEX

INDEX